Alcohol abuse and liver disease

Alcohol abuse and liver disease

EDITED BY

James Neuberger MD, FRCP

Honorary Consultant
Liver Unit
Queen Elizabeth Hospital
Birmingham, UK

Associate Medical Director
Organ Donation and Transplantation
NHS Blood and Transplant
Bristol, UK

Andrea DiMartini MD

Associate Professor of Psychiatry
Associate Professor of Surgery
Medical Director, Psychosomatic Medicine Transplant Program
Starzl Transplant Institute
University of Pittsburgh Medical Center
Pittsburgh, PA, USA

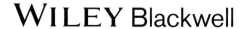

Library of Congress Cataloging-in-Publication Data
Alcohol abuse and liver disease / editors, James Neuberger, Andrea DiMartini.
    p. ; cm.
  Includes bibliographical references and index.
  ISBN 978-1-118-88728-8 (cloth)
I. Neuberger, James, editor. II. DiMartini, Andrea F., editor.
[DNLM: 1. Alcoholism–complications.   2. Liver Diseases, Alcoholic–etiology.   3. Alcoholism–diagnosis.
4. Liver Diseases, Alcoholic–therapy. WI 700]
  RC565
  616.86′1–dc23
                                           2015007953
A catalogue record for this book is available from the British Library.

Set in 8.5/12pt Meridien by SPi Publisher Services, Pondicherry, India
Printed and bound in Singapore by Markono Print Media Pte Ltd

1   2015

Contents

List of Contributors

Omair Abbasi MD
Assistant Professor, Department of Psychiatry
and Human Behavior
Thomas Jefferson University Hospitals
Sidney Kimmel School of Medicine
Philadelphia, PA, USA

Guruprasad P. Aithal BSc, MBBS, MD, FRCP, PhD
Professor of Hepatology, Director, National Institute for
Health Research (NIHR) Nottingham Digestive Diseases
Biomedical Research Unit
Nottingham University Hospitals NHS Trust
and the University of Nottingham
Nottingham, UK

Stephen Atkinson MBBS, MA, MRCP
Clinical Research Fellow, Gastroenterology and Hepatology
Department of Medicine, Imperial College London
London, UK

Thomas P. Beresford MD
Professor of Psychiatry
University of Colorado School of Medicine;
Physician, Laboratory for Clinical and Translational
Research in Psychiatry
Department of Veterans Affairs Medical Center
Denver, CO, USA

Ed Britton MBBS, MRCP
Fellow in Hepatology
Royal Liverpool University Hospital
Liverpool, UK

Patrizia Burra MD
Head, Multivisceral Transplant Unit
Department of Surgery
Oncology and Gastroenterology
Padova University Hospital
Padova, Italy

Chris Day MA, MBBChir, MD PhD, FRCP
Pro-Vice-Chancellor, Faculty of Medical Sciences;
Consultant Physician, Institute of Cellular Medicine
Newcastle University
Newcastle upon Tyne, UK

James Ferguson MD, FRCPE
Consultant Hepatologist, Liver Unit
Queen Elizabeth Hospital Birmingham
Birmingham;
Associate Medical Director
Organ Donation and Transplantation
NHS Blood and Transplant
Bristol, UK

Joaquim Fernández-Solà MD, PhD
Medical Senior Consultant in Internal Medicine
Alcohol Unit, Hospital Clínic, Institut
d'Investigacions Biomèdiques August Pi i Sunyer (IDIBAPS)
CIBEROBN Fisiopatología de la Obesidad y la Nutrición,
Instituto de Salud Carlos III;
Professor of Medicine, University of Barcelona
Barcelona, Spain

Marian Fireman MD
Associate Professor of Psychiatry
Oregon Health and Science University
Portland, OR, USA

Giacomo Germani MD, PhD, FEBTM
Consultant Physician, Multivisceral Transplant Unit
Department of Surgery
Oncology and Gastroenterology
Padova University Hospital
Padova, Italy

Ian Gilmore MD, FRCP
Honorary Professor
Department of Medicine
University of Liverpool
Liverpool, UK;
Adjunct Professor
National Drug Research Institute, Faculty of Health Sciences
Curtin University
Perth, Australia

William Gilmore BSc, MSc
Research Fellow
National Drug Research Institute
Faculty of Health Sciences
Curtin University
Perth, Australia

Jane I. Grove BSc, PhD
Postdoctoral Research Fellow
National Institute for Health Research (NIHR)
Nottingham Digestive Diseases Biomedical
Research Unit
Nottingham University Hospitals NHS Trust
and the University of Nottingham
Nottingham, UK

Peter Hayes PhD, FRCP(Ed)
Professor of Hepatology
Department of Gastroenterology
Royal Infirmary of Edinburgh
Edinburgh, UK

Eileen Kaner PhD
Professor of Public Health Research
Institute of Health and Society
Newcastle University
Newcastle upon Tyne, UK

Stuart Kendrick MA, BMBCh, PhD, MRCP
Consultant Physician
Institute of Cellular Medicine
Newcastle University
Newcastle upon Tyne, UK

Martin Lombard MB, BCh, BAO, MD,
MSc, FRCPI, FRCP
Professor and Consultant Hepatologist
and Gastroenterologist
Gastroenterology and Liver Services
Royal Liverpool University Hospital
Liverpool, UK

Michael R. Lucey MD
Professor and Chief of Division
Department of Medicine
Division of Gastroenterology and Hepatology
University of Wisconsin School of Medicine
and Public Health
Madison, WI, USA

Andrea DiMartini MD
Associate Professor of Psychiatry
Associate Professor of Surgery
Medical Director, Psychosomatic Medicine
Transplant Program
Starzl Transplant Institute
University of Pittsburgh Medical Center
Pittsburgh, PA, USA

Desley A.H. Neil FRCPath, MBBS, PhD, BMedSc
Consultant Histopathologist
Queen Elizabeth Hospital Birmingham
Birmingham, UK

James Neuberger DM, FRCP
Honorary Consultant
Liver Unit
Queen Elizabeth Hospital Birmingham
Birmingham;
Associate Medical Director
Organ Donation and Transplantation
NHS Blood and Transplant
Bristol, UK

John G. O'Grady MD, FRCPI
Professor of Hepatology
Institute of Liver Studies
King's College Hospital
London, UK

Richard Parker MBChB, MRCP
MRC Clinical Research Training Fellow
NIHR Centre for Liver Research and Biomedical
Research Unit
University of Birmingham;
Honorary Hepatology Registrar
University Hospitals Birmingham NHS Foundation Trust
Birmingham, UK

Stephen Potts MA FRCPsych FRCPE
Consultant in Transplant Psychiatry
Department of Psychological Medicine
Royal Infirmary of Edinburgh;
Honorary Senior Clinical Lecturer
University of Edinburgh
Edinburgh, UK

Ulrich W. Preuss MD
Professor of Psychiatry
Kreiskrankenhaus Prignitz, Perleberg;
Department of Psychiatry, Psychotherapy
and Psychosomatic Medicine
University of Halle
Halle, Germany

Jens Reimer MD, MBA
Professor
Department of Psychiatry and Psychotherapy
Center for Interdisciplinary Addiction Research
University Medical Center Hamburg-Eppendorf (UKE)
Hamburg, Germany

Shari Rogal MD, MPH
Gastroenterologist and Transplant Hepatologist
VA Pittsburgh Healthcare System;
Center for Health Equity Research and Promotion
VA Pittsburgh Healthcare System;
Visiting Assistant Professor of Surgery
Division of Gastroenterology
Hepatology and Nutrition University of Pittsburgh
Pittsbugh, PA, USA

John B. Saunders MA, MB, BChir, MD,
FRACP, FAChAM, FRCP
Professor, Faculty of Medicine and Biomedical Sciences
University of Queensland
Queensland;
Disciplines of Psychiatry and Addiction Medicine
Sydney Medical School, University of Sydney
New South Wales, Australia

Terry D. Schneekloth MD
Assistant Professor of Psychiatry
Mayo Clinic
Rochester, MN, USA

Karl-Heinz Schulz MD, PhD
Professor
Institute of Medical Psychology and Center for
Transplantation Medicine
University Medical Center Hamburg-Eppendorf (UKE)
Hamburg, Germany

Stephanie Scott PhD
Research Associate
Human Nutrition Research Centre and Institute
of Health and Society
Newcastle University
Newcastle upon Tyne, UK

Amanda Smith BPharm(hons), MRPharmS,
DipClinPharm
Lead Pharmacist, Liver and Solid Organ
Transplantation
University Hospitals Birmingham NHS Foundation Trust
Birmingham, UK

Julie Taub MD
Assistant Professor of Medicine
University of Colorado School of Medicine;
Hospitalist, Department of Medicine
Denver Health Medical Center
Denver, CO, USA

Benjamin A. Temple
Professional Research Assistant
University of Colorado School of Medicine;
Laboratory for Clinical and Translational Research
in Psychiatry
Department of Veterans Affairs Medical Center
Denver, CO, USA

Natasha Thon MSc
Department for Psychiatry and Psychotherapy II
Christian-Doppler Hospital
Paracelsus Medical University
Salzburg, Austria

Mark Thursz MD, FRCP
Professor of Hepatology
Department of Medicine, Imperial College London
London, UK

Santiago Tomé MD
Professor
Hepatology Unit, Internal Medicine Department
Hospital Universitario de Santiago de Compostela
Santiago de Compostela, Spain

Sandra van Eckert RN, MCommH, MPH, PhD
Research Associate
Institute of Medical Psychology and Center for
Transplantation Medicine
University Medical Center Hamburg-Eppendorf (UKE)
Hamburg, Germany

Wolfgang Weinmann PhD
Professor
Institute of Forensic Medicine
University of Berne
Berne, Switzerland

Robert M. Weinrieb MD, FAPM
Director, Psychosomatic Medicine and Psychosomatic
Medicine Fellowship
Department of Psychiatry
University of Pennsylvania Health System
Perelman School of Medicine
Philadelphia, PA, USA

Michael Williams BMBCh, PhD, MRCP
Specialist Registrar
Department of Gastroenterology
Royal Infirmary of Edinburgh
Edinburgh, UK

Jessica Wong MD
Kreiskrankenhaus Prignitz
Perleberg, Germany

Narin Wongngamnit MD
Addiction Psychiatrist, Substance Abuse Treatment Program
Department of Veterans Affairs;
Instructor in Psychiatry, School of Medicine
University of Colorado Denver;
Laboratory for Clinical and Translational Research
in Psychiatry
Department of Veterans Affairs Medical Center
Denver, CO, USA

Friedrich Martin Wurst MD
Professor, Paracelsus Medical University (PMU)
Salzburg, Austria;
Centre for Interdisciplinary Addiction Research, University
of Hamburg, Germany

Renata Yang MD, MPH
Fellow, Addiction Psychiatry
Oregon Health and Science University
Portland, OR, USA

Michel Yegles PhD
Head of Forensic Toxicology
Laboratoire National de Santé
Division de Toxicologie
Centre Universitaire
Luxembourg, Luxembourg

Preface

First you take a drink, then the drink takes a drink, then the drink takes you. F. Scott Fitzgerald

To alcohol! The cause of … and solution to … all of life's problems. Matt Groening

It is difficult to feel sympathy for these people. It is difficult to regard some bawdy drunk and see them as sick and powerless…. Can there be any other disease that renders its victims so unappealing? Russell Brand

I have taken more good from alcohol than alcohol has taken from me. Winston Churchill

Alcohol and alcohol-related disease is becoming an increasing health issue throughout the world. Patients present in many ways and across the health care services and effective management presents a number of challenges: social, medical, and psychiatric. The issue is further complicated by the ambivalent societal approaches to alcohol and the people suffering its adverse consequences.

The rationale for this volume is to provide a useful resource for both gastroenterologists and hepatologists and for those specialists in mental health and substance abuse and addiction to help the clinicians provide a joined-up, holistic approach to manage those with alcohol-related liver disease effectively. We have brought together hepatologists, addiction and alcohol specialists, epidemiologists and others from the United States, Europe, and Australia to provide what we hope will be a valuable aid.

We are grateful to these international experts for their contribution for their contributions. We are aware that there is some overlap and some differing in views: we have intentionally left them in place to provide the reader with coherent chapters and an understanding of the spectrum of opinion.

We would like to thank the publishers for their help, especially Oliver Walter, Jennifer Seward, and Jasmine Chang. As editors, we have enjoyed working together and hope that the benefits of a psychiatrist and a hepatologist working either side of the Atlantic is reflected in the book. We hope the reader will also find this useful, educational, and enjoyable.

James Neuberger
Andrea diMartini

CHAPTER 1

Epidemiology of alcohol use

Ian Gilmore[1,2] and William Gilmore[2]

[1] *Department of Medecine, University of Liverpool, Liverpool, UK*

[2] *National Drug Research Institute, Faculty of Health Sciences, Curtin University, Perth, Australia*

KEY POINTS

- Alcohol use has been established throughout the world for millennia.
- The alcohol consumed can be assessed from sales and survey data but both have limitations.
- The potential harm caused by alcohol will depend not only on the amount consumed, but also on the pattern of drinking, gender, age, other comorbidities, and other behavioural, cultural, and genetic factors.
- The amount of alcohol consumed depends on both availability and cost.
- Trends in alcohol consumption levels over time have varied considerably between countries.
- While many countries have seen a fall in cases of cirrhosis and deaths from alcohol in recent years, some, such as the United Kingdom, have seen a rise.

Introduction

Alcohol is our drug of choice, not just in the western world but globally. Its use defines societies and often divides them. This complexity of attitudes and behaviors can be traced back to the earliest times of civilization. Written reference to alcohol is as old as writing itself – the cuneiform scripts of Sumerians around 3000 BC – but the wild grapevine was indigenous to current wine-producing countries of Europe and Asia several hundred thousand years earlier and has been cultivated since 6000 BC at least. Neolithic man cultivated barley and it is likely that beer consumption has just as long a history. Inebriation likewise is as ancient as the availability of alcoholic beverages, and in Babylon in 1800 BC it was found necessary to regulate price and availability in "wineshops" or taverns [1]. The Hebrews found the Promised Land fertile for viniculture, and the result was an early temperance or prohibition movement amongst rebel Rechabites who "will drink no wine." But, overall, wine consumption became a positive and symbolic ritual of God's natural gifts in Judaism and early Christianity. However, the New Testament exhorts temperance as a virtue, and St. Paul clearly understood the physical harms associated with alcohol when he stated that drunkenness barred the gates of Heaven and desecrated the body. Chinese literature shows a similar timeline, and an imperial edict around 1000 BC recognized that alcohol in moderation was a gift from heaven.

Medieval life was generously lubricated by alcohol and beer drunk in volumes 10-fold greater than today – although it may have been considerably weaker. The

---

Alcohol Abuse and Liver Disease, First Edition. Edited by James Neuberger and Andrea DiMartini.

principle of distillation was probably known several thousand years ago but was only recognized again in the Middle Ages, initially mainly for the preparation of remedies for ailments. It crept into popular consumption in the sixteenth century, when grain-distilled whisky started in Ireland and spread to Scotland. In England in the seventeenth century it was the spread of juniper-flavored white spirit from Holland, gin, that became the rage, encouraged by an Act of Parliament of 1690 for the "encouraging of the distillation of brandy and gin from corn." However, this was more to do with antagonism towards France and protection of British grain production by William of Orange than of the virtues of alcohol. The seventeenth century American colonies demonstrated the accelerated move of a new society towards regulation and taxation.

The eighteenth century has been much parodied in the United Kingdom as in Hogarth's Gin Lane, and certainly the plethora of Parliamentary Acts and Repeals laid testament to the societal consequences of the ready availability of cheap, strong liquor. The prohibitive taxes introduced in 1736 had to be withdrawn in the face of bootlegging, riots, and smuggling. In hindsight, much of the concern over the next century was about the poorer classes taking up heavy drinking, hitherto a diversion of the landed gentry, and the consequences for productivity and industrialization. In the United States the influential physician William Rush, perhaps the father of modern psychiatry, introduced the concept of alcoholism as an illness and addiction rather than a sin. However, in the eighteenth and nineteenth centuries the power of organized religion in combating the evil of drink and the virtue of abstinence was at its peak. In many countries there was in addition the ebb and flow of regulation and taxation.

The destructive power of alcohol to the national effort was obvious to Lloyd George in Britain during the First World War (although he was no doubt influenced by his Welsh chapel upbringing), and stringent restrictions on availability contributed to the decline in consumption that was reversed only after the World War II. In the second half of the twentieth century, developed countries fell under the influence of large national, and later multinational, producers of alcoholic drinks who discovered the power of marketing developed by motor car, tobacco, and soft drink manufacturers. Increasing globalization has seen developing countries move from local, often unregulated and unmeasured consumption to joining the party with international, heavily marketed products, and it has been only the Islamic religion that has halted alcohol's progress in those parts of the world.

Why monitor alcohol use?

Per capita consumption has been shown to be a relatively reliable proxy measure of the number of heavy drinkers in a population, which can help predict the magnitude of harm associated with alcohol use in that population [2]. As the potential harms associated with alcohol use vary depending on the drinking patterns within populations, it is important to look at not just overall consumption but to dig deeper into the patterns of drinking. There are clear cultural differences in drinking patterns, for instance between northern and southern European countries. There are also differences in pattern between age groups. Even in dependent drinkers there are those who consume a relatively constant amount each day but others who will drink in "benders" for days or weeks but then remain abstinent for long periods.

Methods of measuring alcohol use

Alcohol consumption estimates are usually derived from data on the regulated production, sale, trade, and taxation of alcohol and presented as liters of pure alcohol consumed per adult in a given year. Unregulated production and consumption, more prevalent in developing and Islamic countries, can lead to underestimates. The World Health Organization (WHO) has estimated that 29% of alcohol consumption is unrecorded [3], but within that global figure the unrecorded portion can be as high as 66% in India and 90% in East Africa [4]. Other factors that may affect the accuracy of national consumption estimates include tourist drinking, stockpiling, waste, smuggling, and duty-free sales.

Population level survey data should not be used to calculate per capita consumption and have been found to underestimate consumption levels by 40–60% when compared with estimates from sales data. This gives credence to the doctor's "rule of thumb" of doubling the amount his or her patient admits to. Self-reported estimates will tend to reflect ordinary weeks and ignore special occasions and vacations. However, with these caveats, surveys are essential to provide additional information on patterns of consumption within populations, for example the number that drink alcohol, how often they drink, the way in which they drink, and how much they drink.

National alcohol consumption estimates

According to the WHO [3], worldwide alcohol consumption in 2005 was 6 liters of pure alcohol for every person aged 15 years or older, ranging from 0.02 liters in Afghanistan to 18 liters in the Republic of Moldova. The highest levels of consumption are seen across Europe and the former Soviet Republic; moderate levels are seen in North and South America and South Africa, and the lowest levels seen across North and Central Africa, the Middle East and South-East Asia (Figure 1.1). It is the countries with lower levels of total consumption that tend to have a higher proportion of alcohol that is homemade or illegally produced. These countries are also most likely to have outbreaks of illness and death as a result of contaminated sources of illicit alcohol. For example, 121 people died and 495 were hospitalized in Nairobi, Kenya, in 2000 after consuming homemade drink that contained methanol [5].

The most popular choice of drink varies considerably between cultures (Figure 1.2). In Asia, Eastern Europe, and parts of the Middle East and Caribbean spirits are the predominant alcohol type. Beer is the most consumed alcoholic drink in Australia, New Zealand, most of North and South America and northern Europe, and parts of Africa and South-East Asia. In southern Europe (excluding Spain), Sweden, and the tip of South America wine is the most popular drink. Spain and Sweden are both breaking with tradition and not drinking like their southern and northern European neighbors.

Changes in national alcohol consumption over time

There are remarkable differences between countries in their drinking habits over the last 50 years. Those countries with the highest per capita consumption, such as France and Italy, have seen a remarkable fall in overall consumption (Figure 1.3) and this has been accompanied by falls in deaths from cirrhosis – a very useful surrogate for consumption and general harm [6].

Conversely, the United Kingdom has seen a more than doubling of consumption from historically low levels after the World War II (Figure 1.4) [7]. This rise has almost exactly matched increases in the affordability of alcohol (Figure 1.5) [8] and in deaths from cirrhosis [6].

The rise in alcohol consumption in the United Kingdom is not unique and there is a similar gradient from a lower starting point in China, Thailand, Brazil, and Nigeria [4], where the unrecorded fraction is likely to be larger.

There has been a small but consistent fall in consumption in the United Kingdom since 2005 (Figure 1.4), which is not fully explained. There has been an increase in ethnic diversity, with more abstainers for religious reasons, and there has also been a duty escalator since 2007 that has ensured that duty has risen faster than inflation. The economic downturn is also likely to have been a factor – there was a sharp downturn in consumption during the depression of the late 1920s.

The United States (Figure 1.6), Canada, Australia, and New Zealand have followed a similar trend with increasing total consumption from the 1960s to the 1980s, followed by a decrease and then stabilization [4,9].

Patterns of alcohol use

The presented consumption estimates do not take into account that the proportion of drinkers within countries varies greatly. Rates of abstinence mirror estimates of per capita consumption and it is the countries with higher consumption levels that have a lower prevalence of abstinence. Therefore, countries with low levels of per capita consumption can in fact have high levels of consumption when calculated per drinker.

The WHO patterns of drinking score [3], based on survey data and measured on a scale from 1 (least risky drinking pattern) to 5 (most risky drinking pattern), reflect the way in which people drink and not just the quantity they drink (Figure 1.7) [3]. The more risky patterns of drinking occur in Russia, Ukraine, Belarus, Kazakhstan, South Africa, and Mexico. The less risky patterns occur in southern and central Europe, the United States, Canada, Argentina, North Africa, China, Australia, and New Zealand.

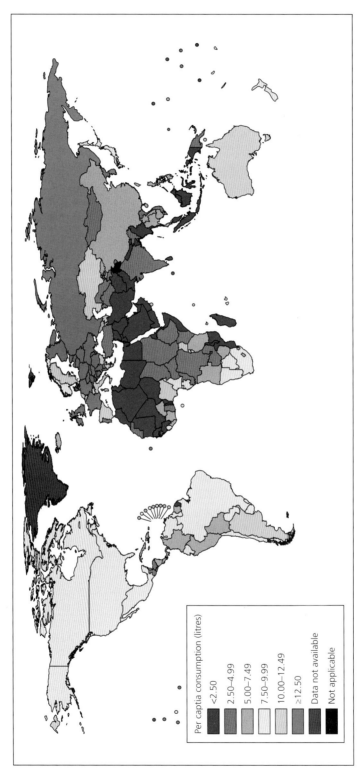

Figure 1.1 Liters of pure alcohol consumed per person aged 15+, from both regulated and unregulated production, 2005. (Source: World Health Organization, 2011 [3]) *(See insert for color representation of the figure)*

Per captia consumption (litres)

- <2.50
- 2.50–4.99
- 5.00–7.49
- 7.50–9.99
- 10.00–12.49
- ≥12.50
- Data not available
- Not applicable

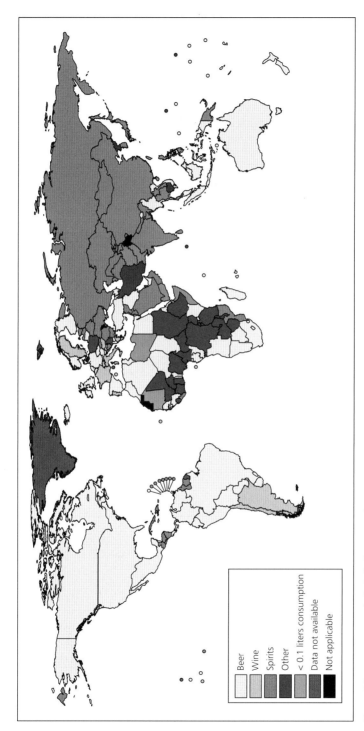

Figure 1.2 Most consumed alcoholic beverages from regulated production in liters of pure alcohol, 2005. (Source: World Health Organization, 2011 [3])
(See insert for color representation of the figure)

Beer
Wine
Spirits
Other
< 0.1 liters consumption
Data not available
Not applicable

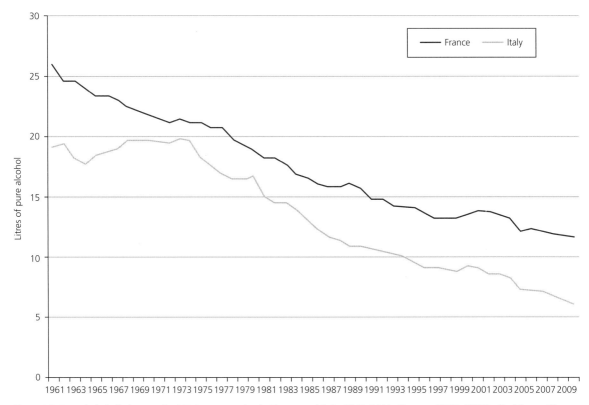

Figure 1.3 Recorded alcohol per capita (15+) consumption in France and Italy, 1961–2010. (Source: OECD (2012), Health at a Glance: Europe 2012, OECD Publishing)

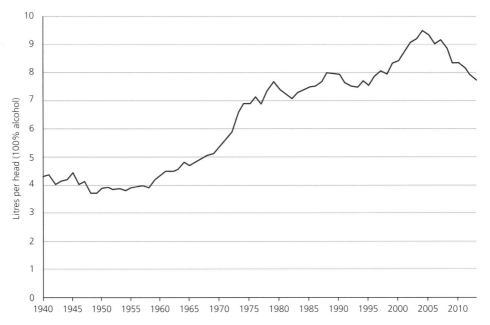

Figure 1.4 Per capita pure alcohol consumption in the UK, 1940–2013. (Source: British Beer and Pub Association Statistical Handbook, 2013 [7]. Reproduced by permission of British Beer and Pub Association)

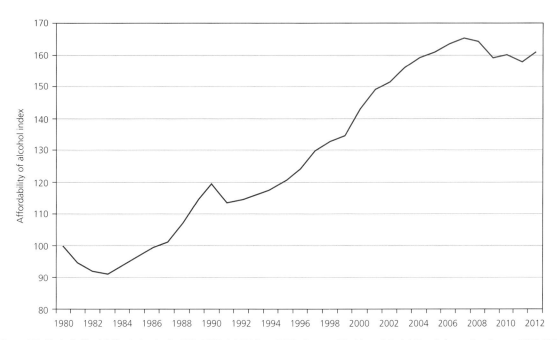

Figure 1.5 Alcohol affordability index in the UK: 1980 (=100%) to 2012. (Source: Health and Social Care Information Centre, 2013 [8])

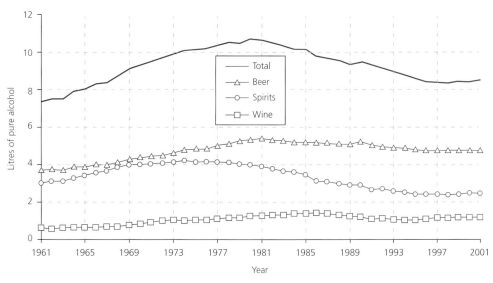

Figure 1.6 Recorded per capita consumption (age 15+) in the United States. (Source: United Nations Food and Agriculture Organization World Drink Trends, 2003 [9]; World Health Organization, 2004 [4])

Within populations there is an uneven distribution of alcohol consumption. Alcohol, like most population variables, fits the Pareto or 80 : 20 principle (Pareto was an Italian economist who pointed out in 1906 that 80% of the wealth in Italy was owned by 20% of the population). Studies have shown that the majority of alcohol in a population is drunk by a minority of heavy drinkers. Thus, when levels of total alcohol consumption increase in a population so does the prevalence of heavy drinking.

Men are more likely to be drinkers than women and, among those that do drink, men tend to drink larger amounts and more frequently than women. Generally,

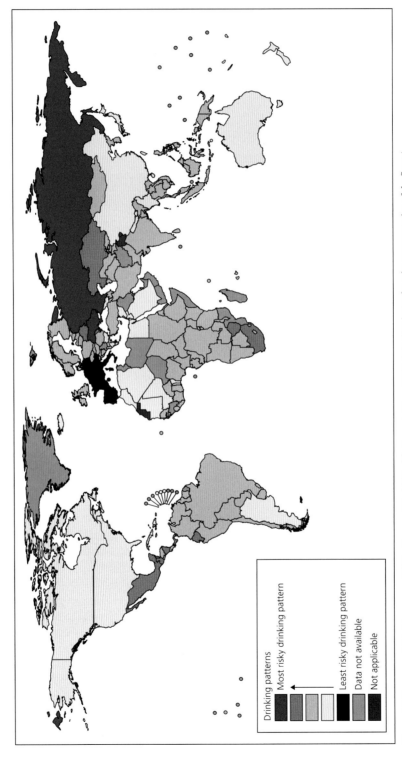

Figure 1.7 Patterns of drinking score, 2005. (Source: World Health Organization, 2011 [3]) *(See insert for color representation of the figure)*

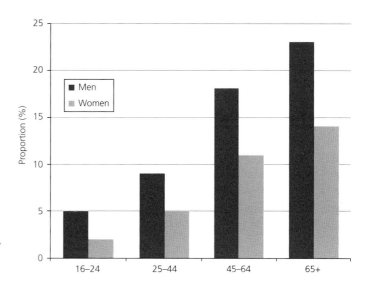

Figure 1.8 Drinking 5 days per week or more by age in the United Kingdom. (Source: Office for National Statistics, 2013 [10])

young adults and adolescents are more likely to engage in occasional heavy drinking than older adults, a pattern of drinking that is more associated with the acute consequences of alcohol such as injury to self or others. The latest data from the UK Office for National Statistics (2012) show that 27% of 16- to 24-year-olds drank very heavily at least once in the previous week compared with only 3% of over-65-year-olds [10]. The corollary of this is that older people drink more often than younger ones (Figure 1.8).

In the United Kingdom and Australia, where large supermarkets and supermarket-owned chains now dominate off-licence sales and can offer heavily discounted drink, drinking at home rather than at a licensed premise is the preferred option.

Among the indigenous populations of North America, Australia, and New Zealand, alcohol consumption levels and associated harms are significantly higher than among non-indigenous populations, despite higher reported levels of abstention [11]. The pattern of drinking among indigenous peoples that drink tends to be infrequent but drinking to intoxication on occasion.

Factors determining use

Clearly, cultural factors are important in determining differences between and within countries, although these factors are becoming less prominent as international travel and globalization erode national custom and practice. There is a similar blurring of national differences as multinational drinks manufacturers promote their products across the world. India is now the biggest market for Scotch whisky, and brands such as Guinness, once so clearly linked to a single country, are available universally.

Marketing has been similarly successful in rebranding products. An example is the way that vodka has been recreated as an attractive drink for young people by introducing a new brand and heavily marketing it [12]. In many parts of the world young people currently drink spirits in preference to the traditional student drink of beer. While there is nothing inherently different about the alcohol in beer and spirits, low volume high strength preparations are likely to encourage heavier consumption.

The ever-increasing size and success of alcohol companies mean that they are very well positioned to influence government policy in favor of the alcohol industry. This is already evident in developed countries with a long history of both alcohol use and policies regulating the availability of alcohol. Developing countries, which are the current target in the global alcohol expansion, are likely to be even more susceptible to industry influence [5].

Both the increased economic and physical availability of alcohol in society are well-known drivers for increased alcohol use [5]. Increases in beverage price, typically through taxation, have been shown to reduce levels of consumption and associated harms in populations. Likewise have measures that aim to reduce the physical availability of alcohol such as restrictions on the age of purchase, number of licensed premises, trading hours, and sale to intoxicated persons.

The burden of alcohol use

Alcohol use has wide-ranging harmful effects (Table 1.1). It is associated with long-term conditions, such as liver disease, as well as short-term health impacts that come with drinking to intoxication, such as injury. Harms not only occur to the individual drinker but there are others to consider. These may be victims of alcohol-related violence or an unborn child exposed to alcohol *in utero*. Finally, there are the wider social impacts, often difficult to measure, affecting families, workplaces, communities, and countries.

Table 1.1 Examples of the health and social harms associated with alcohol use.

Health	Social
Gastrointestinal disease	Violence
Cardiovascular disease*	Vandalism
Cancer	Antisocial behavior
Neuropsychiatric conditions	Family problems
Diabetes*	Work problems
Infectious diseases	Social and economic costs
Alcohol poisoning	
Intentional injury	
Accidental injury	
Fetal alcohol spectrum disorder	

*Both harmful and protective effects shown with different levels of use.

References

[1] Austin G. *Alcohol in Western Society from Antiquity to 1800: A Chronological History*. ABC-Clio Press, Santa Barbara, CA; 1985.

[2] Stockwell T, Chikritzhs T (Eds). *International Guide for Monitoring Alcohol Consumption and Related Harm*. World Health Organization, Geneva; 2000.

[3] World Health Organization. *Global Status Report on Alcohol and Health*. World Health Organization, Geneva: 2011.

[4] World Health Organization. *Global Status Report on Alcohol*. World Health Organization, Geneva: 2004.

[5] Babor T, Caetano R, Casswell S, Edwards G, Giesbrecht N, Graham K, et al. *Alcohol: No Ordinary Commodity. Research and Public Policy*, 2nd edition. Oxford University Press, Oxford; 2010.

[6] Leon D, McCambridge J. Liver cirrhosis mortality rates in Britain from 1950 to 2002: an analysis of routine data. *Lancet* 2006; **367**(9504): 52–56.

[7] British Beer and Pub Association (BBPA). *Statistical Handbook 2013*. BBPA, London; 2010.

[8] Health and Social Care Information Centre (HSCIC). *Statistics on Alcohol: England, 2013*. HSCIC, Leeds; 2013.

[9] Food and Agriculture Organization of the United Nations. *World Drink Trends* 2003.

[10] Office for National Statistics (ONS). *Drinking Habits Amongst Adults, 2012*. ONS Statistical Bulletin; 2013.

[11] Brady M. Alcohol policy issues for indigenous people in the United States, Canada, Australia and New Zealand. *Contemporary Drug Problems* 2000; **27**: 435–509.

[12] Mosher J. Joe Camel in a bottle: Diageo, the Smirnoff brand, and the transformation of the youth alcohol market. *Am J Public Health* 2012; **102**: 56–63.

CHAPTER 2

Epidemiology of alcohol-related liver disease

Ed Britton and Martin Lombard

Royal Liverpool University Hospital, Liverpool, UK

KEY POINTS

- Alcohol accounts for 1.8 million deaths, nearly 500 000 cases of cirrhosis, and 14.5 million disability-adjusted life years lost from alcohol-related cirrhosis annually.

- There is a clear correlation between the global pattern of alcohol consumption and the pattern of liver-related deaths attributable to alcohol both as an incidence and percentage of mortality within that region.

- Alcohol is a factor in one in three (30%) sexual offences, one in three (33%) burglaries, and one in two (50%) street crimes.

- Public health interventions such as increasing alcohol cost with a minimum unit pricing policy by taxation, bans on alcohol marketing, stringent drink driving policies, and reducing alcohol availability offer the biggest public health benefit.

- Binge drinking (>8 units/day) is detrimental to public health because of aggression and violence, mental and behavioral disorders, sudden cardiac death, stroke, self-harm including suicide, road traffic accidents, impaired performance at work, and antisocial behavior because of the effects of alcohol. However, the effect on liver disease is less clear.

- Identifying those at risk of alcohol-induced cirrhosis before the onset of fibrosis is the key to minimizing the health impact of the disease.

- Noninvasive fibrosis tests may identify disease at an earlier stage but do not prevent disease onset.

- Current tools adequately assess alcohol consumption but do not reliably identify those at risk of liver disease.

Introduction

Alcohol-related social and health problems are at the forefront of the medical and political agenda in most countries with both alcohol-related liver disease and mortality on the increase. Globally, in 2010, alcohol-related cirrhosis was the identified cause of 493 300 deaths and 14 544 000 disability-adjusted life years (DALYs) (4 112 000 for women and 10 432 000 for men), representing 0.9% of all global deaths and 0.6% of all global DALYs [1].

The increasing burden of liver disease and liver mortality is on the background of improving age standardized mortality rates for other major chronic illnesses (cancer, chronic heart disease, cerebrovascular and respiratory diseases). Furthermore, increasing prevalence of associated risk factors for liver disease such as obesity, accompanied by changing patterns of alcohol consumption, make this epidemiologic pattern one that is likely to continue.

This chapter focuses on the historical population-based association of alcohol consumption and liver

Alcohol Abuse and Liver Disease, First Edition. Edited by James Neuberger and Andrea DiMartini.
© 2015 John Wiley & Sons, Ltd. Published 2015 by John Wiley & Sons, Ltd.

disease alongside the global burden of alcohol-related disease on mortality health and social care worldwide. The changing patterns of alcohol consumption and associated risk factors increasing the likelihood of chronic liver disease are explored. Finally, population methods to reduce the burden of disease are discussed.

Alcohol and liver disease: a historical perspective

Humans have consumed alcohol since prehistoric times; the links to liver disease have been drawn from population data throughout the last 100 years. The first published insights into the effects of alcohol on health were made in 1920 and published in the *British Medical Journal* in 1924, showing a lower life expectancy in heavy drinkers than in abstainers or moderate consumers of alcohol [2]. Similar observations were noted during the Prohibition era in the United States; when alcohol was in short supply mortality from cirrhosis appeared to fall. Further reinforcing this trend was the observation of an 80% reduction in deaths from cirrhosis during a period of wine rationing in France during World War II. Further studies throughout the decades have demonstrated the association of heavy alcohol consumption with mortality and more specifically cirrhosis [3,4].

Interestingly, however, small to moderate amounts of alcohol consumption are purported to have some health benefits. This was first demonstrated in 1981 in a large study of civil servants where mortality in moderate drinkers was lower than in both abstainers and heavy drinkers (>34 g/day), a so-called U-shaped relationship (Figure 2.1). However, in a recent simulation all data indicated that the optimal level of alcohol intake for its protective effect was only 3–5 g/day, well below the currently recommended "safe limits." The difference in mortality between abstainers and moderate drinkers appeared to be mediated by a reduced risk of cardio-vascular disease mortality whereas the increased mortality of the heavy drinkers was brought about by noncardio-vascular causes. In this study the relationship was independent of differences in smoking, blood pressure, cholesterol, or employment grade [5].

Through these epidemiologic studies, alongside animal model studies that demonstrated liver disease was inducible by feeding large amounts of ethanol to

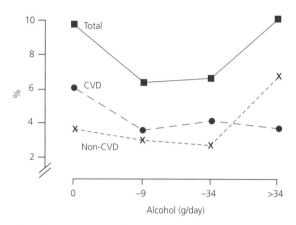

Figure 2.1 10-year mortality (age-adjusted percentage) according to daily alcohol consumption divided into all cause (Total), cardiovascular (CVD), and noncardiovascular (non-CVD) [5].

rats, the case for alcohol as a cause for chronic liver disease and mortality associated with cirrhosis became compelling. As a consequence, a World Health Organization (WHO) funded review was published, reviewing and summarizing the available evidence linking alcohol to mortality and cirrhosis, and concluding that cirrhosis among heavy drinkers was 2–23 times the background population risk.

Despite the accumulation of population-based data, two problems remained, first, trends in per capita consumption of alcohol in the population did not directly mirror those for cirrhosis or liver-related mortality. In fact, cirrhosis mortality appeared to better reflect alcohol consumption of several years previous; the supposition being that liver disease took time to develop. In 1980, a model to explain the relationship between consumption and liver-related mortality in any one year was proposed and labeled the "distributed lag model," confirming the assumption that liver disease developed over time as a consequence of alcohol consumption [6]. However, more recently, epidemiologic data from Russia described how sociologic changes and alcohol regulation resulted in rapid and dramatic reductions in alcohol-related mortality when population consumption was curtailed, so it seems that the "lag" relationship is complex and can be reversed rapidly [7].

A second problem that remains to this day is that despite some early animal models and ultimately compelling epidemiologic data, there are no controlled trials in humans to examine the direct dose-dependent effect of alcohol on the liver, nor is there a clear molecular understanding of why certain individuals develop liver disease related to alcohol while others do not. Associated risk factors for developing chronic liver disease related to alcohol are covered in more detail elsewhere in this chapter (see Associated risk factors for liver disease).

However, recently the impact of alcohol on global health, not just in the form of liver disease, was demonstrated by the WHO global status report for alcohol published in 2004. This found that overall alcohol causes 1.8 million deaths (3.2% of total) and a loss of 58.3 million (4% of total) DALYs. Unintentional injuries alone account for about one-third of the 1.8 million deaths, while neuropsychiatric conditions account for close to 40% of the 58.3 million DALYs (World Health Organization, 2004).

Key points

- Alcohol-related cirrhosis accounts for 493 300 deaths per year worldwide.
- The first association of alcohol to increased mortality was reported by Perl in 1924.
- Periods of enforced population abstinence, including World War II in Europe, Prohibition in the United States, and stringent regulation in Russia, were associated with falls in levels of cirrhosis.
- Currently, there are no controlled studies in humans examining the effects of alcohol; all data are drawn from epidemiologic data.
- Alcohol has a wider effect on global health, being accountable for a total of 1.8 million deaths and 58.3 million DALYs.

Current trends in alcohol consumption and cirrhosis

The current global trends of alcohol consumption are outlined in Figure 2.2 with Table 2.1 defining amounts of alcohol consumption considered as safe, harmful, or hazardous. Reporting of population consumption statistics can be confusing: international convention is to report alcohol consumption in "liters of pure alcohol" to avoid misinterpretation over variations in definition of units. However, one must be somewhat cautious about international comparisons because some use "per capita" for whole adult populations, some for whole

populations including children, and some for drinking populations excluding abstainers. The latter two may appear comparatively low or high, respectively, compared to most reports. Furthermore the proportion of the population who abstain varies widely between countries and cultures. For example, in 2010 Eastern Europe had the highest consumption of alcohol per adult capita of the population of 15.7 L of pure alcohol per person per year and although the consumption per adult capita in sub-Saharan Africa is low they have some of the highest consumption rates per drinker with southern African drinkers consuming a mean of 30.3 L of pure alcohol per year. High levels of alcohol consumption are also seen throughout Europe, Central Asia, and the United States, thus highlighting that the problem of alcohol consumption is not limited to western society.

A potential explanation for the trends in alcohol consumption is affordability. Currently, alcohol within the United Kingdom is proportionally 45% more affordable than in 1980.

Table 2.2 shows the impact of these patterns of alcohol consumption upon liver disease and liver health worldwide. There is a clear correlation between the global pattern of alcohol consumption and the pattern of liver-related deaths attributable to alcohol both as an incidence and percentage of mortality within that region. The global mortality from cirrhosis attributable to alcohol of 493 300 accounts for approximately 47% of mortality from cirrhosis of any cause. Globally, alcohol-related cirrhosis mortality accounts for 7.2 deaths per 100 000 population, a standardized mortality higher than many common cancers.

A further reflection of the increasing burden of cirrhosis worldwide is the increasing incidence of liver cancer exemplified by the UK trend of a 40% rise in the period 2002–2012 alongside declines in incidences of lung, breast, bowel, and many other solid organ malignancies (Cancer Research UK statistics).

While mortality may represent one aspect of a significant ongoing health problem there is also the ongoing health and social care impact of DALYs attributable to alcohol-related cirrhosis. Globally, DALYS related to alcohol-induced cirrhosis alone were more than 14.5 million years representing 211.1 DALYs per 100 000 population and 25% of all DALYs attributable to alcohol consumption. Of further importance is that the population most affected by this are those of working age (35–64 years), 459.4 DALYs per 100 000 within this

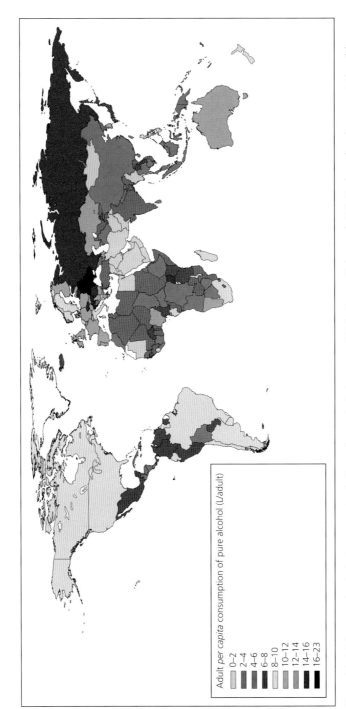

Figure 2.2 Adult per capita alcohol consumption in liters of pure alcohol per year, 2010. (Source: Rehm et al. [81]) *(See insert for color representation of the figure)*

Adult *per capita* consumption of pure alcohol (L/adult)

- 0–2
- 2–4
- 4–6
- 6–8
- 8–10
- 10–12
- 12–14
- 14–16
- 16–23

Table 2.1 Defining drinking levels (1 unit alcohol = 10 g/volume) (UK definition of a unit).

	Safe (units/week)	Hazardous (units/week)	Harmful (units/week)
Male	<21	22–50	>50
Female	<14	14–35	>35

age category, representing a significant social and health care burden.

However, alcohol-related epidemiologic data has some limitations. First, DALYs account for loss due to both years lost as a consequence of premature mortality and of years lost to disability. In those with alcohol-induced cirrhosis the majority of DALYs are attributable to premature mortality.

A further caveat and limitation to the liver disease attributable to alcohol mortality data is that they are drawn from epidemiologic statistics of alcohol consumption, and estimates of mortality are made related to alcohol consumption. This occurs because it is not possible to differentiate reliably between alcohol-related and non-alcohol-related cirrhosis deaths unless alcohol is specifically reported in the notification of death. There may well be a significant proportion of liver disease mortality attributable to alcohol that remains unrecorded.

Further exacerbating these limitations are the potential difficulties in assessing amount of consumption from population surveys. First, there is both reported and unreported consumption, with the reality not always matching what is reported. Second, the definition of a unit of alcohol or a standard drink and the required labeling of alcoholic beverages is not universal, which makes interpretation of consumption data difficult. For example, in the United Kingdom, the amount of alcohol in a beverage is defined by the number of units, with one unit of alcohol defined as 10 mL (7.9 g). A typical drink can therefore be anywhere between 1 and 3 units. In the United States, Australia, Japan, and other countries, the term standard drink is used to quantify the amount of alcohol in a given beverage and this can vary considerably, with one standard drink in the United States representing 0.6 US fluid ounces of alcohol (14 g), in Australia a standard drink contains 12.7 mL (10 g) of alcohol, and in Japan one standard drink is equivalent to 25 mL of alcohol (19.75 g). These varying definitions

make interpretation and comparison of consumption data difficult but, by convention, most studies convert consumption to liters of pure (absolute) alcohol.

Finally, data in this context represent a single snapshot view and will not reflect changes in consumption over time. As a consequence there remains a need for epidemiologic studies to determine the true burden of compensated alcohol-related cirrhosis within populations and the importance of alcohol-related disease as a cause of cirrhosis.

> **Key points**
>
> - The global mortality from cirrhosis attributable to alcohol of 493 300 accounts for approximately 47% of mortality from cirrhosis of any cause.
>
> - Globally, DALYS related to alcohol-induced cirrhosis alone were 14 544 000 years, with the vast majority caused by premature mortality.
>
> - Mortality from alcohol-related cirrhosis accounts for 47% of all cirrhosis mortality.

Changing trends in alcohol consumption

Within western society it had been noted that the mortality from cirrhosis was increasing significantly beyond what would have been expected by general alcohol consumption. As a consequence, studies were set up to examine the effects of binge drinking on risk of liver disease. Binge drinking is defined as the practice of drinking large amounts of alcohol in a short space of time or drinking to get drunk or feel the effects of alcohol. The actual number of units consumed to be considered a binge is less well defined in the literature. However, within the United Kingdom it is defined as binge drinking for men if more than 8 units of alcohol – or about 3 pints of strong beer – are consumed and more than 6 units of alcohol, equivalent to two large glasses of wine, for women.

The culture of binge drinking was recognized by the Chief Medical Officer in the United Kingdom in 2001 as a potential cause of increasing cirrhosis and cirrhosis mortality as well as a threat to public health from its other effects on society; alcohol is a factor in one in

Table 2.2 Liver-related deaths attributable to alcohol [1].

Global burden of disease region	Women			Men			Total		
	Deaths	All deaths (%)	Alcohol attributable deaths (%)	Deaths	All deaths (%)	Alcohol attributable deaths (%)	Deaths	All deaths (%)	Alcohol attributable deaths (%)
Asia, Pacific (high income)	7300	1	15.3	13900	1.7	14.3	21200	1.3	14.6
Asia, Central	5400	2.1	11.7	6800	2	9.8	12200	2	10.5
Asia, East	17100	0.5	8.1	53300	1	9	70500	0.8	8.8
Asia, South	22700	0.4	16.7	64900	0.9	14.6	87500	0.7	15
Asia, South-East	6500	0.4	12.6	27900	1.3	16.2	34500	0.9	15.4
Australasia	400	0.5	4.5	800	0.8	5.8	1200	0.7	5.2
Caribbean	900	0.4	8.7	1600	0.6	8.3	2500	0.5	8.4
Europe, Central	6600	1.1	6.9	16600	2.5	10.3	23200	1.8	9
Europe, Eastern	17000	1.1	3.7	16100	1.1	4.1	33100	1.1	3.9
Europe, Western	19900	1	9	32100	1.6	10.5	52000	1.3	9.9
Latin America, Andean	1700	1.5	21.1	2200	1.7	15.4	3900	1.6	17.5
Latin America, Central	7600	1.5	20.9	23900	3.6	20	31500	2.7	20.2
Latin America, Southern	2300	1.1	12.7	4800	2.1	14.8	7100	1.6	14
Latin America, Tropical	4500	0.8	11.1	13600	1.9	12.2	18100	1.5	11.9
North Africa/Middle East	4500	0.5	18.3	3800	0.3	5.8	8300	0.4	9.2
North America (high income)	13400	0.9	8.2	19700	1.4	9.3	33100	1.1	8.8
Oceania	400	1	23.7	500	1	18.3	900	1	20.4
Sub-Saharan Africa, Central	1700	0.4	16.8	3200	0.5	14.3	5000	0.5	15
Sub-Saharan Africa, Eastern	8500	0.6	21.8	12300	0.8	14.4	20800	0.7	16.7
Sub-Saharan Africa, Southern	1000	0.3	10.9	2400	0.6	6.1	3400	0.5	7
Sub-Saharan Africa, Western	7400	0.5	15.2	15900	0.9	17	23200	0.7	16.4
World	156900	0.7	9.3	336400	1.2	11	493300	0.9	10.4

three (30%) sexual offences, one in three (33%) burglaries, and one in two (50%) street crimes.

There is clear evidence that binge drinking is detrimental to public health for many reasons including aggression and violence, mental and behavioral disorders, sudden cardiac death, stroke, self-harm including suicide, road traffic accidents, impaired performance at work, and antisocial behavior due to the effects of alcohol. However, evidence to support the hypothesis that binge drinking increases the risk of liver disease has not been forthcoming so far. To date the largest study to examine the effects of binge drinking carried out in North America included 22 000 individuals and found that the risk of cirrhosis was twice as high with daily drinking than with intermittent drinking once or twice a week [9].

Interestingly, however, there is evidence that patterns of alcohol consumption are established early in life. Those who undertake risky alcohol consumption with heavy binge drinking in their early twenties are more likely to continue a behavioral pattern of risky alcohol consumption later in life.

Otherwise, although the pattern and context of drinking varies widely in different countries or cultures (e.g. drinking with or without food, or drinking in private or public places), their relationships with the development of liver disease has not been studied.

Key points

- Globally, alcohol consumption is on the rise.
- In the western world a binge drinking culture has a negative effect on public health through accidents and antisocial behavior; however, no clear increased risk of alcohol-related liver disease has been demonstrated.
- Risky alcohol consumption behavior in the early twenties, including binge drinking, is associated with lifelong risky alcohol consumption.

Associated risk factors for liver disease

Trends in alcohol consumption are on the rise and are undoubtedly contributing to the rising levels of global liver disease mortality and morbidity. However, there are a significant number of coexisting factors that increase the risk of alcohol-related liver disease.

Gender

The differences in the effects of gender on risk of liver-related death attributable to alcohol are clear from Table 2.1. However, this epidemiologic phenomenon is largely because men typically drink more than women and also the proportion of heavy drinkers and alcohol dependency among men is higher than in women. However, it is also well recognized that for a given amount of alcohol consumption the risk of a woman developing liver disease is greater than that of a man. This phenomenon is poorly understood although many theories have been put forward. An initial hypothesis reflected proportionally lower body mass, lower body water, and higher body fat, meaning that for a given amount of alcohol consumption circulating levels of alcohol are higher, increasing the risk of liver damage. Studies have shown a reduced first pass metabolism of alcohol by gastric acetyldehydrogenase in females, further contributing to higher circulating levels of alcohol for any given amount consumed. Finally, estrogen has been proposed to have a role in increasing the risk of liver disease by increasing gut permeability, exposing the liver to gastrointestinal tract endotoxins and perpetuating an inflammatory response started by the ethanol.

Ethnicity

Epidemiologic data suggest a significant role for ethnicity. A US study found that the risk of cirrhosis was higher in the Hispanic and Black communities than amongst white drinkers for the same level of alcohol consumption [10]. While this raises the possibility of specific genetic susceptibilities, the phenomenon could also be related to many other socioeconomic factors that affect these groups differentially such as socioeconomic class, rates of employment, education, access to health care and especially access to alcohol support services. An understanding of the factors that affect these population subgroups is key, however, when it comes to public health planning to reduce the effects of alcohol on these at-risk groups.

Obesity

While obesity, and associated type 2 diabetes, may be the next global epidemic, its role and interplay with alcohol-induced liver disease is important. It is well documented that patients with pre-existing liver disease who drink are at higher risk of cirrhosis than the background population. Epidemiologic studies have demonstrated that obesity and the metabolic syndrome exacerbate the progression of alcohol-related disease and increase hepatocellular carcinoma (HCC) incidence and mortality. Furthermore, current evidence also suggests a synergistic relationship between alcohol and obesity in both mortality and HCC incidence. Most notably, a large UK-based epidemiologic study recruiting over 1 million middle-aged women examined the effects of obesity and alcohol on cirrhosis. Obesity (body mass index, BMI, above 22.5) increased the risk of developing cirrhosis by 28%; when coupled with alcohol the absolute risk of developing cirrhosis rose even further. The absolute risk of cirrhosis per 1000 women over 5 years whose alcohol consumption was under 70 g/week was 0.8 for those with a BMI of 22.5–25 and 1.0 for those with a BMI of over 30. With an alcohol consumption of over 150 g/week these figure rose to 2.7 and 5.0, respectively.

Finally, obesity is an independent risk factor for clinical decompensation in patients with established cirrhosis of all etiologies. Therefore obesity impacts upon mortality and DALYs in patients with established liver disease.

Socioeconomic status

Socioeconomic status has been shown to be an independent risk factor in two separate studies in Europe. In the United Kingdom, socioeconomic status is a risk factor for alcohol-related mortality, although it is mediated by age and sex. A Finnish study drew a similar conclusion, showing that alcohol-related mortality was doubled by deprivation [11].

Genetic polymorphisms

There is clear evidence that not all individuals with harmful levels of alcohol consumption develop chronic liver disease. Furthermore, it is apparent that some individuals develop liver disease at a lower level of alcohol consumption than others. While we have already highlighted other associated risk factors that may account for this, genetic polymorphisms are also likely to have a role although they are not fully understood at present. While many genetic polymorphisms associated with cirrhosis and HCC have been examined, the sensitivity of individuals to alcohol mediated by abnormalities of the aldehyde dehydrogenase allele are probably the best understood with those with a

heterozygous or homozygous deficiency being at increased risk of developing alcohol abuse-related end organ damage. Polymorphisms at other loci including tumor necrosis factor alfa (TNF-α) and transforming growth factor beta (TGF-β) being implicated in HCC risk related to alcohol cirrhosis.

> **Key points**
> - Gender, ethnicity, and lower socioeconomic class have an effect on incidence and mortality from alcohol-attributable liver disease.
> - Pre-existing liver disease plus excess alcohol consumption increases the risk and accelerates the progression to cirrhosis.
> - The global obesity epidemic will increase the incidence of pre-existing steatosis.
> - Obesity is an independent risk factor for clinical decompensation of cirrhotic liver disease of all etiologies.

Methods for reducing the burden of liver disease attributable to alcohol

In essence, the burden of liver disease from alcohol is preventable. However, as we have established, this would rely on accurate detection of those patients at risk of developing liver disease and being able to offer effective treatment for dependence. Methods for reducing the health burden of alcohol itself, but more specifically alcohol-induced liver disease, can be grouped into two distinct strategies: those targeted at the population as a whole and those targeted at the individuals at risk from their alcohol consumption.

Population strategies to reduce the burden of disease

Population strategies to reduce the burden of alcohol-related liver disease are likely to require significant cultural changes within the western world to move away from a longstanding heavy drinking culture. In 2011, as part of a global status report on alcohol and health, the WHO published a global strategy to reduce the harmful use of alcohol. The WHO recommended 10 areas for national action to minimize the harmful effects of alcohol.

1 *Leadership, awareness, and commitment:* appointing lead institutions responsible for setting, implementing, and following up national strategies.

2 *Health services' response:* health services need to respond and treat any alcohol dependence issues as well as minimize the harmful effects of alcohol excess.

3 *Community action:* empowerment of communities to impart cultural change of attitude to alcohol consumption rather than focusing on the individual.

4 *Drink-driving policies and countermeasures:* promoting stringent drink drive laws and minimizing risk to intoxicated pedestrians.

5 *Availability of alcohol:* establishing, operating, and enforcing an appropriate system to regulate production, wholesaling, and serving of alcoholic beverages by introducing a licensing system for retailers, allowing regulation of modes and days of alcohol sale.

6 *Marketing of alcoholic beverages:* setting up regulatory frameworks to reduce the effect of marketing of alcohol on young people.

7 *Pricing policies:* minimum unit pricing (MUP) policies through taxation. Alongside policies to limit price promotion on alcoholic beverages as well as offer price incentives on nonalcoholic beverages.

8 *Reducing the negative consequences of drinking and alcohol intoxication:* increasing consumer awareness of the negative effects of alcohol. Policies to regulate the drinking context to reduce incidences of antisocial behavior associated with intoxication.

9 Reducing the public health impact of illicit alcohol and informally produced alcohol.

10 Monitoring and surveillance to assess the efficacy of interventions.

Minimum alcohol prices (Canada and Australia) and consumption restriction policies (Russia) have been used sporadically to address risky alcohol consumption and the effect on public health over recent years. The effect of MUP on alcohol consumption has been shown in British Columbia, Canada, where prices have been adjusted intermittently over the last 20 years. By comparing alcohol pricing with reported statistics for household consumption it has been estimated that for a 10% increase in the minimum price of an alcoholic beverage, consumption of all alcoholic drinks reduces by 3.4%. However, more strikingly, the consumption of beverages favored by those with risky consumption

including spirits and alcoholic soda and ciders reduced by 6.8% and 13.9%, respectively [12].

Large public health interventions such as increasing alcohol cost with a MUP policy by taxation, bans on alcohol marketing, stringent drink driving policies, and reducing alcohol availability offer the biggest public health benefit. However, they are less popular with politicians as evidenced by the recent failure of the MUP bill in England to be considered by parliament although Scotland has passed such a bill but not yet enacted it. Political interventions often prefer education and community empowerment schemes to potentially unpopular interventions, although there is little evidence that they are effective.

Individual strategies to reduce the burden of disease

As already established, identifying those at risk of developing alcohol-related disease from their drinking behavior prior to the onset of disease is the key to reducing the burden of alcoholic liver disease. It is estimated that 20–30% of patients who attend primary care are either harmful or hazardous drinkers and once these individuals have been identified different interventions have been assessed. The best-studied intervention is that of screening and brief intervention (i.e. the harmful or hazardous drinkers are identified and then undergo a brief intervention aimed at reducing their alcohol consumption). A brief intervention has been classified as anything from a single session to up to four sessions. There is evidence that a brief intervention for those with harmful or hazardous drinking does reduce the consumption of alcohol although at 1 year the effect was only seen in men and not in women [13]. Within this large meta-analysis there was no benefit from longer interventions. Furthermore, in the United Kingdom, cost-effectiveness modeling showed that screening and brief intervention offered by a physician (general practitioner) would incur an incremental net cost of £108 million, with health gains equivalent to 92 000 QALYs, giving an incremental cost-effectiveness ratio of £1175 per QALY gained compared with current practice [14]. Unfortunately, however, this is yet to become a standard requirement for primary care physicians in the United Kingdom.

A potential barrier to mandating screening and brief intervention in primary care settings is the current lack of agreement on the best intervention. Recent studies have shown no difference in effect on drinking, assessed by AUDIT-C score (Alcohol use disorder identification test -AUDIT), between patient information leaflets and a structured lifestyle advice consultation. As a consequence, future research should focus on identifying a structured, clinically effective, and cost-effective intervention for these at-risk patients to reduce the burden of alcohol-related liver disease in the population. Furthermore, it is well known that not all those with harmful, hazardous, or dependent patterns of alcohol consumption will develop chronic liver disease related to their drinking behavior. Therefore future research to improve understanding of either the demographics and risk factors or molecular processes predisposing to alcohol-induced chronic liver disease is needed such that interventions can be targeted at those at greatest risk.

Those with patterns of alcohol dependency are at greatest risk of developing alcohol-related disease. There are an estimated 76 million people worldwide with a diagnosable alcohol use disorder (alcohol abuse or dependence) including 18 million Americans and 1.6 million people dependent on alcohol in England alone. However, only 6.4% of those dependent on alcohol access treatment and only 108 906 adults were in structured alcohol treatment in England in 2011–2012 (64% male, 36% female).

The problems with treatments of alcohol use disorders are that they represent a complex interplay between genetic, socioeconomic, and mental health conditions. Therefore the phenotypes of those individuals who have an alcohol use disorder and alcohol dependence vary significantly. As a consequence, planning treatment has to be individualized and any one intervention certainly does not fit all.

There is good evidence that effective withdrawal treatment in alcohol dependence can be achieved safely on either an inpatient or outpatient basis. Following successful detoxification there is evidence to support both the use of psychosocial (e.g. 12-step facilitation therapy and cognitive behavioral therapy) and pharmacologic interventions to facilitate abstinence. Abstinence is the hallmark of preventing disease development, progression, and mortality. Five-year mortality for patients with alcoholic cirrhosis who cease drinking decreases to 10%, compared with 30% for patients who continue to drink. Unfortunately, current pharmacologic interventions including naltrexone, acamprosate, and baclofen can reduce craving and facilitate abstinence but they do

not work for all. With alcohol use disorders currently costing the US health care system $30 billion annually and a wider cost to society of $235 billion, interest in alternative treatments for alcohol use disorders and streamlining the process of bringing them to market has been proposed in the United States [15].

Key points

- Population methods to reduce alcohol consumption can be effective. Evidence for MUP suggest that although total alcohol consumption is reduced, the greatest effect is on cheap high strength alcohol typically consumed by high risk drinkers.
- Approximately 20–30% of patients presenting to primary care settings have hazardous or harmful levels of alcohol consumption. Screening and brief intervention will offer cost-effective health benefits in this care setting.
- Abstinence is the key to reducing mortality in alcohol-related disease and can be achieved with detoxification alongside therapies to maintain abstinence.

Methods for early detection of liver disease

The crucial aspects to managing liver disease attributable to alcohol occur before the onset of cirrhosis. While current tools including screening questionnaires like AUDIT (alcohol use disorder identification test) and latter modifications including AUDIT-C have been effective in identifying those patients with alcohol use disorders, they have significant limitations. First, the prescribed cutoff to define unhealthy alcohol use has been the subject of debate, with initial WHO algorithms suggesting a score of 8 compared to some clinical studies showing an ideal cutoff of 4 for men or 3 for women. The current score used by Public Health England is 5. "High level of alcohol problems" is defined by the WHO as a score of 16–19 and dependence is defined as above 20. These screening tools identify those with high alcohol consumption but they are not mandated regularly at primary care visits where hazardous levels of consumption could be identified and support implemented (see Methods for reducing the burden of liver disease attributable to alcohol). Furthermore, they do not take into account other risk factors for the development of chronic liver disease and will therefore not allow clinicians to target therapy for abstinence to those at greatest risk.

Once hazardous consumption has been identified, a robust method for screening for liver fibrosis would allow intervention to assist abstinence and, it is hoped, reduce disease progression. Many technologies have been investigated for this and are covered elsewhere in this textbook. However, this will not prevent the onset of disease and only with a better understanding of epidemiologic and molecular risks for developing alcohol-related disease will we be able to identify those who are at risk of cirrhosis from their alcohol consumption.

Key points

- Identifying those at risk of alcohol-induced cirrhosis before the onset of fibrosis is the key to minimizing the health impact of the disease.
- Noninvasive fibrosis tests may identify disease at an earlier stage but do not prevent disease onset.
- Current tools adequately assess alcohol consumption but do not reliably identify those at risk of liver disease.

References

[1] Rehm J, Samokhvalov AV, Shield KD. Global burden of alcoholic liver diseases. *J Hepatol* 2013; **59**: 160–168.

[2] Pearl R. Alcohol and life duration. *Br Med J* 1924; **1**: 948–950.

[3] Mann RE, Smart RG, Anglin L, Adlaf EM. Reductions in cirrhosis deaths in the United States: associations with per capita consumption and AA membership. *J Stud Alcohol* 1991; **52**: 361–365.

[4] Pell S, D'Alonzo CA. A five-year mortality study of alcoholics. *J Occup Med* 1973; **15**: 120–125.

[5] Marmot MG, Shipley MJ, Rose G, Thomas B. Alcohol and mortality: A U-shaped curve. *Lancet* 1981; **317**: 580–583.

[6] Skog OJ. Liver cirrhosis epidemiology: some methodological problems. *Br J Addict* 1980; **75**: 227–243.

[7] Rehm J. Russia: lessons for alcohol epidemiology and alcohol policy. *Lancet* 2014; **383**: 1440–2.

[8] Rehm J, Taylor B, Mohapatra S, et al. Alcohol as a risk factor for liver cirrhosis: a systematic review and meta-analysis. *Drug Alcohol Rev* 2010; **29**: 437–445.

[9] Dawson DA, Li T-K, Grant BF. *A Prospective Study of Risk Drinking: At Risk for What?* NIH Public Access 2008: 1–20.

[10] Stinson FS, Grant BF, Dufour MC. The critical dimension of ethnicity in liver cirrhosis mortality statistics. *Alcohol Clin Exp Res* 2001; **25**: 1181–1187.

[11] Mäkelä P, Paljärvi T. Do consequences of a given pattern of drinking vary by socioeconomic status? A mortality and hospitalisation follow-up for alcohol-related causes of the Finnish Drinking Habits Surveys. *J Epidemiol Community Health* 2008; **62**: 728–733.

[12] Stockwell T, Auld MC, Zhao J, Martin G. Does minimum pricing reduce alcohol consumption? The experience of a Canadian province. *Addiction* 2012; **107**: 912–920.

[13] Kaner EFS, Beyer F, Dickinson HO, et al. Effectiveness of brief alcohol interventions in primary care populations. *Cochrane Database Syst Rev* 2007; **2**: CD004148.

[14] Purshouse RC, Brennan A, Rafia R, et al. Modelling the cost-effectiveness of alcohol screening and brief interventions in primary care in England. *Alcohol Alcohol* 2013; **48**: 180–188.

[15] Litten RZ, Egli M, Heilig M, et al. Medications development to treat alcohol dependence: a vision for the next decade. *Addict Biol* 2012; **17**: 513–527.

CHAPTER 3

Alcoholism: diagnosis and natural history in the context of medical disease

Thomas P. Beresford,[1,3] Narin Wongngamnit,[1,2,3] and Benjamin A. Temple[1,3]

[1] Laboratory for Clinical and Translational Research in Psychiatry, Department of Veterans Affairs Medical Center, Denver, CO, USA
[2] Substance Abuse Treatment Program, Department of Veterans Affairs Medical Center, Denver, CO, USA
[3] University of Colorado School of Medicine, Denver, CO, USA

KEY POINTS

- To the psychiatrist alcoholism is a disorder that is diagnosed empirically from observable behaviors, while other sets of observations inform treatment prognosis.

- Those with alcoholism present to other health care professionals because of medical sequelae.

- Alcoholism is a medical disease comprising many aspects of the model of medical illness with associated symptoms and a natural history of onset, course, and recovery.

- Alcohol **dependence** may be divided into type 1 or late onset alcoholism and is associated with just alcohol use; type 2 or early onset alcoholism is associated with polydrug dependence (addiction to two or more substances, including alcohol but not nicotine).

- Interventions claiming to change the natural history of alcoholism can be assessed from systematically gathered data.

- Alcohol **use disorder** is diagnosed using the DSM-5 criteria that are based on a variety of clinical patterns.

- Understanding of prognosis is now much more advanced but medications to treat dependence are still inadequate.

Natural history and clinical assessment

Alcoholism frequency

Alcoholism, known clinically in its most severe form as Alcohol Dependence (AD), and in its early course as Alcohol Abuse, affects as many as 7–10% of persons in the United States [1]. It directly affects nearly one in every three families in the United States and carries with it considerable negative social stigma. Those suffering from it often appear to reject any help from others, or even to ignore the presence of the condition itself, in their struggle to give up alcohol use.

Large population studies may offer background insights to the practicing clinician but may not carry sufficient specificity to inform the care of individual patients. For example, the National Institute on Alcohol Abuse and Alcoholism (NIAAA) conducted a two-stage prevalence study, the National Epidemiologic Survey on Alcohol Related Conditions (NESARC), in 2001–2002 and 2004–2005 [2]. Criteria for AD and Alcohol Abuse were borrowed from the *Diagnostic and Statistical Manual of Mental Disorders*, fourth edition (DSM-IV, 1994; DSM-IV-TR, 2000) [3]. The NESARC data were compared with a previous investigation, the National Longitudinal Alcohol Epidemiologic Survey (NLAES, 1991–1992). Owing to differing methods used in each, even though by the same researchers, they only approximate each other in offering prevalence comparisons at different times. In the NLAES, the percentage of Americans with

Alcohol Abuse and Liver Disease, First Edition. Edited by James Neuberger and Andrea DiMartini.

AD was 4.38 while the percentage of those with Alcohol Abuse was 3.03. In the NESARC, the corresponding figures were 3.81 – 13% fewer – and 4.65 – 53% more – than in the NLAES, suggesting a disunion of clinical and epidemiologic assessments of individual cases. The combined percentage point prevalence totals for AD plus Alcohol Abuse are NLAES = 7.41 and NESARC = 8.46, however, suggesting an estimated *increase* in prevalence of problematic alcohol use of 1.5% of the population between the two surveys, from 1992 to 2005. According to our calculations from these frequency data, this increase of 1.5% accounts for some 4.4 million Americans, allowing for the estimated increase in the US population itself over those years. If the same rate persists today, the estimated increase for combined AD and Alcohol Abuse in the United States would be 5.9 million people. Added to the 2005 NESARC base of 25 million, this results in a total of nearly 31 million AD or alcohol abusing persons in the United States, or about 10% of the present population. These figures speak to the magnitude of the problem.

Differentiation by natural course

It is important to keep in perspective that alcoholism has been viewed in many model systems over many centuries, ranging from moral failing to medical illness with many other models between (see Beresford's Science Update installments on the website of the National Council on Alcoholism and Drug Dependence, beginning in October 2013, for a brief historical overview). The present discussion refers to alcoholism in the disease model and as an illness that courses over decades, rather than a few weeks, months, or even years. This occurs for two practical reasons:

1 It allows application of the methods of clinical science to a ubiquitous, and deadly, condition; and
2 It provides patients with an all-important sense of hope. Quoting one, "It is much easier to think of myself as an ill person trying to get better than as a bad person trying to become good." Nonetheless, it is important to recall that other models provide useful discussions from other points of view with helpful contributions from time to time. Physicians have a particularly critical role in applying the principles of clinical science with respect to diagnosis and prognosis, both of which inform specific treatments.

For the hepatologist, transplant surgeon, and psychiatrist working as a team, an approach modeled in *Liver Transplantation and the Alcoholic Patient* [4], and for other health professionals the more practical, disease course-based characteristics of AD carry more pertinence. The vast majority of AD cases, for example, involve alcohol as the primary, and often only, drug of sustained, uncontrolled use. Research reports refer to this as primary AD; it has accrued other synonyms such as or type 1 [5], type A [6], or late onset [7] alcoholism. By contrast, polydrug dependence – that is, addiction to two or more substances, not including nicotine, that may include alcohol as one of the dependence substances – affects about 0.5% of adults in the United States. Viewed from the perspective of alcoholism research, this group refers to type 2, type B, or early onset alcoholism. Although the distinction between the two clinical groups with respect to their abstinence prognoses has been known for many years, clinical programs frequently fail to take this distinction into account. For example, among the early outcome reports on post-transplant abstinence frequencies those liver transplant programs that separated the two types at evaluation demonstrated high rates of abstinence in the primary AD group [8,9] while those that did not make this distinction reported much lower abstinence rates [10,11]. Prior research on nontransplant samples demonstrated that the much more common primary AD group will enjoy a better prognosis than the polydrug-dependent group [1]. Table 3.1 summarizes some of the characteristic differences between the two in brief form.

More recently, in a report on the controversial topic of liver transplant for those with severe alcoholic hepatitis that is refractory to medicinal treatment [12] the authors reported postoperative alcohol abstinence for a minimum of 24 months in 23 of 26 cases in their sample, with two returning to some level of alcohol use at 24 months and a third at 38 months. Unfortunately, that report does not provided data on how many of their sample met criteria for the AD diagnosis, let alone subtype data; all 26 qualified for clinical diagnosis of alcoholic hepatitis refractory to steroid treatment, 23 of whom had tissue biopsies consistent with this.

At about the same time, a longitudinal prospective study [13] again corroborated the prior reports on the expected course of the two AD subtypes in a sample followed prospectively after liver grafting. As expected, those with a history of polydrug dependence fared far

Table 3.1 Alcohol dependence clinical subtypes.

Primary alcohol dependence	Polydrug dependence
• 7–10% US population	• 0.5% US population
• Alcohol primary dependence	• Polysubstance dependence
• Normal childhood	• Deprivation and/or abuse in childhood
• No CD	• CD symptoms before age 15
• Regular use: late teens, twenties	• Polydrug dependence: teens
• No characteristic personality diagnosis before addictive use	• Adult personality disorder diagnoses concurrent with use
• Natural remission: 30% per year	• Natural remission: 10% per year
• With treatment: 45% per year	• With treatment: 10% per year

CD, conduct disorder.

Box 3.1 ICD-10 guidelines for a dependence diagnosis

> **1** Evidence of tolerance, such that increased doses of alcohol are required to achieve effects originally produced by lower doses.
> **2** Physiological withdrawal state when alcohol use has ceased.
> **3** A strong desire or sense of compulsion to drink alcohol, during abstinence periods.
> **4** Difficulties in controlling alcohol drinking behavior, when once begun, whether in onset, termination, or levels of use.
> **5** Progressive neglect of alternative healthy activities because of alcohol use.
> **6** Persistence in alcohol drinking despite clear evidence and prior knowledge of harmful consequences.

worse than any of the other subgroups that the study tracked. The present chapter discusses this in more detail in respect to pretransplant evaluation and the process of clinical decision making in the setting of AD. To do that, let us first examine the steps in diagnosing AD that lead to prognostic assessment.

Alcohol use history

Clinically, two general concepts guide the assessment of alcohol use, with or without other drugs of abuse. First, the interviewer is assessing an addictive disorder and AD is a form of this phenomenon. Alcohol addiction is second in prevalence only to nicotine addiction in the general population.

Second, AD and other forms of substance dependence are clinical diagnoses based on specific *behaviors*, rather than attempted quantifications of amounts and frequencies of alcohol use. Box 3.1 lists the World Health Organization's current diagnostic guidelines (Tenth Revision of the International Classification of Diseases and Health Problems, or ICD-10 [14]) edited by the primary author to focus on AD. They begin with the stipulation that diagnosis of AD requires evidence for three or more of the six criteria and that these must have occurred together at some time during the previous year.

The ICD-10 criteria describe AD as a diagnostic syndrome, that is, as a grouping of concurrent, associated symptoms. Very recently, the American Psychiatric Association abandoned the syndrome approach used

in previous editions of its Diagnostic and Statistical Manuals (DSM) [3,15,16]. Ostensibly to gain better statistical resolution of the lesser Alcohol Abuse diagnosis in large population samples, the new DSM-5 [17] in this same series adopts a more generally stated Alcohol Use Disorder terminology construed on a continuum of mild, moderate, and severe, rather than the syndrome approach. This is discussed further on in this chapter. For clarity when referring to medical diagnosis, we will retain the ICD-10 version for AD syndrome diagnosis as the most commonly used in clinical settings.

Making a diagnosis

Viewed in its most basic form, the diagnosis of AD requires specific evidence of phenomena in three clinical domains:

1 Physiologic dependence – including tolerance or withdrawal;
2 Loss of Control of alcohol use – often erroneously referred to as "craving"; and
3 A resultant decline in either physical or social functioning, or both.

For practical purposes, this discussion will leave questions of alcohol abuse – defined here as evidence of alcohol use problems in the absence of the Loss of Control phenomena – and "caseness" for the judgments taken from further independent empirical evidence. Instead, the workaday medical, surgical, and mental health specialists may best serve their patients by focusing on the three large symptom domains as offering a brief, practical way of assessing symptoms in clinic settings.

Physiological dependence: tolerance and withdrawal (ICD-10 categories 1 and 2)

Tolerance

Tolerance, more specifically acquired tolerance, refers to the ability of the central nervous system (CNS) to approximate normal functioning in the presence of ever-increasing doses of ethyl alcohol. Clinically, the person reports an acquired need for more alcohol to obtain the same effect once noticed at a much lower dose earlier in the natural history of drinking. To assess this, the clinician must establish a baseline drinking effect that has changed over time. This necessitates careful attention to the details of the drinking history.

One useful approach is to ask what effect the alcohol had when a person first began drinking on his or her own. Results include such reports as nausea, feeling high, or perhaps other unique descriptors in the patient's own words: what they noticed after one or two standard alcohol drinks. A standard drink, each containing roughly ¾ oz of ethyl alcohol, may be approximately defined as a 12-oz can or bottle of beer, a 6-oz glass of table wine, or a 1.5-oz shot of whisky or other spirits.

After establishing a baseline, for example "In high school I got high after one or two cans of beer," the interviewer may then ask how many standard drinks the person noticed achieved the same effect at the time when their drinking was at its greatest. Some formal criteria require a 50% increase. In the case of alcohol, most heavy drinkers will describe a doubling or more of the amount used for an initial effect. Many patients with AD will describe amounts several times greater than those drunk in the state naïve to alcohol, such as "Back then I got high after two beers. Now I don't notice anything until after I drink a six pack and I need a case (24 12-oz cans or bottles of beer) to feel drunk." This signals that the CNS has adapted to heavy alcohol use, that is, developed a tolerance.

While most forms of tolerance are acquired over time with repeated drinking, research has demonstrated that a minority of individuals have a very high *innate tolerance* to ethyl alcohol as part of their neural make-up. In research paradigms this is currently referred to as low response (LR) to alcohol [18]. Clinically, LR can be approached through questions such as "Some people tell me that they didn't notice an effect of the alcohol when they first began to drink. What was your experience?"

This same subjective insensitivity to alcohol in a drinking-naive state is mirrored in reduced neuroendocrine responses and in a lack of neurologic impairment on such tasks as maintaining balance [18]. More ominously, follow-up studies of innately alcohol-tolerant persons indicate a much higher AD prevalence rate, estimated as high as 29–50%, far higher than the control group estimated frequency of 11% [19]. In such cases, the body appears to lack a "built-in" negative feedback mechanism for the effects of ethanol. This tendency runs in families and serves as a focus of ongoing genetic explorations as to its cause. Whether LR carries the same diagnostic weight as an acquired tolerance may be argued. Clinically, however, it serves as a risk factor for AD.

Alcohol withdrawal syndrome

Defined clinically as an excessive activity of the sympathetic nervous system triggered by a rapid decline in alcohol blood level, withdrawal symptoms accompany tolerance in the great majority of individuals. In those who report no withdrawal symptoms despite a history of clear tolerance to alcohol the clinician must ask whether the patient is drinking in the morning before withdrawal symptoms manifest themselves, or is regularly taking some other CNS depressant, such as a benzodiazepine, an anticholinergic agent, or another sedative drug that covers withdrawal symptoms, especially in the morning. On occasion, the clinician will encounter patients who have few or no withdrawal symptoms despite a clear alcohol tolerance. Although relatively infrequent, this recognized clinical phenomenon appears most likely due to a genetically based constitutional invulnerability to withdrawal [20].

As ethanol is a short-acting CNS depressant, its quick removal after constant and heavy exposure triggers CNS hyperactivity both centrally, as for example expressed by a subjective sense of jitteriness or impending disaster (anxiety), and peripherally through the symptoms of sympathetic nervous system discharge. Table 3.2 lists acute withdrawal symptoms that patients commonly report.

Of note, neither headache nor blackout are symptoms of alcohol withdrawal. The former, a component of "hangover" often may have to do with fluid shifts in the brain that are thought to activate pain sensors in the arachnoid layer of the brain's coverings. The latter is a state-dependent amnesia that occurs when reaching acutely high levels of ethanol. While these can indicate

Table 3.2 Patient reported symptoms and clinical signs of early alcohol withdrawal.

Anxiety	Palpitations (pulse ≥110 bpm)
Tremor	Rapid breathing (tachypnea >20/minute)
Nausea with vomiting	Low grade fever (>99.5°F, 37.5°C)
Sweating	High blood pressure (≥90 mmHg diastolic)

acute heavy drinking with or without AD, they are not diagnostic for AD.

Later and more severe occurrences, however, such as generalized grand mal seizures on or after the first day of withdrawal and Delirium Tremens (the DTs) occurring after the third day, make up the most severe and most dangerous withdrawal phenomena. Both are often preceded by either or both of two *clinical signs*: hyperreflexia and ankle clonus, both indications of the severely irritated CNS.

The DTs, characterized by the clinical triad of (i) confusion, (ii) usually visual or tactile hallucinations, and (iii) extreme rises in vital signs, such as malignant hypertension or tachycardia, presents a true medical emergency and often results in hospitalization. Because of his or her confusion during the DTs, the patient may not appreciate the significance of a hospitalization for withdrawal. A corroborating third party can provide clinically crucial information in that instance.

In epidemiologically vulnerable populations, such as those admitted to general hospitals, withdrawal seizures and DTs may occur as frequently as 7% or 5%, respectively [21]. Both should be regarded as emergencies. Active seizures indicate attention to assuring open airway status via standard mandibular extension or, if needed, intubation when continued airway compromise occurs. Both isolated convulsions and status epilepticus respond to parenteral benzodiazepine administration of agents such as diazepam or lorazepam, the same agents used to treat alcohol withdrawal. Most regard admission to an intensive care unit as the best site of treatment for the DTs, a condition with reported death rates in the range of 10–15% when left untreated [22]. Adequate doses of benzodiazepine agents to relieve targeted symptoms, followed by a tapering of those agents over the next few days, constitute the standard treatment of withdrawal symptoms in the United States.

Loss of control phenomenon (ICD-10 category 4)

The essence of any addiction, and certainly of AD, loss of control (LOC) refers to the *inability* of the affected person to predict with any degree of certainty how much alcohol they will drink from one episode to the next [1]. Clinically, once the drinking episode starts, the person with AD will be unable to stop in the middle of the drinking bout without a very great struggle. Useful questions at interview include the phrasing presented in Box 3.2.

Indirect phrasing of this kind, with the reference to "some people," displaces the patient's concern at being accused of some form of vice and allies both interviewer and patient in looking at one phenomenon – the patient's experience. This lessens the likelihood of an implied adversarial setting in which the interviewer examines the patient as if under a microscope. Experience suggests that an allying approach gains much more detailed, and more useful, information than an adversarial confrontation.

At the same time, it is important to distinguish the LOC phenomenon from "craving" (ICD-10 category 3). The former has to do with the inability to stop drinking *once started*. Craving refers to the episodic and often intense desire or compulsion to drink while in an alcohol or drug-free state, that is, *between* bouts of use. Craving may also be confused with the patient's intense search for alcohol to relieve withdrawal symptoms, a separate

Box 3.2 Assessing loss of control.

> Introductory statement: "Some people tell me they notice these things when they drink and I would like to know if you've ever noticed them."
>
> Specific items:
>
> 1 Some find it very hard to stop drinking, once they start. They feel that they are "off to the races" where drinking is concerned.
> 2 Some people find themselves drinking more than they wanted to drink or had planned to drink.
> 3 Some notice that they try to make rules to control their drinking, such as by drinking only certain types of beverages and avoiding others or by restricting drinking to a specific time of day.
>
> Note the indirect phrasing using simple declarative sentences that invite the patient to agree or disagree. The same items can be phrased as questions.

phenomenon. The distinction can be made accurately in the clinical setting by paying attention to what occurs during episodes of use and what occurs between them. LOC during use is a hallmark of addiction while craving between use episodes appears to be a much more complex phenomenon involving brain–environment interactions. The ICD-10 diagnostic guidelines include both. DSM-5 now includes mention of craving whereas prior editions did not.

Social or physical decline (ICD-10 categories 5 and 6)

The combination of physical addiction and LOC usually results in a patient spending a large portion of time and effort to sustain heavy drinking or to manage or recover from its effects. To assess this, the clinician asks whether drinking has become a problem with respect to family relationships, legal status, work, friendships, or physical health. Physicians and surgeons will be especially attuned to the last of these because the physical illness sequelae of AD result in frequent clinic visits and hospitalizations. However, the patient's family relationships usually offer the most sensitive indications of social difficulties resulting from alcohol or drug use. A change in work status is usually one of the last occurring indicators of social problems because income provides the basis for continued use.

AD, then, may be reliably diagnosed when evidence in all three domains presents. None of the current or immediately past sets of DSM diagnostic criteria require evidence in all three domains and therefore may cast a somewhat wider diagnostic net. The ICD-10 guidelines add the dimension of craving use among their six symptom categories. While either approach is defensible, the physician will do well to choose one or more of the standard definitions and use it consistently over time [3,10].

Assessing prognosis

As noted in Table 3.1, drinking remission rates for primary AD persons range from about 30% per year without clinical treatment to about 45% per year when clinical treatment is added. However, this figure is complicated by high relapse rates. Some studies note relapse rates of 70% or higher in the first year with a gradual reduction in relapse frequency to the single digit range after 6 years [1]. Clearly, patients with primary AD require treatment aimed at relapse prevention and alcohol-free living. Achieving this has to do with patients resolving a sense of underlying ambivalence about their alcohol use. For those with polysubstance-dependent AD, however, outcome studies are much less sanguine. Annual abstinence rates approximate 10% and show little in the way of an incremental response to treatment. For this group, some argue that harm reduction – maintaining life and health until the person "matures out" of their polydrug addictions that include alcohol – offers the best treatment goal. The natural courses of both variations of AD invite us to consider the specific phenomena that predict recovery and abstinence.

Positive versus negative

How can the physician go about the task of assessing the prognosis for alcohol-free living [23]? While each individual patient and their social network provide unique considerations, a series of general factors, gleaned from prospective, longitudinal research on populations of alcohol or drug-dependent persons, offer useful windows on prognosis. In the great majority of cases these include:

1 The AD diagnosis;
2 An understanding of the patient's ambivalence towards continuing use;
3 Measures of personal social stability; and
4 A series of four empirically based factors that Vaillant [1] found to predict stable abstinence in prospective research studies.

In addition, those with a co-occurring diagnosis of a major psychiatric disorder require: (i) an evaluation of psychoactive medication response to the primary disorder; and (ii) a medication adherence history in addition to the factors already mentioned.

Some clinical programs focus more on what they see as negative prognostic predictors – those that predict a return to drinking – rather than positive factors such as those that predict continued abstinence. The negative factors often include: (i) mention of alcohol or other drug use in the past 6 months – the infamous "Six Month Rule" that has not been borne out either in follow-up or in prospective research [13]; and (ii) counting previous "recidivist" episodes, a term that calls to mind criminal incarceration and punishment rather than a remitting–relapsing medical condition.

In most cases, a focus on the positive prognostic factors that predict abstinence offers the more sound clinical approach.

Diagnosis is prognosis

The diagnostic procedure described provides the basis for important prognostic distinctions bearing on continued abstinence. Practically speaking, health professionals must evaluate AD type as a clinical guide to prognosis. While the Six Month Rule has little justification for use in primary AD [24], a history of recent use of *any* dependent drug – including alcohol – in a person with polydrug-dependent AD predicts the limits of targeting only abstinence in treatment. Empirical data on the polydrug group suggests that continuous, stable abstinence comes only after the emotional growth of many years, often not until the person's late thirties or early forties [1]. In a person with polydrug-dependent AD, demonstration of a corroborated, sustained, stable abstinence from both drugs *and* alcohol for a significant period of time – often measured by one or more years rather than by months – affords confidence in providing medical treatments, including that of a scarce resource such as liver graft for which clinical need far exceeds the graft supply.

Abuse rather than dependence

When diagnosing primary AD, it is important to establish whether the LOC phenomenon exists in each case. Its absence, even in the face of a clear history of tolerance or alcohol-related social or physical problems, strongly suggests a lesser diagnosis of Alcohol Abuse or, in DSM-5 terms, mild or moderate alcohol use disorder. As an example of specific importance, in our clinical series [4] about 10% of those applying for a liver transplant for alcoholic cirrhosis did not meet AD criteria but could clearly be considered in the Alcohol Abuse category. Abuse generally suggests that behavioral processes moving towards LOC and AD appear to be in place but that the clinical line into AD has not yet been crossed. Even though a lesser diagnosis than AD [25], Alcohol Abuse may still indicate asking the patient to cease alcohol use. In that case, two phenomena often occur:

1 The person achieves and maintains abstinence without a struggle; and
2 The risk of relapse over the long term appears considerably lower.

Generally speaking, Alcohol Abuse offers a much better prognosis with respect to natural course than does AD.

While the lesser diagnosis is sometimes more difficult to define, it is a generally more optimistic diagnosis to make.

Behavioral versus hepatic diagnosis

A significant portion of those candidates referred to as "alcoholic" on the basis of liver disease or other alcohol-related conditions will not merit the AD diagnosis. In our previous series [4], only about 75% of those with a tissue diagnosis of alcoholic liver disease fit the behavioral AD diagnosis. Conversely, only about 80% of those referred as "alcoholics" met the AD diagnosis. Of the remaining 20%, half fit the Alcohol Abuse diagnosis and half did not merit either. This was especially true of women who, because of a well-known gender-specific vulnerability to alcoholic liver disease, may injure the liver without ever reaching AD. This limited overlap emphasizes the need for diagnostic precision in establishing the presence of AD.

Assessing ambivalence and continuing LOC risk

Clinically, longitudinal studies of abstinence make it clear that once the control of drinking behavior departs, it does not return in the great majority of cases [1]. Longitudinal studies over several years have established that once lost, controlled alcohol or drug use cannot be relearned or reconstituted. In this sense a diagnosis of AD signals a permanent condition – including a permanent risk of uncontrolled drinking or use. One component of the interview therefore requires review of this risk with the patient and a third party. Poor understanding, or ambivalent acceptance, of drinking relapse risk in a patient with normal cognition may indicate an unresolved ambivalence toward AD itself and therefore the need to refer for alcohol or other drug-focused behavioral treatment.

Social stability

This is the foundation upon which ongoing medical adherence and favorable prognosis are built. While several social stability scales exist, the simplest comes from the work of Strauss and Bacon [26] who found that the presence of any two of four social factors predicted clinic appointment compliance among those with AD:

1 Being married;
2 Not living alone;

3 Stable employment for 3 years; and

4 A stable residence for 2 years.

Viewed teleologically, falling below the cut point suggests, but does not establish, the likelihood of insufficient social resources to support treatment efforts. These may include social isolation and homelessness, two conditions that raise the likelihood of both drinking relapse and medical noncompliance. When present, the specialized involvement of a treatment clinic program aimed at increasing social resources offers the next step towards AD recovery.

Vaillant's four prognostic factors

In the best available prospective, longitudinal study of AD prognosis, Vaillant's 8-year study noted four operating factors, any two or more of which, when present, predicted long-term sobriety – defined as 2 years or more in his study. One or none indicated a return to drinking within 1 year [1]. A proper prognosis evaluation includes them.

1 *Structured time:* because AD style drinking requires a lot of time and effort, newly abstinent persons often encounter considerable "dead," or unstructured, time that can itself foster a relapse. Structuring that time corrects this concern and is a frequent ingredient in specialized clinic and self-help group (such as Alcoholics Anonymous) formats. Any setting that fills time with productive and engaging activity – that the person's "heart is in" – fits the need. At interview, a brief assessment of how the patient spends his or her day addresses whether they engage in active projects that involve other people, or live an isolated existence such as in filling the time with endless television viewing.

2 *A rehabilitation relationship:* sustained, heavy drinking or drug use serves to isolate the person from others and to create the need in those who come into social contact, such as family members, to "fix" the drinking or use. Direct intervention, such as telling the person not to drink or use, generally results in an interpersonal struggle that works against continued abstinence. Rather, abstinence sets the stage for proper boundaries between person and social network. In brief, the family, a clinic, and a self-help network communicate the same approach to the person: "You can stay but the drinking has to go." Clinic personnel, other professionals, seasoned self-help group members, and family members who have learned to set boundaries on drinking behaviors may qualify as providing these kinds of healthy relationships to AD patients.

3 *Sources of hope or self-esteem:* regretful thoughts about having hurt others during drinking days frequently return to most AD people during abstinence periods. Ruminating on them has the effect of lowering hope and self-confidence and thereby promoting a return to drinking: "I am a terrible person, I may as well drink." In assessing prognosis, the interviewer enquires after mechanisms that help a person through such periods. These include hope for the future ("What keeps you going in life? What do you look forward to?") and sources of accomplishment or self-esteem ("What helps you to feel good about yourself? What gives you a sense of usefulness or accomplishment?"). The evaluator may also note "Most people run into regrets about their drinking days. Does this happen to you?" If the answer is positive, "What helps you get past regretful thoughts without drinking?" For some it may be religious beliefs, for others the "higher power" without religion as Alcoholics Anonymous describes it, and for others a concentration on items of hope and accomplishment, such as "another day behind me without drinking." Clinically, the absence of forces that counterbalance regretful ruminations presents an ominous sign toward relapse and indicates further specialized treatment to focus on that.

4 *A negative behavioral reinforcer:* in other words "Is there something very painful that will happen to you, without doubt, the very next time you drink alcohol?" Very few circumstances meet these criteria; severe pancreatic pain and the disulfiram–ethanol reaction qualify and are the most frequently encountered. Neuropathies, seizures, cardiomyopathy, liver failure, and most other alcohol-related medical conditions do not fulfill the criteria because of their subtlety and lack of predictability on each occasion. While the others of Vaillant's factors can be considered positive changes in the path to sustained abstinence, this is the only negative one and is generally the least frequently encountered except in the clinic setting. Disulfiram treatment often results in low adherence rates in most instances unless it is involuntary, as when ordered by a court. Cooperation between court and clinic results in much higher disulfiram assisted abstinence rates [27,28]. This medication is not

Box 3.3 Addressing prognostic factors systematically.

Physical diagnosis

Cognitive impairment: add lactulose or other treatment and re-evaluate.

Substance use diagnosis

1 *Primary AD:* proceed to further prognostic evaluation
2 *Polydrug dependence with AD:* verify either lengthy sustained abstinence and the "maturing out" process or verify continued effective treatment as for example in methadone maintenance for opiate dependence
3 *Abuse:* verify or corroborate cessation and abstinence
4 *No diagnosis:* corroborate and proceed to other treatments as medically or surgically indicated.

Substance use prognosis

1 *Unresolved ambivalence toward use:* focused treatment on this aspect of abstinence; re-evaluate in 3–6 months.
2 *Unstable social adjustment:* establish viable social resources; 3–6 month follow-up reassessment.
3 *One or none of Vaillant's factors:* focused treatment referral; 3–6 month follow-up assessment.

without risk, however, and must be given with frequent, careful monitoring, especially during the first 3 months of prescription.

Summing up prognosis

While none of the factors listed under Prognosis may singly offer absolute certainty in respect to sustained abstinence in each individual case, their combination of variables offers a prognostic pattern that appears useful. Our early algorithm [29], for example, predicted high rates of abstinence in AD liver transplant recipients who present a series of good prognostic factors and this has been borne out in subsequent studies [11]. This approach can be applied to any concurrent disease entity, such as in a clinic specializing in alcoholic liver disease, with similar results. The individual factors summed in Box 3.3 can be addressed in the initial evaluation and re-evaluated longitudinally.

Other psychiatric assessment

Psychiatric diagnoses

The foregoing discussion relates to the great majority of persons with alcohol or substance use histories who do not have other pre-existing psychiatric conditions.

One critically important feature of this patient group recalls that AD can *mimic* all of the major psychiatric disorders including Major Depressive Disorder, Bipolar Disorder, Psychosis, several Anxiety Disorders, and Obsessive Compulsive Disorder, as well as other entities such as sleep discontinuity and anorexia. These and others can be assessed through a series of standard screening questions. When addressing them, the evaluator must keep one truly important factor in mind: other psychiatric disorders cannot be established with certainty during periods of heavy drinking, alcohol withdrawal or, to a large extent, during periods of other drug use. Diagnostic clarity for the listed psychiatric disorders requires evidence *during* abstinence periods, generally exceeding 1 month. Failing to observe this may lead to misdiagnosis and misutilization of treatments, most often seen in psychoactive medications given gratuitously.

Nicotine dependence

With long-term study of liver graft recipients, the higher-than-expected occurrence of lung and other smoking-related cancers has highlighted the need to assess smoking histories in liver transplant candidates. Like AD, nicotine dependence can be diagnosed and it can be successfully treated by knowledgeable treatment programs. Similar to AD, treatment often requires time and attention to the concerns about LOC and ambivalence. For the purposes of this chapter, it is important to note that AD and nicotine dependence co-occur in higher than expected rates. It is to be hoped that treatment studies of co-occurring disorders in transplant samples will shed light on the role of nicotine treatment in liver graft candidates.

DSM-5 and alcoholism diagnosis: evolution of the new diagnostic criteria

Since 1952, the DSM has been updated five times, the last in 1994, DSM-IV-TR [3]. In 2007, the American Psychiatric Association formed a workgroup whose findings led to the changes found in DSM-5 in 2013 [17]. For perspective, the Diagnostic and Statistical Manual of Mental Disorders in their various editions were intended as a classification guide. For many, however, they have become less of a guide and more of a diagnostic cookbook.

It is best to remember that they were never intended to supplant clinical judgment in making a diagnosis. In the practical world, the clinician of any discipline best serves his or her patients by adopting one of the standard approaches and using it consistently over time, creating the core of systematized clinical experience that results in consistent diagnosis on the one hand and accounting for the variation among individuals on the other.

The most substantial change in DSM-5 over previous editions is that it replaces Alcohol Abuse and AD with a spectrum disorder: "alcohol use disorder." This appears driven by the hope of better statistical validity for the Alcohol Abuse diagnosis, beyond the robust validity seen for AD consistently across the DSM editions. Some claim observation of cases in which Alcohol Abuse appeared more "severe" than AD, adding to the complexity of the discussion. From these considerations, the workgroup looked at combining abuse and dependence criteria in favor of a severity rating [30].

The DSM-5 also added Craving, defined as a strong desire or urge to drink, although the workgroup data revealed limited utility to this addition in respect to validity or reliability. This criterion was added because craving had served as a target for some attempts at pharmacotherapy and may relate to a subgroup of persons with AD. Interestingly, the ICD-10 guidelines had already incorporated this concept in its syndrome approach (see Box 3.1).

The DSM-5 outlines that in order to meet a Mild severity level, 2 of 11 criteria must be met. The DSM-5 supporters acknowledged this as a low threshold but claim that this would not add to the diagnosed population. Rather, it might allow for identification of mild cases of alcohol use disorder in the primary care setting, or other settings, perhaps where Screening, Brief Intervention, Referral to Treatment (SBIRT) may be implemented. To define Moderate and Severe cases, weighing of individual criteria appeared to add no benefit and a numeric strategy was implemented: Moderate, 4–5 criteria; Severe, 6 or more criteria.

The DSM-5 diagnostic model aims to recognize the range of persons with alcohol use disorders more efficiently than the previous models and to align criteria with some newer conceptualizations of the disorder. As always is the case in science, independent verification studies will assess whether the new model is useful. In the meantime, syndromal alcoholism, formally defined

as AD, offers the best predictive properties in respect to course and prognosis of the most severe form of alcohol drinking disorders.

Does liver transplant change the natural history of alcoholism?

Many different liver transplant teams at different points in time have noted similarly sustained and high rates of abstinence from alcohol and concomitantly low rates of relapse to uncontrolled, addictive style drinking among the Primary or type 1/A alcoholic graft recipients. While medieval authors regarded the liver as the home of the soul, and while modern research notes brain effects from endogenous agents synthesized in the liver, there is no direct evidence to suggest that replacement of one liver with another "cures" alcoholism as it does in supplying the missing molecular machinery that can eliminate hemophilia or Wilson's disease among affected recipients. In respect to addictive alcohol use as mediated by behavioral, rather than enzymatic or signaling molecules under the liver's control, current evidence offers no clear insight as to the existence of any structural differences between the livers of those who become alcohol dependent and those who do not. Even alcoholic cirrhosis occurs only in about 15% of heavy drinkers and there are no reliable ways to predict who will be affected.

With no direct "cure" for alcoholism emanating from a transplanted liver, how do we explain the high abstinence rates and low return rates to addictive drinking [24]? Case selection offers a first, and most obvious, answer: only the AD cases with the best prognosis for continued AD remission receive a liver graft. Although clearcut decision-tree approaches such as that presented in Box 3.3 have existed for many years [29], evaluative approaches are by no means uniform across transplant groups and do not match the high rates of recovery in Primary AD cases after transplant.

Another explanation invokes psychology: all liver graft recipients receive at least three of Vaillant's four factors in the care they receive from the liver transplant team [31]. The care teams:

1 Provide a caring relationship in which the person is welcome but alcohol is not;
2 Provide a way of structuring time with the new interest of continued graft health, as for example in

structuring the day around anti-immune agent doses, along with follow-up medical contacts; and

3 Providing a strikingly large source of hope in continuing to live rather than die of liver failure.

Contrary to this, however, the transplant medical team recesses into the background of the graft recipient's life over the first year of care with less and less contact. Yet the AD remissions go on for much longer periods. A number of post-transplant factors may play into this including social stability and Vaillant's prognostic factors, but in the absence of clear systematic evidence there remain more questions than answers [23].

Faced with these alternative explanations, neither particularly satisfying from the evidence, our group wondered about a third possibility: an antidrinking effect of the immunosuppressant agents needed to protect the liver graft from its host's own immune-mediated destruction. We first asked whether those agents exhibited a preference effect in a rodent model of alcohol consumption and found a positive effect when comparing cyclosporine to vehicle injections [32]. The same effect was obtained with cyclosporine and tacrolimus, but not with sirolimus, in another drinking model [33]. Present efforts focus on mechanisms that may account for these observed behavioral effects. While liver transplant may not "cure" alcoholism, it may provide useful insights from biological study for better understanding alcohol addiction itself.

Conclusions

Alluding to an ancient Chinese saying: alcoholism clinicians, scientists, and patients, and their communities, large and small, all live in interesting times. On the one hand there is much debate on formulations, reformulations, and rereformulations of diagnosis. On the other, our understanding of prognosis is much better than ever before. At the same time, medications to treat AD are generally regarded as largely ineffective – a complicated perception that this chapter has not discussed. Meanwhile, the US economy takes a significant beating at the hands of alcoholism and every day many thousands of people fall ill, die, or lose their families owing to this preventable, treatable illness. There is much work to be done, much more to learn, and many more lives to be saved and families preserved.

References

[1] Vaillant GE. *The Natural History of Alcoholism, Revisited.* Harvard University Press, Cambridge, MA;1995.

[2] Hasin DS, Stinson FS, Ogburn E, Grant BF. Prevalence, correlates, disability, and comorbidity of DSM-IV alcohol abuse and dependence in the United States: results from the National Epidemiologic Survey on Alcohol and Related Conditions. *Arch Gen Psychiatry* 2007; **64**(7): 830–842.

[3] American Psychiatric Association. *Diagnostic and Statistical Manual of Mental Disorders: DSM-IV-TR.* American Psychiatric Association, Washington, DC; 2000.

[4] Lucey MR, Merion R, Beresford T. *Liver Transplantation and the Alcoholic Patient.* Cambridge University Press, Cambridge; 1994.

[5] Cloninger CR, Bohman M, Sigvardsson S. Inheritance of alcohol abuse: cross-fostering analysis of adopted men. *Arch Gen Psychiatry* 1981; **38**(8): 861–868.

[6] Brown J, Babor TF, Litt MD, Kranzler HR. The type A/type B distinction: subtyping alcoholics according to indicators of vulnerability and severity. *Ann N Y Acad Sci* 1994; **708**: 23–33.

[7] Wetterling T, Veltrup C, John U, Driessen M. Late onset alcoholism. *Eur Psychiatry* 2003; **18**(3): 112–118.

[8] Everson G, Bharadhwaj G, House R, et al. Long-term follow-up of patients with alcoholic liver disease who underwent hepatic transplantation. *Liver Transpl Surg* 1997; **3**(3): 263–274.

[9] Lucey MR, Carr K, Beresford TP, et al. Alcohol use after liver transplantation in alcoholics: a clinical cohort follow-up study. *Hepatology* 1997; **25**(5): 1223–1227.

[10] Tang H, Boulton R, Gunson B, Hubscher S, Neuberger J. Patterns of alcohol consumption after liver transplantation. *Gut* 1998; **43**(1): 140–145.

[11] Lucey MR. Liver transplantation for alcoholic liver disease: past, present, and future. *Liver Transpl* 2007; **13**(2): 190–192.

[12] Mathurin P, Moreno C, Samuel D, et al. Early liver transplantation for severe alcoholic hepatitis. *N Engl J Med* 2011; **365**(19): 1790–1800.

[13] DiMartini A, Dew MA, Day N, et al. Trajectories of alcohol consumption following liver transplantation. *Am J Transplant* 2010; **10**(10): 2305–2312.

[14] World Health Organization (WHO). *ICD-10 Classifications of Mental and Behavioural Disorder: Clinical Descriptions and Diagnostic Guidelines.* WHO, Geneva; 1992, revised 2010.

[15] American Psychiatric Association. *Diagnostic and Statistical Manual of Mental Disorders: DSM-III-R.* American Psychiatric Association, Washington, DC; 1987.

[16] Schuckit MA. DSM-IV: was it worth all the fuss? *Alcohol Alcohol Suppl* 1994; **2**: 459–469.

[17] American Psychiatric Association. *Diagnostic and Statistical Manual of Mental Disorders: DSM-5.* American Psychiatric Association, Washington, DC; 2013.

[18] Schuckit MA, Smith TL, Anderson KG, Brown SA. Testing the level of response to alcohol: social information processing model of alcoholism risk: a 20-year prospective study. *Alcohol Clin Exp Res* 2004; **28**(12): 1881–1889.

[19] Schuckit MA, Smith TL. An 8-year follow-up of 450 sons of alcoholic and control subjects. *Arch Gen Psychiatry* 1996; **53**(3): 202–210.

[20] Crabbe JC, Kendler KS, Hitzemann RJ. Modeling the diagnostic criteria for alcohol dependence with genetic animal models. *Curr Top Behav Neurosci* 2013; **13**: 187–221.

[21] Kaim SC, Klett CJ, Rothfeld B. Treatment of the acute alcohol withdrawal state: a comparison of four drugs. *Am J Psychiatry* 1969; **125**(12): 1640–1646.

[22] Clark BJ, Keniston A, Douglas IS, et al. Healthcare utilization in medical intensive care unit survivors with alcohol withdrawal. *Alcohol Clin Exp Res* 2013; **37**(9): 1536–1543.

[23] Beresford TP. Probabilities of relapse and abstinence among liver transplant recipients. *Liver Transpl* 2006; **12**(5): 705–706.

[24] DiMartini A, Day N, Dew MA, et al. Alcohol consumption patterns and predictors of use following liver transplantation for alcoholic liver disease. *Liver Transpl* 2006; **12**(5): 813–820.

[25] Schuckit MA, Smith TL, Danko GP, et al. Prospective evaluation of the four DSM-IV criteria for alcohol abuse in a large population. *Am J Psychiatry* 2005; **162**(2): 350–360.

[26] Straus R, Bacon SD. Alcoholism and social stability: a study of occupational integration in 2,023 male clinic patients. *Q J Stud Alcohol* 1951; **12**(2): 231–260.

[27] Martin B, Clapp L, Bialkowski D, et al. Compliance to supervised disulfiram therapy: a comparison of voluntary and court-ordered patients. *Am J Addict* 2003; **12**(2): 137–143.

[28] Martin BK, Clapp L, Alfers J, Beresford TP. Adherence to court-ordered disulfiram at fifteen months: a naturalistic study. *J Subst Abuse Treat* 2004; **26**(3): 233–236.

[29] Beresford TP, Turcotte JG, Merion R, et al. A rational approach to liver transplantation for the alcoholic patient. *Psychosomatics* 1990; **31**(3): 241–254.

[30] Hasin DS, O'Brien CP, Auriacombe M, et al. DSM-5 criteria for substance use disorders: recommendations and rationale. *Am J Psychiatry* 2013; **170**(8): 834–851.

[31] Beresford TP, Schwartz J, Wilson D, Merion R, Lucey MR. The short-term psychological health of alcoholic and nonalcoholic liver transplant recipients. *Alcohol Clin Exp Res* 1992; **16**(5): 996–1000.

[32] Beresford HF, Deitrich R, Beresford TP. Cyclosporine-A discourages ethanol intake in C57bl/6j mice: a preliminary study. *J Stud Alcohol* 2005; **66**(5): 658–662.

[33] Beresford T, Fay T, Serkova NJ, Wu PH. Immunophyllin ligands show differential effects on alcohol self-administration in C57BL mice. *J Pharmacol Exp Ther* 2012; **341**(3): 611–616.

CHAPTER 4

Alcohol and other substance misuse

John B. Saunders

Faculty of Medicine and Biomedical Sciences, University of Queensland, Queensland; Disciplines of Psychiatry and Addiction Medicine, Sydney Medical School, University of Sydney, New South Wales, Australia

Everything is poison; it only depends on the dose.

Paracelsus, 1493–1541

Introduction

Alcohol-related liver disease has been a major cause of morbidity and mortality in most developed countries for more than three centuries. It continues to pose challenges for prevention, diagnosis, and treatment. Management of patients is often more complex nowadays because their repertoire has extended to other forms of substance use. This chapter briefly summarizes the status of alcohol as a cause of liver disease and then explores the causation and mechanisms of repetitive alcohol consumption, and its association with other types of psychoactive substance use. There follows an account of how the extent and impact of alcohol and other substance use can most conveniently be assessed in clinical practice.

This chapter has been guided by developments in scientific knowledge in areas that are somewhat removed from the mainstream of hepatology, as summarized in the following statements.

1 Liver disease and other physical sequelae do not reflect simply a person's self-determined excessive consumption of alcohol; rather, there are disorders of regulation of alcohol consumption that underpin them.

2 These disorders need to be recognized and managed in their own right for maximum therapeutic benefit.

3 Alcohol consumption is often combined with use of other psychoactive substances (including tobacco and illicit drugs), and an understanding of the range of substances the patient is taking is key to accurate assessment.

4 Common mechanisms and antecedents exist with respect to all psychoactive substances and explain in part the association with other forms of psychoactive substance use.

Alcohol and liver disease

Alcohol consumption has been known to be a cause of liver disease for over 2000 years. Accounts exist of the features of cirrhosis in heavy drinkers in Ancient Greek medical writing and in the works of Paracelsus in the sixteenth century. Detailed descriptions of alcoholic liver disease are found in the nineteenth century textbook of Budd [1]. In the twentieth century, alcoholic liver disease reached epidemic proportions in many western countries, as a result of increasing alcohol consumption in the general population. The exceptions were the periods of World Wars I and II when alcohol consumption was greatly restricted, and also in many states in the United States during the 1920s era of Prohibition. Since the 1960s there has been resurgence in alcoholic liver disease, and now in several Asian countries it is a leading cause of morbidity and mortality.

Although the epidemiologic data demonstrating the link between alcohol consumption and the occurrence of liver disease are compelling, laboratory evidence as to the mechanism was lacking for decades. There was considerable debate as to whether alcohol was the direct cause of liver disease or whether liver disease seen in heavy drinkers was a disorder of malnutrition – using the analogy of choline deficiency-induced liver disease – plus the fact that malnutrition is very common in heavy drinkers. The work of Lieber [2] in the 1960s left little doubt that alcohol was a sufficient cause of a spectrum of liver disease, ranging from minimal changes (essentially microstructural changes reflecting the enzyme-inducing effects of alcohol), alcohol-induced fatty liver, fatty-fibrotic liver, alcoholic hepatitis, and alcoholic cirrhosis. Experimental studies in primates showed that this spectrum could be reproduced, even when nutrition was excellent. The mechanisms of alcohol-induced liver disease are several and include toxic effects of its principal metabolite, acetaldehyde, generation of excess hydrogen equivalents, free radical generation, and immune-mediated mechanisms.

Alcohol may also be a cofactor in hepatitis B and C virus infection (often acquired from injecting drug use), and with hepatotoxic agents such as paracetamol (acetaminophen), and organic solvents (e.g. carbon tetrachloride). Tobacco smoking accentuates centrilobular hypoxia, which may be a mechanism of hepatic cell necrosis and fibrogenesis. Alcohol consumption also seems to contribute to liver disease that occurs in the metabolic syndrome and obesity.

Disorders of alcohol regulation

Spectrum of alcohol use and misuse

Alcohol consumption exists as a continuum in most societies. Some people drink alcohol sparingly, for example only on special occasions such as a birthday; others are infrequent users or limit their consumption to small amounts. However, some drink on a regular daily (or near-daily) basis, and others drink large quantities periodically, while others consume large amounts on a regular basis.

Alcohol consumption is influenced by cultural norms and religious observance. In most western societies and in Russia, 80% of the population consumes alcohol, in general men more than women. In Asian countries where alcohol consumption has traditionally been low or restricted to certain demographic groups (young and middle-aged men), drinking has increased many-fold over the past 30 years. In Islamic countries, alcohol consumption is typically a minority pursuit, reflecting the proscription of alcohol in the Koran.

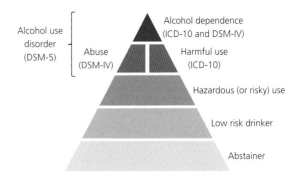

Figure 4.1 The spectrum of substance use and misuse in the general population.

The continuum of alcohol consumption is illustrated in Figure 4.1. For most people who drink alcohol, it is a pleasant social activity and most drinking takes place in the company of others. In approximately 15–20% of adults in western countries the level or pattern of alcohol consumption may be described as "risky" or "hazardous," in that epidemiologic studies show increased morbidity and mortality if it continues like this. For many conditions there appears to be a threshold of approximately 40 g/day for men and 20 g/day for women, above which physical and mental harm increases in a dose–response relationship. This level of consumption is termed "hazardous alcohol consumption." Consumption of alcohol (irrespective of dose or pattern) that has caused harm is termed "harmful alcohol consumption" in the International Classification of Diseases, tenth revision (ICD-10 [3]). Where this has led to social problems it is termed "alcohol abuse" in the Diagnostic and Statistical Manual of Mental and Behavioural Disorders, fourth edition (DSM-IV [4]), and is within the rubric of "alcohol use disorder" in DSM-5 [5]. In approximately 4–5% of adults in western societies the psychobiologic syndrome of alcohol dependence develops. This diagnosis occurs in both ICD-10 and DSM-IV. It is in this group that alcoholic liver disease is most common and becomes most severe, although it is also well represented among those with lesser alcohol use disorders.

Nature of alcohol use disorders

All these types of unhealthy alcohol use are influenced by social and psychologic factors. In turn, neurobiologic changes develop, typically insidiously, which transform voluntary patterns of consumption to a more stereotyped, internally driven activity.

Nonhazardous drinking is influenced by opportunity and social context; a social gathering will tend to increase the group's alcohol consumption and therefore the consumption of each person present. Parties, certain sporting occasions, reunions and the like are often the setting for higher than usual consumption.

Repetitive consumption also tends to be driven by processes that have been well defined by social and behavioral psychologists. Urges to drink can be triggered by associations of drinking with certain environments or companions, on the basis of classical (Pavlovian) conditioning. Operant conditioning processes inform us how positive and negative consequences of drinking influence subsequent consumption. Social cognitive theory developed in particular by Bandura [6] emphasizes the iterative pathways whereby the anticipated effects of drinking combined with the social environment result in characteristic patterns of consumption in individuals, which can become harmful and maladaptive. Alcohol intake is also influenced by the person's internal psychologic milieu, such as low mood, frustration, and perceived stress after a day's work. Thus, repetitive alcohol consumption is strongly influenced by well-known and powerful psychologic processes. By the stage of harmful alcohol consumption or alcohol abuse it cannot be considered to represent simply a "voluntary" or self-determined action.

Recent developments in our knowledge of the neurobiology of substance dependence (addiction) inform us of how physiologic processes convert patterns of alcohol consumption that have the capacity for variation (upwards or downwards) over time to types of drinking that are increasingly stereotyped and are "internally driven." In essence, repeated consumption of alcohol induces allostatic changes in several neurocircuits in the mid and lower forebrain that lead to the clinical syndrome of alcohol dependence.

Alcohol dependence has (according to the ICD-10) six central features, which are listed in Box 4.1 and reflect the "internal driving force." Three or more of the six

Box 4.1 The central features of alcohol dependence.

1 **A strong desire to use** the substance, sometimes called a craving or a compulsion, which is an experience that the person has and recognizes. It is described as one of the cognitive features of dependence.
2 **Impaired control** over alcohol consumption. This may be manifested as drinking alcohol in inappropriate settings and circumstances, being unable to stop drinking once one or two drinks have been consumed (this is known as the "priming effect"), and ceasing consumption only when the supply of alcohol has been exhausted or the person becomes intoxicated. This is a very characteristic of the central features of alcohol dependence and is one of its behavioral manifestations.
3 **Salience** (prioritization) of alcohol consumption over other activities. This refers to the altered priorities in an alcohol-dependent person whereby alcohol consumption becomes central in that person's life and relegates other interests, activities, and responsibilities to the periphery. Excuses are made why responsibilities have to be jettisoned in favor of drinking although this may be explained in quite subtle ways.
4 **Increased tolerance.** There is a characteristic increase in tolerance to the effects of alcohol such that the effects that were once experienced are no longer experienced at the same dose and more is required to achieve the desired effect. Sometimes this experience is explained by a suspicion that the alcoholic drink has been diluted, sometimes it is obscured by the fact that drinking often takes place in settings where heavy drinking is the norm. The type of tolerance is an acquired tolerance and may need to be distinguished from a greater "natural" or "primary" tolerance that is also recognized in some people.
5 **Withdrawal symptoms.** As dependence develops, the person becomes increasingly likely to experience withdrawal symptoms. Usually, these occur most commonly on the morning after a period of especially heavy drinking. Withdrawal symptoms include tremor of the hands, sweating, anxiety, agitation, and often gastrointestinal disturbances such as nausea, retching, and diarrhea. A distinction should be made between a withdrawal state which typically lasts for some hours or longer, and hangover symptoms which may include minor manifestations as described above, together with headache and a "muzzy" feeling but abate spontaneously within 30 minutes to 2–3 hours and are not particularly clustered or syndromal as a withdrawal state is. The criterion is also fulfilled if the person consumes alcohol for the purpose of alleviating or preventing a withdrawal state. Some people do not experience overt withdrawal because of constantly "topping up" and maintaining the requisite blood alcohol concentration.
6 **Continued use despite harm.** This feature essentially means that the person has repeatedly consumed alcohol and has experienced harm as a result – and then continues drinking despite that harm. The harm may be physical illness, mental health disturbance, or social and personal or occupational problems. The existence of such consequences is not sufficient in itself for this criterion to be fulfilled. The essential element is that despite the occurrence of consequences such as these, consumption of alcohol persists.

central features need to occur together and repeatedly (typically over 12 months or more) for the diagnosis to be made.

The severity of alcohol dependence may not be as great in patients with alcoholic liver disease as with patients who present for psychiatric treatment. This partly reflects a pattern of longstanding consumption which has often been integrated into the person's life. Sometimes the most obvious feature of dependence in patients with alcoholic liver disease is "continued use despite harm." This criterion is also relevant in patients with many chronic physical complications of alcohol consumption. Overt craving for alcohol or spectacular loss of control over consumption may be little evident. Withdrawal symptoms may not be particularly prominent. The clue to the diagnosis of dependence in patients with alcohol-induced physical disorders is the continuation of consumption *despite* the presence of disease – when logic would suggest that consumption should cease to alleviate symptoms and to encourage recovery from the illness. When this feature is identified, the other central features of dependence often become evident.

Neurobiology of alcohol dependence

Repeated consumption of alcohol results in fundamental and enduring changes in key neurocircuits, coursing in the tegmental area of the mid-brain and nuclei of the lower forebrain and with "iterative loops" that extend into the prefrontal gyrus and the cingulate gyrus. These subserve the sensation of reward, the level of alertness (essentially the balance between the excitatory and antistress systems), the circuits that govern salience or prioritization of activities, and cognitive control of these somewhat primitive drives [7]. Box 4.2 outlines the characteristics of these neurocircuits and how they are affected by repetitive alcohol consumption. It should be noted that many of the behaviors that are driven by these changes are essentially at the subconscious level.

Implications of dependence
Short term

In the short term, the diagnosis of alcohol dependence is important because such a patient is at risk of developing an alcohol withdrawal syndrome when alcohol intake is interrupted, as would happen following hospitalization.

Box 4.2 The neurobiology of alcohol dependence.

1 **Resetting of the reward pathways.** Initially, alcohol induces a sense of euphoria and relaxation but that experience (obviously desired by the drinker) fades with the passage of time and as blood alcohol levels decline. Adaptive changes occur in the reward circuitry that results in a blunting of the effect (termed "tolerance"), so that more alcohol is required to achieve the desired effect. The adaptive changes progress so that the person begins to develop a sensation of need for larger amounts of alcohol and that consumption increases over time to overcome the effects of increased tolerance. Correspondingly, changes in the reward neurocircuitry result in an internal increasing strong desire or "craving" to consume alcohol. Without it the person feels increasingly low in mood and lacking in motivation. The reward circuitry has become reset so that the person now experiences a persistently low mood and lack of motivation, relieved only by repeated consumption of increasing doses of alcohol.

2 **Enhancement of the alertness (stress) pathways.** Alcohol when taken acutely suppresses the alertness system by inhibiting transmission of glutamate, the principal excitatory neurotransmitter in this region of the brain. As a consequence of adaptive processes, repeated alcohol consumption increases the degree of alertness and subsequently the sensation of increased tension and stress becomes apparent. GABA-induced sedation, which normally is a predictable response to alcohol, occurs now only with larger and larger doses. The person increasingly has a state of heightened stress and is also particularly easily triggered by alcohol-associated cues such as the sight of a pub, club, or alcohol sales outlet. The sensation of stress is also increased by internal sensations such as anxiety or fear.

3 **Perturbation of the salience (prioritization) pathways.** As alcohol consumption develops into dependence, the act of drinking alcohol and also acquiring it and experiencing and recovering from its effects takes up more and more of the individual's time. Alcohol can now be described as increasingly occupying the "center stage" of the person's life. Other interests, activities, and responsibilities are shifted to the periphery and tend to be ignored.

4 **Impairment of the behavioral control pathways.** Control mechanisms on behavior. Although the behaviors that are part of the human rapid response set are under imperfect cognitive control even in healthy persons, in alcohol-dependent individuals the behavioral control system is substantially impaired. This means that the heightened reactivity to alcohol-associated cues is not modified through cognitive processes. Hence, impulsive and often ill-thought decisions can be made and translated into action to the person's detriment rather than being modified and possibly prevented in the cognitive domains.

The occurrence of a withdrawal state may not be recognized as such, and the patient may be merely considered to have an anxiety state or be rather distractible or generally "nervous." An unrecognized and untreated withdrawal state increases morbidity and the length of hospitalization, and it can progress to withdrawal seizures and delirium tremens. Making a diagnosis of alcohol dependence therefore alerts the treating team to the considerable risk that the patient will develop a withdrawal state. The patient can be monitored from the time of admission using a suitable withdrawal rating scale such as the Clinical Institute Withdrawal Assessment – Alcohol, Revised (CIWA-Ar) or the shorter Alcohol Withdrawal Scale (AWS). Identifying and treating an alcohol withdrawal state at an early stage is known to reduce the risk of withdrawal complications.

Longer term

The diagnosis of alcohol dependence is important in the longer term because moderated or controlled use of alcohol is very unlikely to be achieved. The reason for this is the "reinstatement phenomenon" which reflects some of the central features of dependence such as craving and impaired control over consumption. Reinstatement means that when a person who has had a period of abstinence from alcohol resumes drinking the level of consumption rapidly returns to what existed before the period of abstinence. There is a cascade effect whereby the first one or two drinks lead to an urge to drink and further consumption; there is a strong tendency for drinking to escalate as the hours or days go by. A person with severe alcohol dependence can return to their previous level of consumption and experience dependence symptoms within 24 hours of resuming drinking. The average reinstatement period is 3–4 days. It may be extended to several weeks when the person has a moderate severity of dependence or attempts to rein in their drinking during this period.

The importance of the reinstatement phenomenon is that a person with alcoholic liver disease who also fulfills the criteria for alcohol dependence should be advised to abstain from alcohol for the foreseeable future irrespective of the severity of their liver disease. It is common practice for medical practitioners to advise long-term abstinence from alcohol to patients with alcoholic cirrhosis or clinically significant alcoholic hepatitis. However, patients with lesser degrees of damage such as fatty liver should also be advised on long-term abstinence if they have concomitant alcohol dependence. If there is no diagnosis of alcohol dependence, but for example harmful alcohol use or another nondependent disorder, the duration of abstinence should be determined by the known recovery time for the particular grade of liver disease. For alcoholic fatty liver this would typically be 3 months.

Alcohol and other substance use

Historically, physicians managing patients with alcoholic liver disease have had one substance to consider: alcohol or at the most two, tobacco being the other one – and smoking being particularly common in heavier drinkers. Nowadays, patients with alcohol use disorders have a more extended repertoire of substance use. This is particularly evident in the younger age groups [8]. Multiple or polysubstance use is therefore to be expected. There are several reasons for this, the first being that there is a greater range of psychoactive substances available in the community than hitherto. Other reasons are addressed after a brief summary of the commonly used substances.

Types of substance use
Cannabis

The last half century has seen successive waves of substances entering circulation and being taken up, especially by young people. The mid to late 1960s saw cannabis (marijuana) being smoked widely as part of the youth counterculture. Cannabis use has waxed and waned since then but it remains the most common of the illicit substances, being smoked at some stage by more than one-third of the adult population. It used to be smoked as small cigarettes ("joints") but the predominant means nowadays is using a water-cooled pipe or "bong." This cools and filters the smoke, allowing the user to inhale more deeply and achieve greater absorption into the systemic circulation. Increasingly potent forms of cannabis produced by selective breeding techniques or hybridization combined with more efficient delivery mean that typical doses taken have increased compared with a generation ago. Synthetic cannabinoids are now available and these have a predominance of psychotomimetic effects over relaxing and sedating ones.

Sedative hypnotics

Sedative hypnotics encompass: (i) the barbiturates, (ii) "nonbarbiturate sedatives" such as methaqualone, (iii) the benzodiazepines, (iv) "z-drugs" such as zolpidem, and (v) miscellaneous sedatives such as chloral hydrate. These drugs were introduced as prescription medications for anxiety states, insomnia, and have a place in the pharmacopeia, though a more restricted one these days. Their relaxing and disinhibiting effects make them popular as recreational drugs and their dependence-inducing properties serve to perpetuate their use. Over time, increased doses are needed to maintain therapeutic plasma levels and dependence develops through rather similar mechanisms to alcohol.

There are, broadly, three populations of sedative hypnotic users. The first are those aged over 35 years who are typically prescribed them for anxiety, insomnia, or for more nebulous indications such as "stress." This group consists of women more than men and the doses tend to be moderately but consistently supratherapeutic but not to escalate greatly with the passage of time. The second group comprises young people who tend to take them periodically, often to deal with personal crises, when they may be taken in overdose. The third group is made up largely of men in their twenties and thirties who tend to take particularly high but often variable amounts. Dependence may be severe but sometimes the expected withdrawal syndrome does not occur, probably because of inconsistency in dosage.

Opioids

Opioid use, be it smoked, inhaled, injecting, or taking tablets, used to be a niche activity, seen predominantly in artistic and bohemian subcultures, with a second group comprising patients with chronic pain. From the 1960s onwards, heroin injecting increased in prevalence among young people. It often followed a phase of cannabis use (hence, cannabis was considered to be a "gateway" drug). However, it came to be the drug of choice of many, especially in victims of abuse and others who had become disaffected and disaffiliated from society. Property crime and prostitution became the most common ways for users to fund their drugs and this resulted in a vicious circle of criminality and drug use, and an absence of viable alternative ways of life. Sharing injecting equipment led to successive epidemics of blood-borne virus infection, notably hepatitis B, hepatitis C, and HIV.

Heroin use has become less common as a result of a decline in global heroin production around 2000, but it would be premature to conclude that it will remain a low-prevalence drug. More common nowadays is abuse of prescription and over-the-counter opioids. These include various codeine preparations, oxycodone (particularly a formulation of Oxycontin, since modified to reduce the risk of injecting). There are two main populations using these agents, a younger one who are involved in the illicit drug scene and who use it, often by injecting, as a substitute for heroin when this is not available, and an older population who were originally prescribed opioids for repeated or chronic pain.

Psychostimulants

Psychostimulants are commonly found in nature and certain drugs of this type are used traditionally by many peoples. For example, cocaine (in the form of coca leaf) is taken to increase stamina among people living at high altitudes (e.g. in the Andes mountains in South America). Betel nut is used for similar reasons but also recreationally and in ceremonies in Pacific Ocean nations. The other source of psychostimulants is therapeutic preparations, of which the amphetamines, introduced into medicine in the 1930s, are the best known.

Waves of psychostimulants use have occurred in western countries since the late 1970s and 1980s. Often this occurred when the drugs were transplanted to regions where they were not indigent. The most striking example is this is the surge in cocaine use in the United States in the late 1970s, which was in the form not of coca leaf but purified coca paste and then freebase cocaine and "crack" cocaine, which is typically smoked. In these higher potency forms cocaine use spread in epidemic proportions through the United States, initially in wealthier sectors of the population and then into poor and minority groups. Since the mid 1980s cocaine use has spread to much of Europe.

In other parts of the world, notably Asia and Australia, the amphetamines are the most common psychostimulants, with methylamphetamine being dominant, in the form of "crystal meth" or "ice," which is smoked or may be injected. This is now commonly used in Europe and North America too. The derivative methylenedioxy methylamphetamine (MDMA or "Ecstasy") is popular worldwide among young people, being the classic "party drug."

Tobacco (nicotine)

Tobacco smoking reached epidemic proportions in the western world in the early twentieth century with the development of the automatic cigarette rolling machine, a good example of how technologic advances often have deleterious health consequences, in this case leading to escalating mortality rates from coronary heart disease, stroke, chronic airways disease, carcinoma of the bronchus, and multiple other carcinomas. Alcohol-induced liver disease is also exacerbated by smoking, caused, it seems, by greater centrilobular hepatic hypoxia. Cigarette smoking has been in decline in many western countries from a majority phenomenon to under 20% of some adult populations. However, in China and other Asian countries it has a strongly upwards trajectory.

Reasons for multiple substance use

Availability of a range of new substances, both naturally grown and sometimes imported from producer countries and synthetic, is one reason for the modern trend to multiple substance use. Common groupings of substances are illustrated in Figure 4.2.

Another reason is a pharmacologic one; combinations of substances have desirable effects for the user or can regulate or terminate a drug experience at will. An example of the former is the addition of a benzodiazepine to boost the disinhibiting effects of alcohol, especially when the aim is to make a female more sexually

available. Other examples are combinations of alcohol and cocaine, which increases the sense of exhilaration by combining sedating and energizing effects.

Perhaps more commonly, psychoactive substances are used in sequence to regulate or terminate a drug effect. For example, the effects of the long-acting amphetamines are often terminated by the use of a sedating drug several hours (or days) later; these include alcohol, benzodiazepines, and cannabis.

Sometimes multiple substances are taken with the aim of changing the person's mental state, but without consideration of the direction of that change. People with this pattern of substance use may have alcohol as the predominant substance. Mental health and personality disorders are particularly common in this group.

Substances are also used sequentially to ameliorate the effects of a withdrawal state. Benzodiazepines may be taken to self-manage an alcohol withdrawal syndrome, while stimulants may be taken to avoid or treat withdrawal-induced dysphoria.

Pathways to alcohol and other substance use

There are well-recognized risk factors, conditions, disorders, and experiences that underlie alcohol and other substance use. For alcohol dependence (and in all likelihood less severe forms of alcohol use disorder) genetic predisposition is the single most powerful influence. The influence is a polygenic one and includes variants of genes coding for:

1 Alcohol metabolizing enzymes (alcohol dehydrogenase and aldehyde dehydrogenase, but also some cytochrome P450 species), and

2 Receptors and transport mechanisms subserving neurotransmission with gamma-aminobutyric acid (GABA), glutamate, glycine, noradrenaline, serotonin, and dopamine.

Space does not allow a full exposition of these, but it should be noted that with the exception of the alcohol metabolizing enzymes, all the recognized variants regulate neurotransmission affected by numerous psychoactive substances. Other genetic variants associated with substance use are involved with intracellular signal transduction and cell microstructure and it is more difficult to link these associations with the downstream mechanisms.

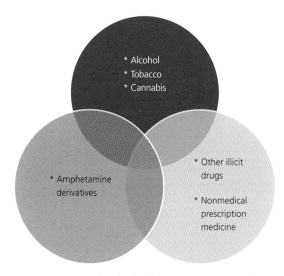

Figure 4.2 Patterns of multiple substance use in a general population.

The second most potent influence, especially on the development of illicit drug use disorders, is the experience of abuse in childhood. This takes many forms and it is often underdiagnosed, but it may also be overdiagnosed. Abuse, be it physical, sexual, or emotional, exists on a continuum and thresholds need to be established for abuse of clinical significance. A history of abuse is commonly found in people diagnosed subsequently as having certain forms of personality disorder. Self-medication of the memories of abuse or the psychologic sequelae is a well-recognized mechanism for the development of substance use disorders. Trauma, usually defined as occurring in young or later adult life (and which may be military trauma, physical, or emotional trauma in police, and ambulance crew, or interpersonal violence) is also recognized as an antecedent to alcohol and other substance use disorders – as well as a forerunner of post-traumatic stress disorder.

Several psychiatric disorders are associated with alcohol and other substance use disorders. The strength of the association differs among the psychiatric disorders. It is particularly strong for bipolar disorder and schizophrenia (with odds ratios of approximately 4 to 10), and of moderate strength for major depression and some of the anxiety disorders (approximately 1.5 to 4). It is often assumed that the relationship is a causal one with the psychiatric disorder leading to a secondary alcohol and/or other substance use disorder. However, the nature of the association and its directionality differs in different studies. It is also well-recognized that psychoactive substance use can lead to a range of psychiatric disorders. Among daily methamphetamine users, 70% report experiencing psychotic symptoms (paranoia being the most common) in any 12-month period and one-third require hospitalization, if only overnight, for a psychotic syndrome. Alcohol and cannabis-induced psychoses are well recognized. With regard to anxiety disorders and depression, the direction of the relationship is often less clear. However, irrespective of what comes first, substance dependence and anxiety and depression exacerbate each other in a "vicious circle" mechanism.

Personality disorders (formerly listed in Axis II of the DSM multiaxial classification system) are strongly associated with many forms of substance use and substance use disorders. Although they are multifactorial in etiology, there has been growing recognition in recent years of the association of personality disorders with prior abuse and neglect.

Physical disorders associated with substance use are typically those causing repeated or chronic pain, and the association is particularly strong with alcohol, prescribed or over-the-counter opioids, and with benzodiazepines.

Making the diagnosis of alcohol and substance use disorders

Approaches to the history

The great majority of diagnostic information is obtained from a careful history. The accuracy of the information is dependent on the setting and context of the interview and the interactional style of the clinician. With an empathic approach and in a clinical (as opposed to a custodial setting), a high level of accuracy can be achieved, as judged by inter-rater and test–retest reliability assessment, and validation against collateral information and (in the Nordic countries) social security data.

Among the approaches that enhance the quality and accuracy of the history are to:
1 Show empathy and understanding;
2 Establish a good therapeutic rapport with the patient;
3 Be nonjudgmental; and
4 Be sensitive to the patient's cultural background.

Experienced practitioners may employ what are termed "enhancement techniques," such as:
1 Placing the onus of denial of substance use on the patient;
2 Suggesting high levels of intake, the "top high technique"; and
3 Being aware of diversionary tactics, and not being diverted from line of questioning.

These techniques should be employed only by experienced clinicians as their use may rebound on the practitioner and lead to termination of the interview.

In addition, collaborative information should be sought from family members, the family physician, and the patient's medical records, with due care paid to ethical and privacy issues.

Three domains of enquiry

To structure the enquiry about alcohol and other substance use it is helpful to subdivide it into three conceptual domains: (i) intake, (ii) dependence, and (iii) consequences (or problems). These domains are applicable to all psychoactive substances and so the

Table 4.1 Quantification of substance use.

Substance	Measures of use
Alcohol	Grams
	Standard drinks[1]
	Standard units[2]
Tobacco	Number of cigarettes
	Ounces of tobacco
Sedative hypnotics	Dose (per tablet)
	Number of tablets per day
Cannabis	Joints
	Cones (when a pipe or "bong" is used)
	Number of bongs
Heroin	Weights
	("Street") grams
	Cost (e.g. dollars)
Amphetamines/ methamphetamine	Points (0.1 g)
	Grams
	Cost (e.g. dollars)
MDMA	Number of tablets
Cocaine	Lines
	Grams
	Cost (e.g. dollars)

[1] The amount in grams differs from country to country. In most European countries it is 10 g, in Australia and New Zealand 10 g, in the United States 14 g, in Canada 13 g.
[2] The UK standard unit is 8 g.

following outline should help in generic terms. Different emphases apply to the various substances, the most obvious being the mode of administration. For certain substances such as the opioids, the amphetamines, and cocaine (and to an extent, sedative hypnotics), specific enquiry should be made as to whether there is any injecting use of the drug.

Intake

Quantification of the amount of a substance that is used is a key aspect of the history. This is relatively easy with legal substances such as alcohol, tobacco, and prescribed medication but still feasible with illicit drugs (Table 4.1). Amongst the information that should be obtained is the following:

- Quantity;
- Frequency;
- Cost (especially useful to quantitate illicit drug use);
- Mode of administration (specific enquiry about injecting use should be made of illicit drugs such as heroin, prescribed opioids, and psychostimulants);

- Duration of use (months, years);
- Pattern or variability in use;
- Time of last use (especially relevant to gauge the likelihood of intoxication or a withdrawal syndrome); and
- Periods of abstinence.

Dependence

Establishing whether a patient has a dependence syndrome is the next step. Although this is typically suggested by the quantity and frequency of substance use, these measures are not diagnostic criteria in themselves. The experienced practitioner will assess whether the history points to dependence from information provided about the circumstances and intensity of use, whether this continued despite harm, and the extent to which the person's life is shaped around the substance. Questions reflecting the individual diagnostic criteria for dependence may then be asked. The diagnosis of the dependence syndrome is made on the basis of three out of the six (ICD-10) or seven (DSM-IV) central criteria occurring repeatedly in that person over a period of 12 months or more (or, alternatively, continuously for 1 month).

Consequences (problems)

The adverse consequences of a substance use disorder are legion. At this stage in the interview, the practitioner will likely have identified several that are uppermost in the patient's (or relatives') mind. Physicians and general medical practitioners should focus on identifying or excluding the important physical sequelae, and whether the patient has serious psychiatric problems, including suicidal ideation. It is easy to become overwhelmed by the chaos in some patients' lives and their multiple needs. Where a comprehensive assessment of the patient's psychosocial problems is necessary, this can be undertaken by a practice nurse, allied health professional, or (when there is a concern about comorbid mental disorder) by a consultation liaison psychiatrist.

Areas for enquiry typically include:
- Known comorbid psychiatric disorders;
- Current symptoms of mental disorder;
- Interpersonal difficulties;
- Financial problems;
- Work-related problems or unemployment;
- Prostitution (highly relevant for injecting drug-using females); and
- Legal and/or forensic – drink driving, assault, criminal charges.

Screening, assessment, and diagnostic schedules

There are several well-validated screening, assessment, and diagnostic interview schedules. For alcohol, the most widely employed is the Alcohol Use Disorders Identification Test (AUDIT [9]), a 10-item questionnaire developed for the World Health Organization. It covers the domains of intake (Q 1–3), dependence (Q 4–6), and problems (Q 6–10). Each question is scored 0–4 and the total score ranges 0–40. A score of 8 or more indicates hazardous or harmful alcohol consumption or alcohol abuse. Scores of 13 or more (and even more so, 15 or more) suggest alcohol dependence. The AUDIT can be employed to help structure further enquiry about these aspects of the alcohol history. Another WHO instrument, the ASSIST [10], assesses the range of substance use. It is complex, but as a brief assessment instrument it can help to structure the interview.

More complex assessment and diagnostic interview schedules are available, but these are, for practical purposes, outwith the scope and time availability of the physician. They are most commonly used by members of a multidisciplinary substance disorders clinic or a mental health consultation liaison service: they include the Addiction Severity Index (ASI), the Diagnostic Interview Schedule (DIS), the Composite International Diagnostic Interview (CIDI), and the Alcohol Use Disorder and Associated Disabilities Interview Schedule (AUDADIS).

Key aspects of physical examination

The alert practitioner can often elicit clues to underlying (and sometimes unstated) substance use during the physical examination. These are summarized in Table 4.2.

Laboratory tests

Considerable effort has been devoted to development of laboratory tests of substance use and substance use disorders. For alcohol there are numerous "biologic markers" that reflect a range of physiologic processes, including liver enzyme induction and liver cell damage, suppression of hematopoiesis and metabolic disturbances (such as hyperuricemia). For further details the reader is referred to a companion chapters 12 and 13 in this book.

There are essentially no equivalents for other substances, and detection of recent drug use is based on identification of the parent drug or a metabolite in urine, saliva, blood, or another body fluid. Hair analysis can provide a chronologic picture of drug use over

Table 4.2 Findings on physical examination.

Alcohol	Alcohol on breath
	Features of intoxication or of withdrawal
	Facial and/or periorbital puffiness
	Facial flushing/telangiectasia
	Old scars
	Conjunctival injection
	Scleral jaundice
	Trauma
	Chronic liver disease
	Gastritis/duodenitis/gastric bleeding
	Pancreatitis
	Hypertension
	Atrial fibrillation
	Rib fractures
	Nystagmus
	Peripheral neuropathy
	Head injury
	Cognitive impairment
Tobacco	Nicotine-stained fingers
	Chronic airways disease
	Cardiovascular disease
Cannabis	Smell of marijuana
	Conjunctival injection
	Features of intoxication
Sedative hypnotics	Drowsy, slurred speech (overdose)
	Anxious and agitated (withdrawal)
Injecting drug users in general	Malnutrition
	Poor self-care
	Needle track marks (fresh or old)
	Tattoos
	Jaundice (viral hepatitis C and B)
	Thrombophlebitis
	Cellulitis
	Lymphedema
	Skin abscesses
	Pneumonia
	Septic arthritis
	HIV/AIDS and STIs
Heroin	Overdose or withdrawal
	Pupillary size:
	– pinpoint (overdose)
	– dilated (withdrawal)
	Low blood pressure
	Low respiratory rate
	Noncardiogenic pulmonary edema
Psychostimulants	Underweight and emaciated
	Pupil size – dilated
	Excoriations (formication)
	Clenched jaws (bruxism)
	Caries/broken teeth
	Repetitive stereotypic movements
	Bruxism
	Nasal septal necrosis (cocaine)

STI, sexually transmitted infection.

several months but is fraught with problems in interpretation because of environmental contamination of hair.

No commonly available biologic test can specifically denote dependence on a substance, which remains a clinical diagnosis. Neuroimaging techniques such as functional magnetic resonace imaging (MRI), positron emission tomography (PET), and single-photon emission computed tomography (SPECT) scanning are currently illuminating some of the central neurobiologic mechanism of dependence. As yet they are not part of routine clinical assessment but this may well change with greater experience of these techniques over the next decade.

References

[1] Budd G. *Diseases of the Liver*. Blanchard and Lea, London; 1857.

[2] Lieber CS. Alcoholic fatty liver: its pathogenesis and mechanism of progression to inflammation and fibrosis. *Alcohol* 2004; **34**: 9–19.

[3] World Health Organization. *ICD-10 Classification of Mental and Behavioural Disorders: Clinical Descriptions and Diagnostic Guidelines*. WHO, Geneva; 1992.

[4] American Psychiatric Association. *Diagnostic and Statistical Manual of Mental Disorders, Fourth Edition (DSM-IV)*. American Psychiatric Association, Washington, DC; 1994.

[5] American Psychiatric Association. *Diagnostic and Statistical Manual of Mental Disorders, Fifth Edition (DSM-5)*. American Psychiatric Association, Washington DC; 2013.

[6] Bandura A. *Social Learning Theory*. Prentice-Hall, Eaglewood Cliffs, NJ; 1977.

[7] Koob GF, Volkow ND. Neurocircuitry of addiction. *Neuropsychopharmacology* 2010; **35**: 217–238.

[8] Connor JP, Gullo MJ, White A, Kelly AB. Polysubstance use: diagnostic challenges, patterns of use and health. *Curr Opin Psychiatry* 2014; **27**: 269–275.

[9] Saunders JB, Aasland OG, Babor TF, de la Fuente JR, Grant M. Development of the Alcohol Use Disorders Identification Test (AUDIT): WHO Collaborative Project on Early Detection of Persons with Harmful Alcohol Consumption II. *Addiction* 1993; **88**: 791–804.

[10] World Health Organization. *The Alcohol, Smoking and Substance Involvement Screening Test (ASSIST)*. WHO, Geneva; 2004.

CHAPTER 5

Risk factors for alcohol-related liver disease

Stuart Kendrick and Chris Day

Institute of Cellular Medicine, Newcastle University, Newcastle upon Tyne, UK

KEY POINTS

- Even amongst those with the highest alcohol intakes, liver disease is present in less than half, indicating that other factors modify the risk of liver disease.

- Environmental factors influence the risk of alcohol-related liver disease and are amenable to modification to improve individual outcomes and population health.

- Genetic factors influence the risk of alcohol-related liver disease and their study may advance future therapeutic strategies.

- The identification of additional risk factors does not diminish the prime importance of reducing alcohol consumption to improve individual and population health.

Evidence for risk modifiers in ARLD

At first glance, alcohol-related liver disease (ARLD) appears to have a single, obvious risk factor: the consumption of alcohol. However, deeper study reveals evidence of a more interesting and complex interplay of genetic, environmental, and social factors contributing to the development, progression, and consequences of the ARLD phenotype.

The crucial first piece of evidence is that liver disease is by no means universal, even in the groups with the highest alcohol consumption. Indeed, only a minority of those consuming alcohol at levels established to be hazardous will develop clinically apparent liver dysfunction. For instance, in an Italian cohort study of unselected heavy drinkers, only 20–30% displayed steatohepatitis on liver biopsy and cirrhosis was present in 10% with even fewer suffering symptomatic disease [1]. Another study demonstrated that even in those consuming over 200 g/day, only

20% had evidence of cirrhosis after 13 years and 50% after 20 years. Of course, this does not mean that the majority of heavy drinkers can consider themselves "safe" from the harmful effects of alcohol; although liver disease has the closest association with alcohol intake, it accounts for a minor portion of the total alcohol-related harm, which includes injuries, neuropsychiatric disorders, cardiovascular disease, stroke, and cancers. Second, amongst heavy drinkers, liver disease assorts with a variety of other characteristics including sex, ethnic background, and body composition, with identified groups having an increased risk of liver disease, or developing liver injury at a lower total cumulative dose of alcohol than others.

These observations identify ARLD as a typical "complex" disease in which a number of different factors can modify risk, and the clinical phenotype is determined by the aggregate of a variety of pathogenic and protective factors, both genetic and environmental. This is supported by observational studies in twins which indicate that 50%

Alcohol Abuse and Liver Disease, First Edition. Edited by James Neuberger and Andrea DiMartini.
© 2015 John Wiley & Sons, Ltd. Published 2015 by John Wiley & Sons, Ltd.

of the risk of developing alcohol-related cirrhosis by age 61 is heritable and the other 50% is environmental [2].

Despite the complexity of risk, it is important to emphasize that once ARLD is established and clinically apparent, the one risk factor that can be modified and the only one consistently demonstrated to improve prognosis is to abstain from further alcohol.

Environmental risk factors

The most obvious environmental risk factors for ARLD are those related to alcohol consumption (Figure 5.1). The effect of alcohol dose can be demonstrated at a population level in the relationship between countries' total alcohol consumption and their liver disease mortality rates. A difference in annual absolute alcohol consumption of 1 liter per capita is associated with a difference in national cirrhosis death rates of 14% for males and 8% for females [3,4]. National changes in alcohol consumption are also closely correlated with cirrhosis death rates, as demonstrated by the fall in cirrhosis deaths in 1940s France when war interrupted the supply of alcohol [5], and the rising liver-related mortality in the United Kingdom and Eastern Europe which parallels increases in alcohol consumption in the last 25 years [3,4].

This relationship has also been demonstrated at an individual level, with large cohort studies in several countries establishing a correlation between the number of standard drinks per day and the incidence of ARLD. These data display a threshold effect with risk of liver disease rising once intake exceeds 1–2 standard drinks per day for women and 2–3 standard drinks per day for men, a finding that is the basis for current guidance on "safe" alcohol limits for healthy people [1].

However, dose is not the only aspect of alcohol consumption demonstrated to modify liver disease risk. Epidemiologic data have also demonstrated an effect of pattern of alcohol consumption. In a Swedish study, for a given total alcohol dose, those who drank only at the weekends were less likely to develop liver disease than those who drank every day [6]. This suggests that frequent "recovery" periods can mitigate the damaging effects of high alcohol intake, and supports the advice that drinkers should have two or more nondrinking days per week. The Dionysus study of two northern Italian communities also suggested a protective effect of food, with those who consumed alcohol only with meals apparently protected from liver disease relative to

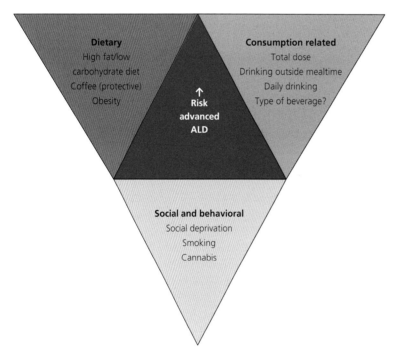

Figure 5.1 Environmental factors influencing the course of alcohol-related liver disease (ARLD).

those who drank outside mealtimes [1]. This is likely to be because of the slowed gastric absorption of alcohol taken with food, leading to lower peak blood (and hence liver) alcohol concentrations.

Investigation of the effect of the type of alcoholic beverage consumed has produced interesting results. A study of 30 630 citizens of Copenhagen confirmed increased liver disease in consumers of any alcohol-containing beverage, but demonstrated that those who drank wine appeared to have a lower risk than those who drank beer or spirits [7]. Compared with those who drank no wine, the relative risk of cirrhosis in those whose alcohol intake was 16–30% wine was 0.4, and in those consuming more than 50% of their alcohol in the form of wine it was 0.3. At first, these data appear to support a "protective" effect of wine or one of its constituents, and there is biochemical evidence for antioxidant and tissue-protective effects of some flavonoids which are more abundant in wine than in beer or spirits. However, an elegant Danish study suggested there might be other variables contributing to the different prevalence of cirrhosis in wine and beer drinkers. This research examined 3.5 million supermarket transactions and demonstrated that people who purchased wine were more likely to also purchase items associated with a healthy diet, such as fruit, vegetables, and low-fat produce, while those who purchased beer were more likely to have bought sugar, chips, soft drinks, and high-fat foods [8]. It is possible that the apparent "protective" effect of wine is more to do with associated variables in the lifestyle of wine drinkers than an effect of the beverage itself. In most countries, the proportion of alcohol consumed as wine increases with higher educational level and social background, which raises the possibility that wine consumption is also associated with better chances of receiving and acting on health improvement information in general.

Evidence from a number of sources supports the assertion that dietary factors may be independent risk factors for liver disease in heavy drinkers. High-fat diets have been shown to assort with more advanced disease. All stages of alcohol-related liver injury (steatosis, steatohepatitis, cirrhosis) are more common in biopsies from heavy drinkers with obesity than in those without [9], and multivariate analysis identified obesity and high blood glucose measurements as the strongest predictors of cirrhosis in this group [10]. A study of 9559 Scottish men followed up for 23 years quantified the relative contributions of alcohol and obesity to liver-related mortality in the population [11]. Relative to

those with neither problem, men with obesity had a relative risk of liver mortality of 1.29, while those with alcohol excess had a relative risk of 3.66. However, those with both problems had a relative risk of liver disease mortality of 9.53, emphasizing that the interaction of fat and alcohol is more damaging than the sum of their individual effects. The physiologic basis for this interaction is likely to lie in the similarities between the biochemical pathogenesis of alcohol- and fat-related liver injury. Both occur in the context of hepatic metabolic overload with NAD^+ depletion, *de novo* lipogenesis and increased free fatty acid flux, associated with oxidative, endoplasmic reticulum, and cytokine-mediated stress, and characterized by enhanced proinflammatory responses to gut-derived bacterial endotoxins. Obesity is also associated with enhanced expression of profibrogenic factors that may accelerate the development of advanced liver disease; these include elevated circulating angiotensin, norepinephrine, insulin and glucose, and imbalanced adipokine profiles, all implicated in the direct activation of hepatic myofibroblasts.

Dietary factors can also have a favorable impact on ARLD risk. A study of 125 580 health care plan participants in the western United States followed for over 15 years identified an apparent dose-dependent protective effect of coffee drinking on the development of ARLD [12]. When data were adjusted for age, weight, smoking, gender, and ethnicity, an intake of four cups of coffee per day reduced the relative risk of ARLD to 0.2. These findings have been replicated in several large cohorts in different countries but the mechanisms of the protective effects of coffee have yet to be firmly established. Possible mechanisms of protection include antagonism and upregulation of anti-inflammatory adenosine A2 receptors, phosphodiesterase inhibition, or enhancement of antioxidant defenses.

Cigarette smoking has been associated with increased risk of cirrhosis in large cohort studies, with 20 cigarettes a day trebling the relative risk [12].

Of particular importance to the public health impact of alcohol is the observation that ARLD mortality is significantly higher in areas of increased social deprivation, and this difference cannot be accounted for by differences in alcohol consumption alone [13]. There is little to support the suggestion that this is due purely to "social drift" of those with ARLD into lower social strata. It is likely that in the context of lower incomes, reduced education, and limited social support, some or all of the factors above combine to enhance the harmful effects of alcohol on the liver.

Genetic risk factors

Evidence for a genetic component to ARLD risk comes from observation of the ethnic variation in incidence when corrected for other variables. Furthermore, study of 15 924 male twin pairs aged 51–61 identified differences in twin–twin concordance rates between dizygotic and monozygotic twins, suggesting that the tendency to drink to excess ("alcoholism") has a genetic basis but that the risk of cirrhosis has an independent genetic component over and above the risk of alcoholism [2]. Interestingly, when the same twin pairs were studied again 15 years later, the incidence of both alcoholism and cirrhosis had increased by 25%, but the genetic risk of cirrhosis was no longer independent, being fully accounted for by the risk of alcoholism [14]. A suggested interpretation of these findings is that genetic factors have an impact on the development of cirrhosis at an earlier age or a lower total cumulative dose, but that sustained drinking over years can eventually lead to cirrhosis even in those with more favorable genetic backgrounds.

The most obvious genetic risk factor for ARLD is female sex. Women are more likely to develop cirrhosis at a given total cumulative dose of alcohol than men, and so recommended limits on alcohol intake are lower for women than for men. Diet does not appear to be responsible for these sex differences. The principal physiologic basis is thought to be the lower percentage water and the higher percentage fat in female body composition. Alcohol is highly soluble in water and distributes through this body compartment. In women the relative volume of distribution of alcohol is lower so in a woman a given dose of alcohol will achieve a higher peak blood alcohol concentration than the same dose in a man. There is rodent evidence of differential effects of male and female sex hormones on inflammatory responses, but this has not been established in humans [15].

Study of non-sex-linked genetic associations of ARLD can be by one of two approaches. The more traditional, hypothesis-based approach is to identify a candidate gene based on existing theories of pathogenesis and then examine whether allelic variants of that gene assort with ARLD cases and controls. In complex diseases, the typical effect of a gene variant is to increase relative risk to 1.5. If the frequency of the rarer allele is 15% then 600 cases and controls would be required to achieve 80% power to detect an association when

$p = 0.05$. By these principles, almost all published candidate gene case–control studies in ARLD have been underpowered and at risk of failing to detect true associations (type 2 error). There is also a risk of reporting false positive associations (type 1 error) due to small sample sizes, failure to control for multiple variables, and publication bias. The selection of control groups for these studies is particularly important, and the controls should have documented persistent heavy drinking but confident exclusion of liver disease. If an unselected "normal" control population is used instead the study may identify gene variants associated with alcoholism rather than liver disease, or the presence of nondrinkers with high-risk alleles in the control group might obscure a significant effect of that allele in the ARLD group [16].

The alternative approach to identifying genetic risk loci is a hypothesis-generating genome-wide association study (GWAS). This requires large numbers of well-characterized patients and controls to mitigate the effects of multiple testing of a large number of genetic variants. These approaches can generate robust data and have the potential to uncover risk loci and pathways outside the previously postulated pathogenic mechanisms but are financially and logistically challenging. No GWAS data in ARLD haves been published at the time of writing, although a multicenter international GWAS study, GenomAlc, is currently recruiting.

Published candidate gene case–control studies focus on four components of ARLD pathogenesis: drinking behavior, oxidative stress, inflammatory response, and tissue fibrosis (Figure 5.2).

The identified genetic associations of drinking behavior include the gamma-aminobutyric acid receptor subunit alfa-2 (GABRA2) which has a role in reward pathways in the central nervous system and which has been shown to be associated with a variety of addictive behaviors. Other variants in this group are in genes encoding enzymes responsible for alcohol metabolism, alcohol dehydrogenase (ADH), and aldehyde dehydrogenase (ALDH). Rapid conversion of alcohol to acetaldehyde by ADH2*1 and ADH3*2 variants, or slowed clearance of acetaldehyde by ALDH2*2, leads to accumulation of acetaldehyde that causes uncomfortable sensations and flushing when alcohol is consumed. Heavy drinking is less common in groups with these variants, and the incidence of liver disease is correspondingly lower.

One of the major mechanisms of alcohol-related liver injury is the generation of reactive oxygen species (ROS)

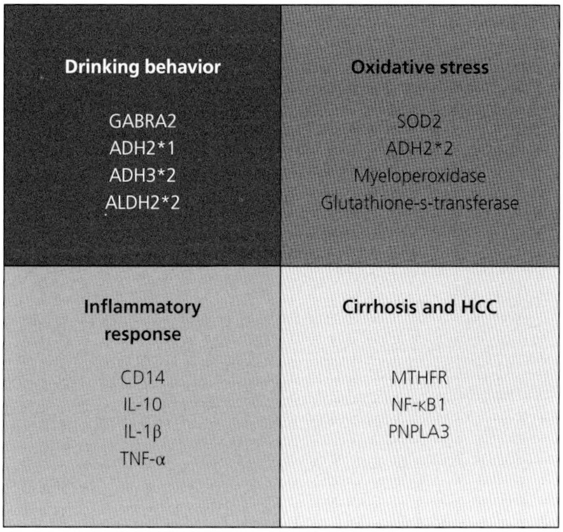

Drinking behavior	Oxidative stress
GABRA2 ADH2*1 ADH3*2 ALDH2*2	SOD2 ADH2*2 Myeloperoxidase Glutathione-s-transferase
Inflammatory response	Cirrhosis and HCC
CD14 IL-10 IL-1β TNF-α	MTHFR NF-κB1 PNPLA3

Figure 5.2 Genetic polymorphisms implicated in the development of ARLD. ADH, alcohol dehydrogenase; ALDH, aldehyde dehydrogenase; GABRA2, gamma-aminobutyric acid receptor subunit alfa-2; HCC, hepatocellular carcinoma; IL, interleukin; MTHFR, methylenetetrahydrofolate reductase; NF-κB1, nuclear factor of kappa light polypeptide gene enhancer in B-cells 1; PNPLA3, patatin-like phospholipase domain-containing 3; SOD2, manganese superoxide dismutase; TNF-α, tumor necrosis factor alfa.

during alcohol metabolism. Variants that produce ROS more readily such as those in myeloperoxidase or ADH2*2 have demonstrated associations with liver disease, as do variants that reduce the cells normal protective ROS clearance mechanisms such as superoxide dismutase 2 (SOD2) and glutathione-s-transferase. Three studies of SOD2 variants as risk factors for ARLD produced inconsistent results, but a study of these variants within a population of ARLD patients revealed improved survival and reduced incidence of hepatocellular cancer in those with normal SOD2 function.

The other major component of alcohol-related liver injury is an inflammatory response mediated by cytokines and chemokines that recruit inflammatory cells to the liver and promote hepatocyte death. Studies of a common variant in tumor necrosis factor alfa (TNF-α) from the United Kingdom, Spain, and Portugal produced variable results but in two studies suggested an association with ARLD. However, mechanistic studies suggest that the variant reduces TNF-α release and have not uncovered a biologically plausible explanation for its role in pathogenesis. Variants in genes for cytokines

IL-1β and IL-10 and in the bacterial lipopolysaccharide co-receptor CD14 have also been described in association with ARLD in small studies.

Genetic variation in tissue fibrogenesis has also been examined in small studies, with early data suggesting a role for methylenetetrahydrofolate reductase (MTHFR) and NF-κB variants. Interest in the patatin-like phospholipase A3 (PNPLA3, encoding the protein adiponutrin) arose when it was identified as a risk allele for nonalcoholic fatty liver disease (NAFLD) in several GWAS. Candidate gene studies in ARLD identified an association with ARLD in general, and also with cirrhosis and the incidence of hepatocellular cancer [17]. The pathogenic mechanism of this association is still under investigation in both NAFLD and ARLD but appears to be consistent with a role for an excess of lipid-derived metabolic intermediates in the cellular stress that characterizes both conditions.

Gene–environment interactions

In recent years our understanding of risk in complex disease has expanded to include the effects of gene–environment interactions in which exposure to environmental factors can modulate the expression of disease-associated genes by modifying DNA and its associated proteins with, amongst others, acetylation, methylation, or ubiquitination. These epigenetic modifications can be transmitted from one generation to the next and modify disease susceptibility. Alcohol has already been shown to influence DNA methylation and histone acetylation in rodent models and human cells. This leads to the intriguing possibility that exposure to excess alcohol in a parent might influence ARLD susceptibility in the offspring.

Relevance to practice

It is unlikely that genetic testing will assume a significant role in the general management of ARLD when the removal of the principal environmental cause, alcohol consumption, is so fundamental to effective therapy. However, in advanced disease an understanding of an individual's genetic and epigenetic background may assist the personalized selection of therapies that specifically target oxidative stress, inflammatory responses, or lipid metabolism as

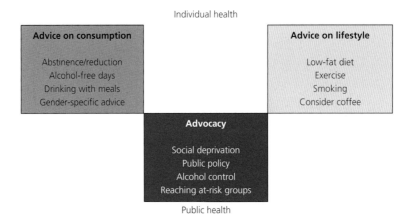

Figure 5.3 Strategies to influence the course of ARLD.

appropriate. Furthermore, an increased understanding of the genetic basis of ARLD progression may guide the development of future therapeutic strategies.

In contrast, our understanding of the environmental risk factors influencing the development of ARLD has the opportunity to influence clinical practice immediately, providing patients, physicians, and policymakers with strategies to slow disease progression and reduce population prevalence in addition to minimizing alcohol intake (Figure 5.3). Individuals can be advised to reduce total alcohol consumption and also to increase the number of alcohol-free days in a week and to take their alcohol with meals rather than outside mealtimes. Improving lifestyle factors, including low-fat diets, weight loss, exercise, and smoking cessation is likely to have a significant effect on disease progression and general health, and this may be combined with consideration of increasing coffee intake. At the public health level the greatest benefits are likely to come from interventions that minimize the impact of social deprivation on health outcomes including reducing inequalities, improving educational provision, minimizing social exclusion, and controlling the ready availability of cheap alcohol [18].

References

[1] Bellentani S, Saccoccio G, Costa G, et al. Drinking habits as cofactors of risk for alcohol induced liver damage. The Dionysos Study Group. *Gut* 1997; **41**(6): 845–850.

[2] Hrubec Z, Omenn GS. Evidence of genetic predisposition to alcoholic cirrhosis and psychosis: twin concordances

for alcoholism and its biological end points by zygosity among male veterans. *Alcohol Clin Exp Res* 1981; **5**: 207–215.

[3] Corrao G, Ferrari P, Zambon A, et al. Trends of liver cirrhosis mortality in Europe, 1970–1989: age-period-cohort analysis and changing alcohol consumption. *Int J Epidemiol* 1997; **26**(1): 100–109.

[4] Leon DA, McCambridge J. Liver cirrhosis mortality rates in Britain from 1950 to 2002: an analysis of routine data. *Lancet* 2006; **367**: 52–56.

[5] Ledermann S. *Alcool, Alcoolisme, Alcoolisation: Mortalite, Morbidite, Accidents du Travail*, 2nd ed. Travaux et Documents, Institut National d'Etudes Démographiques. Presses Universitaires de France, Paris; 1964.

[6] Stokkeland K, Hilm G, Spak F, Franck J, Hultcrantz R. Different drinking patterns for women and men with alcohol dependence with and without alcoholic cirrhosis. *Alcohol Alcohol* 2008; **43**(1): 39–45.

[]7 Becker U, Grønbaek M, Johansen D, Sørensen TI. Lower risk for alcohol-induced cirrhosis in wine drinkers. *Hepatology* 2002; **35**(4): 868–875.

[8] Johansen D, Friis K, Skovenborg E, Grønbaek M. Food buying habits of people who buy wine or beer: cross sectional study. *BMJ* 2006; **332**(7540): 519–522.

[9] Rotily M, Durbec JP, Berthézène P, Sarles H. Diet and alcohol in liver cirrhosis: a case–control study. *Eur J Clin Nutr* 1990; **44**(8): 595–603.

[10] Naveau S, Giraud V, Borotto E, et al. Excess weight risk factor for alcoholic liver disease. *Hepatology* 1997; **25**(1): 108–111.

[11] Hart CL, Morrison DS, Batty GD, Mitchell RJ, Davey Smith G. Effect of body mass index and alcohol consumption on liver disease: analysis of data from two prospective cohort studies. *BMJ* 2010; **340**: c1240.

[12] Klatsky AL, Morton C, Udaltsova N, Friedman GD. Coffee, cirrhosis, and transaminase enzymes. *Arch Intern Med* 2006; **166**(11): 1190–1195.

[13] Effiong K, Osinowo A, Pring A. *Deaths from liver disease: implications for end of life care in England,* 2012. National End of Life Care Intelligence Network.

[14] Reed T, Page WF, Viken RJ, Christian JC. Genetic predisposition to organ-specific endpoints of alcoholism. *Alcohol Clin Exp Res* 1996; **20**(9): 1528–1533.

[15] Enomoto N, Yamashina S, Schemmer P, et al. Estriol sensitizes rat Kupffer cells via gut-derived endotoxin. *Am J Physiol* 1999; **277**(3 Pt 1): G671–677.

[16] Stickel F, Hampe J. Genetic determinants of alcoholic liver disease. *Gut* 2012; **61**(1): 150–159.

[17] Trepo E, Guyot E, Ganne-Carrie N, et al. PNPLA3 (rs738409 C>G) is a common risk variant associated with hepatocellular carcinoma in alcoholic cirrhosis. *Hepatology* 2012; **55**(4): 1307–1308.

[18] Room R, Babor T, Rehm J. Alcohol and public health. *Lancet* 2005; **365**(9458): 519–530.

CHAPTER 6

Mechanisms of alcohol toxicity*

Guruprasad P. Aithal and Jane I. Grove

NIHR Nottingham Digestive Diseases Biomedical Research Unit, Nottingham University Hospitals NHS Trust and the University of Nottingham, Nottingham, UK

KEY POINTS

- Toxic alcohol is usually removed by oxidation in the liver which leads to altered cellular metabolic pathways.

- Steatosis, the initiating step in alcoholic liver disease (ALD), arises as a consequence of the sequestration of resulting excessive fatty acids, as lipids.

- Alcohol causes increased gut permeability to endotoxin which leads to inflammation and production of reactive oxygen species (ROS).

- Oxidative stress arises from ROS generation during ethanol oxidation and from subsequent responses.

- Infiltration of inflammatory immune cells into the liver gives rise to alcoholic steatohepatitis.

- The effect of alcohol on inflammation and fibrosis is coordinated by Kupffer cells, activated by endotoxin, which release cytokines and chemokines, notably TNF-α.

- The transformation of hepatic stellate cells to myofibroblasts that overproduce collagen is a central feature of alcohol-induced progression of ALD to fibrosis through to cirrhosis.

- The cellular changes induced by alcohol are also, in part, dependent on genetic factors (influencing metabolic and immunologic processes) and, in part, are modulated by the presence of comorbid conditions.

The association of alcohol and liver disease has long been known but the pathogenic mechanisms of alcoholic liver disease (ALD) involving genetic, environmental, metabolic, and immunologic factors is poorly understood. Chronic alcohol intake results in damage to the liver where it is primarily detoxified in hepatocytes. This progresses from simple steatosis (fatty liver), through stages of steatohepatitis, followed by fibrosis and then cirrhosis to hepatic failure. In addition, alcohol abuse can contribute to the development of hepatocellular carcinoma and causes injury to the brain, cardiovascular system, and other organs. The fate of alcohol, its metabolites and by-products, and the cellular responses to these molecules, is central to elucidating the component pathways involved in disease development and progression as well as for the identification of therapeutic targets.

Alcohol metabolism and impact

Most ingested alcohol is detoxified by oxidation reactions in the liver (Figure 6.1). The first step is mainly catalyzed by alcohol dehydrogenase (ADH) in the cytosol which converts ethanol to acetaldehyde using

---

*The views expressed are those of the authors and not necessarily those of the NHS, the NIHR, or the Department of Health.

Alcohol Abuse and Liver Disease, First Edition. Edited by James Neuberger and Andrea DiMartini.
© 2015 John Wiley & Sons, Ltd. Published 2015 by John Wiley & Sons, Ltd.

nicotinamide adenine dinucleotide (NAD). An alternative enzyme, cytochrome P450 2E1 (CYP2E1), in the microsomal ethanol oxidizing system of smooth endoplasmic reticulum (ER), can also catalyze this reaction when its expression is induced following chronic alcohol consumption. Catalase can also oxidize some ethanol in the peroxisomes (estimated to detoxify 25%). Acetaldehyde produced in this first metabolic step is then oxidized to acetate in the mitochondria by aldehyde dehydrogenase (ALDH). CYP2E1 can also convert acetaldehyde to acetate via a NADPH-dependent pathway. Acetate is nontoxic; it enters the circulatory system and can break down to CO_2 and H_2O [1].

Experimental models have shown that alcohol is pathogenic through mechanisms including increasing oxidative stress and induction of Kupffer cells by gut-derived endotoxins. Ethanol can alter the fluidity of cell membranes, thereby altering the activity of membrane-bound enzymes and transport proteins causing changes to cell signaling. It also causes mitochondrial dysfunction and triglyceride accumulation.

Acetaldehyde produced in the first oxidation step (Figure 6.1) is considered more toxic and carcinogenic than ethanol. It can interact with DNA directly affecting gene expression and causing lesions and adducts that can contribute to liver cell damage and carcinogenesis. Acetaldehyde also forms adducts with proteins involved in DNA repair, enzymes (including CYP2E1), structural proteins such as cytoskeletal elements, and collagen (contributing to scar tissue formation), impairing cell activities. Acetaldehyde also binds glutathione inhibiting its ability to scavenge hydrogen peroxide reducing defense against damaging free radicals. The deleterious effects of acetaldehyde include impairment of the mitochondrial β-oxidation of fatty acids and covalently binding of hepatic macromolecules, triggering an immune response.

Reactive oxygen species (ROS), such as the superoxide anion and hydroxyethyl radical produced when alcohol is metabolized by CYP2E1, are highly reactive and form adducts with lipids, proteins, and DNA forming the basis of oxidative stress. Lipid peroxidation products generated by ROS are thought to be the predominant mediators of alcohol-induced cirrhosis and cancer pathologies. In particular, malondialdehyde and 4-hydroxynonenal lipid peroxidation products, which have been detected in alcoholics with high levels of CYP2E1 activity, can react with DNA giving adducts associated with chronic liver injury. These peroxidation products also elicit an immune response [1].

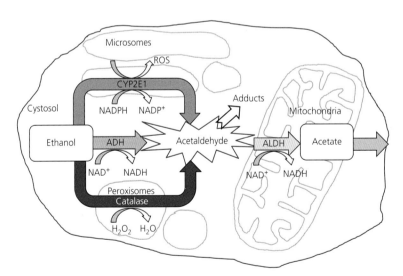

Figure 6.1 Routes of liver ethanol oxidation. Ethanol can be metabolized to acetaldehyde by alcohol dehydrogenase (ADH) in the cytosol using NAD^+. Alternatively, the inducible cytochrome P450 2E1 (CYP2E1) in the microsomal ethanol oxidizing system can catalyze the reaction resulting in the generation of NADPH and reactive oxygen species (ROS) or peroxisomal catalase can be used. The resulting acetaldehyde, which can form damaging adducts with cell components, is detoxified by acetaldehyde dehydrogenase (ALDH) in the mitochondria to produce nontoxic acetate (which subsequently enters circulation) and more NADH. Increased cellular NADH: NAD^+ ratio, ROS, and acetaldehyde adducts initiate cellular processes that contribute to alcoholic liver disease.

As alcohol, acetaldehyde, and ROS all contribute to ALD pathology, genetic variation influencing the relative rates of the different metabolic pathways may influence disease development. Differences in ethanol elimination rates may be the consequence of which variant ADH isoforms are present: fast-metabolizing isoforms more rapidly producing high levels of toxic acetaldehyde may have a greater pathogenic effect. Individuals with a low-activity ALDH*2 isoform accumulate higher levels of acetaldehyde giving effects that prohibit alcohol consumption and an increased risk for malignancy. The severity and duration of alcohol use alters CYP2E1 expression, affecting the proportion of alcohol metabolized via this ROS-producing pathway, contributing to the disease progression. For example, expression of CYP2E1 has been estimated to be 5–20 times higher in patients with alcoholic steatohepatitis. Elimination kinetics of alcohol also varies with its dose and duration leading to differences in associated pathologic mechanisms for acute and chronic alcohol exposure.

Pathologic mechanisms

Metabolic impact and lipotoxicity

Alcohol metabolism results in concomitant excessive reduction of NAD to NADH (Figure 6.1) causing a NAD–NADH imbalance that leads to altered carbohydrate and lipid metabolism. The increasing amount of NADH in the cytosol is transferred to mitochondria which induces the electron transport components to assume a reduced state thus promoting the formation of ROS by facilitating the transfer of an electron to oxygen [2]. NADH-induced inhibition of mitochondrial β oxidation and the diversion of acetyl-CoA into *de novo* fatty acid synthesis results in lipid accumulation thus promoting steatosis [3]. Furthermore, ethanol has also been shown to activate SREBP 1c (sterol regulatory element binding protein-1) which results in the transcriptional activation of numerous genes involved in lipogenesis [4].

Altered lipid homeostasis is the initiating step for ALD. Fatty acids are generated either by increased lipogenesis following alcohol intake, or in response to a dietary energy excess directly as well as from lipolysis of adipose. Lipotoxicity occurs as a consequence of fatty acid interaction with lipid membranes and other cellular components, causing damage directly, and by disrupting cell signaling. Levels of free fatty acids have been shown to be 10-fold higher in liver biopsy samples from patients with ALD. *In vitro* experiments have found that saturated fatty acids are able to promote inflammation by activating Toll-like receptor 4 (TLR4) expressed on macrophages and by activating hepatocyte inflammasomes and chemokine production.

Degradation of surplus fatty acids by oxidation in mitochondria, peroxisomes, and microsomes is potentially hepatotoxic [5]. Hepatocyte uptake of fatty acids is regulated by fatty acid transport proteins (FATPs), fatty acid translocase (CD36), fatty acid binding proteins (FABPs), and adipokines including adiponectin [3]. β-Oxidation of fatty acids in hepatic mitochondria produces superoxide and oxidation in peroxisomes generates hydrogen peroxide contributing to oxidative stress. ROS are also produced by microsomal ω-oxidation of fatty acids, along with dicarboxylic acids which cause mitochondrial dysfunction and contribute to hepatotoxicity. β-Oxidation is controlled by peroxisome proliferator-activated receptor α (PPAR-α) which is inhibited by alcohol consumption. Ethanol also inhibits AMPK (adenosine monophosphate-activated kinase), promoting lipid metabolism [6]. Lower levels of circulating adiponectin further decrease AMPK. The overall impact of fatty acid oxidation depends on the ability of the various metabolic systems and compartments to "cope" with the toxic products of oxidation which otherwise result in various degrees of hepatocyte injury.

Storage of fatty acids as triglycerides protects hepatocytes from toxic effects of fatty acids: the accumulation of triglycerides is not hepatotoxic [3]. So steatosis resulting from excessive accumulation of triglyceride in hepatocytes can be considered as a protective response to fatty acid build-up arising from alcohol intake. The triglycerides are usually packaged into lipoproteins in the hepatocyte ER before export to adipose stores. However, if this system is overwhelmed, excess triglycerides accumulate. The stress placed on the ER can result in altered protein and membrane synthesis which impact on lipid homeostasis and contribute to hepatotoxicity. The "unfolded protein response" is triggered when unfolded proteins accumulate as a consequence of ER stress. This results in reduced protein synthesis and increased protein degradation and activation of Nfr-2-mediated apoptosis. It is further aggravated by the accumulation of protein adducts and ROS. ER stress can subsequently lead to apoptosis of hepatocytes and endothelial cells and sustained activation of the wound-healing response thus promoting fibrosis.

Energy metabolism is altered in liver cells engaged in alcohol detoxification via a number of cellular processes [2]:

- Reduced activity of mitochondrial complexes;
- Abnormalities of respiratory chain resulting in generation of superoxide anions (ROS);
- Lowered rate of ATP synthesis;
- Enhanced oxygen uptake because more is required for ethanol detoxification. However, despite an increased blood flow, it remains insufficient particularly in centrilobular area leading to hypoxia;
- Fatty acid metabolism increases leading to steatosis; and
- ER stress resulting from excessive triglyceride processing.

Steatosis, along with inflammation and fibrosis are the core pathologies in the development and progression of ALD. Preventing steatosis is often sufficient to block inflammation in experimental ALD. With abstinence from alcohol, the normal redox state is restored, the lipid is mobilized, leading to resolution of steatosis.

Oxidative stress

The metabolism of alcohol and lipids generates ROS (oxygen-containing free radicals known as reactive oxygen species) in hepatocytes [3]. Activated Kupffer cells also secrete ROS [7] and ROS are produced by phagocytic cells via a respiratory burst during phagocytosis. Alcohol-induction of NOX (NAD(P)H oxidase) and iNOS (inducible nitric oxide synthase) in hepatocytes, Kupffer cells, and inflammatory cells also generates increasing amounts of ROS [5]. If ROS are not detoxified by antioxidant systems, oxidative stress ensues, causing damage to cellular molecules (e.g. DNA enzymes, transcription factors, cytokines, and membranes), directly modulating their activities [8]. Oxidative stress gives different responses depending on the level of oxidants and exposure duration and cell type.

Oxidative stress leads to:

- Mitochondrial damage/dysfunction;
- ER stress and subsequent apoptosis;
- Increased lipid synthesis resulting from disruption of signaling pathways involved in the regulation of lipid and glucose metabolism;
- A free radical chain reaction between ROS and unsaturated fatty acids which produces toxic lipid intermediates;
- Lipid peroxidation;

- Formation of Mallory bodies due to protein breakdown;
- Apoptosis and necrosis. Necrotic cells can then induce an inflammatory response;
- Disruption of glutathione synthesis and impairment of homocysteine conversion to methionine disabling the redox balance;
- Activation of ERK1/2 (extracellular signal-regulated kinases 1 and 2), p38, MAPK (mitogen-activated protein kinase), and NF-κB (nuclear factor kappa-light-chain-enhancer of activated B cells) by ROS acting as signaling intermediates stimulating TNF-α production, further oxidative stress and inflammation; and
- Activation of hepatic macrophages (Kupffer cells) adding to the inflammatory cascade.

Oxidant stress is a critical factor in the pathogenesis of ALD. It can be measured indirectly through markers including depletion of antioxidants and levels of protein, lipid, or DNA oxidation which have been shown to correlate with the severity of alcohol-induced liver injury. Chronic alcohol use has been found to deplete glutathione levels, especially in the mitochondria of pericentral (zone 3) hepatocytes [8]. Increased free radical formation arising in alcohol infused *in vivo* models results in lipid peroxidation. Markers of oxidative stress are higher with acute alcohol intake and in patients with alcoholic steatohepatitis. Overexpression of endogenous antioxidant proteins reduced levels of alcohol-induced liver injury in animal models. Treatment with antioxidants or inhibitors of alcohol oxidation inhibits alcohol-induced toxicity.

Lipopolysaccharide and endotoxemia

Chronic alcohol exposure increases gut permeability and facilitates translocation of endotoxin, also known as lipopolysaccharide (LPS), derived from intestinal Gram-negative bacteria into the portal circulation in patients with ALD [8]. This is due to:

- Ethanol-mediated microbial proliferation;
- Mucosal membrane damage by alcohol;
- Acetaldehyde-mediated opening of tight junctions in the gut mucosal epithelium due to protein redistribution and disruption of protein interactions thus impairing adhesion;
- Alteration of regulatory microRNAs which affects junction proteins; and
- Cytoskeletal damage in epithelial cells due to induction of nitric oxide synthase.

Subsequently, a "leaky gut" can lead to endotoxemia when LPS is recognized by the immune system which then mounts a response. Bacterial translocation has been correlated with liver dysfunction and clearance of LPS was shown to decrease in cirrhosis. Circulating endotoxin that reaches the liver is normally detoxified by resident macrophages called Kupffer cells and by hepatocytes where it is recognized by the TLR4 complex expressed on the cell surface via the co-receptors, CD14 or MD-2 (Figure 6.2) [8].

Several cellular mechanisms are capable of removing LPS from circulation without significant inflammatory cell activation preventing systemic reactions to LPS by:

- Molecules that can bind to LPS blocking interactions with TLR4;
- Enzymes degrading the lipid A moiety rendering it less potent;
- Inactivation of the signaling pathway following uptake;
- Cellular adaptations that modify subsequent target cell responses; and
- Neutralization by serum lipoproteins.

However, when LPS levels are high and it is not effectively removed, a coordinated immune response is launched which includes the activation of Kupffer cells. Malondialdehyde–acetaldehyde adducts produced during ethanol metabolism and lipid peroxidation further sensitize macrophages to LPS. Production of proinflammatory cytokines and other chemokines and ROS by activated Kupffer cells is central to the pathogenesis of alcoholic steatohepatitis. Administration of antibiotics abrogated the *in vivo* effects of acute alcohol on Kupffer cells, indicating that circulating endotoxin resulting from a "leaky gut" had a key role in mediating the effects of alcohol. Prolonged alcohol sensitization of Kupffer cells to LPS has been proposed in ALD where an alcohol-induced gut-derived endotoxemia results in proinflammatory cytokine induction. When the liver is damaged, less LPS is removed by liver cells, so circulating levels increase as exemplified by the prevalence of endotoxemia in cirrhotic patients.

TLR4-mediated activation

TLR4 is considered to be a major mediator of Kupffer cell activation in alcoholic liver injury: both CD14- and TLR4-deficient mice are protected from alcoholic liver injury [8]. TLR4 is also upregulated in response to LPS and increased expression is seen in mice with ALD.

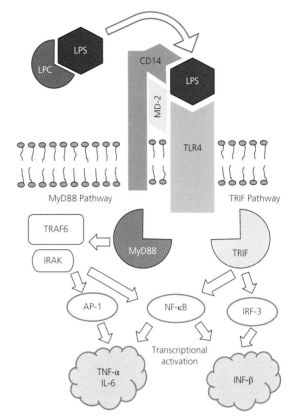

Figure 6.2 Lipopolysaccharide (LPS) induced activation of inflammatory responses via the Toll-like receptor 4 (TLR4). LPS translocated from the gastrointestinal lumen to the portal vein binds to lipopolysaccharide-binding protein (LBP). CD14 expressed on the surface of Kupffer cells recognizes and binds the LPS component and combines with TLR4 and MD-2 on the surface of these cells. This activates an intracellular signaling pathway via the recruitment of either myeloid differentiation factor 88 (MyD88) or MyD88-independently via TIR-domain containing adaptor inducing IFN-β (TRIF). The MyD88 pathway involves the activation of IRAK kinases which activate the transcription factors AP-1 and NF-κB (nuclear factor kappa-light-chain-enhancer of activated B cells). The TRIF pathway results in activation of interferon regulatory factor-3 (IRF-3) and NF-κB. In this way, both pathways can cause upregulation of expression of proinflammatory cytokines, TNF-α, IL-6, and IL-1β, and type 1 interferon.

Ligand binding by TLR4 activates two cellular signaling cascades (Figure 6.2) [6,7]. The MyD88 pathway, in which IRAK (interleukin-1 receptor-associated kinase) and TRAF6 (TNF receptor-associated kinase) are recruited to the receptor by MyD88, leads to the expression of proinflammatory cytokines including TNF-α (tumor necrosis factor α), and apoptosis transcription factor, AP-1, via the activation of NF-κB. The alternative TRIF (TIR-domain containing adaptor inducing IFN-β) pathway activates interferon regulatory factor 3 (IRF-3) which leads to the production of IFN-β and TNF-α. Mice lacking MyD88 are not protected from alcoholic steatosis and inflammation whereas those deficient in IRF-3 were protected for ALD, suggesting the TRIF pathway has the major role in pathogenesis. Studies using chimeric mice also pointed to IRF-3 in parenchymal cells being protective via the upregulation of IFN and IL-10 but detrimental through the upregulation of TNF-α in Kupffer cells.

TLR4 is also expressed by hepatocytes, hepatic stellate cells, and sinusoidal epithelial cells which may also be important in ALD. In hepatocytes, LPS can promote apoptosis [8]. LPS binding to TLR4 on hepatic stellate cells has been found to activate Jnk kinase and NF-κB inflammatory signaling and result in the induction of fibrosis. Monocytes and macrophages of the innate immune system cells also respond to LPS via TLR4 resulting in TNF-α/proinflammatory cytokine production which promotes infiltration of inflammatory cells including neutrophils. In this way LPS contributes to the development of steatohepatitis.

Immunologic mechanisms inducing inflammation

Cells of the innate immune system such as monocytes and macrophages are equipped with a broad range of pattern recognition receptors that sense "danger" signals from pathogens and injury. Acute inflammation is a homeostatic mechanism for protection against dangers by mediating the processes that remove damaged cells and tissue repair. However chronic inflammation, often involving adaptive immune cells, arises if the danger or damage is not resolved and the persistent presence of cytotoxic immune cells contributes to disease development.

Proinflammatory cytokines are produced by the combined activities of various liver cell types in response to chronic alcohol intake; for example, activated Kupffer cells produce TNF-α, IL-6, and IL-10. Alcoholic steatohepatitis is characterized by the infiltration of inflammatory cells into the liver as a result of cytokine and chemokine activation. Active alcoholic hepatitis often persists for months after cessation of drinking. In fact, its severity may worsen during the first few weeks of abstinence. This observation suggests that an immunologic mechanism may be responsible for perpetuation of the injury.

Several studies have demonstrated extremely high levels of TNF-α and several TNF-inducible cytokines, such as interleukins IL-1β, IL-6, and IL-8, in the sera of patients with alcoholic hepatitis. Human macrophages exposed to alcohol not only produce a proinflammatory response, but also become sensitized to LPS-induced proinflammatory signals. Inflammatory cytokines (TNF-α, IL-1β, IL-8), NF-κB activation, and hepatic acute-phase cytokines (IL-6) have been postulated to have a significant role in modulating certain metabolic complications in alcoholic hepatitis, and are probably instrumental in the liver injury of alcoholic hepatitis and cirrhosis.

The discovery that mice deficient in complement C3 were protected from alcoholic liver injury indicates that complement also has a role in disease possibly by promoting inflammation and by modulating transcription of lipogenic genes.

Serum immunoglobulins levels, especially IgA, are increased in patients with alcoholic hepatitis. Antibodies directed against acetaldehyde-modified cytoskeletal proteins can be detected in some individuals. Patients have decreased peripheral lymphocyte counts with an associated increase in the ratio of helper cells to suppressor cells, signifying that lymphocytes are involved in a cell-mediated inflammatory response [4]. This causes necroinflammation and leads to hepatocyte ballooning and apoptosis. Alcohol also functionally suppresses cells of the innate immune system and decreases clearance of bacteria.

TNF-α

Progression from steatosis to steatohepatitis (alcoholic hepatitis) is promoted by increased TNF-α levels (3). TNF-α:

- Activates kinases that block insulin signaling, leading to insulin resistance and metabolic changes;
- Inhibits adiponectin expression and activity exacerbating the accumulation of fatty acids in hepatocytes;
- Alters metabolism leading to increased mitochondrial ROS production;
- Induces IL-8 and other chemokines which cause inflammatory cell infiltration into the liver.
- Causes hepatocyte injury;
- Promotes programmed cellular death (apoptosis); and
- Induces phagocytosis of injured cells by Kupffer cells.

This phagocytic activity in turn activates the Kupffer cells and increases their secretion of inflammatory cytokines amplifying the inflammatory cascade [7].

Despite success in various animal and cell culture disease models, agents that block TNF-α have not proved effective in humans. The reason for this is unclear, but may be related to interspecies differences in injury severity. Anti-TNF antibody, infliximab, showed some efficacy but, in patients with severe alcoholic steatohepatitis, TNF-α antagonism led to systemic TNF-α deficiency, subsequent infections, increased morbidity, and mortality [3]. Inhibition of TNF-α transcription by pentoxifylline has proven beneficial, but it has not been shown to reduce serum TNF-α and may exert its effect by inhibiting other cytokines and phosphodiesterases and by reducing fibrosis [7].

Other proinflammatory factors

NF-κB is a transcriptional regulator that mediates gene expression responses to cellular stress in liver cells, hence regulating the immune response to chronic and acute inflammation. Patients with ALD demonstrated increased plasma IL-17 which can activate NF-κB and stimulates proinflammatory cytokine release by non-parenchymal hepatic cells. When activated, it causes an increase in expression of IL-1, IL-6, and IL-8 as well as TNF-α. IL-8 induces neutrophil infiltration during alcoholic liver injury and perpetuates inflammation leading to alcoholic hepatitis. IL-8 is elevated in alcoholic steatohepatitis, but only minimally in alcoholics without significant liver disease, and in alcoholic cirrhotics. Expression of IL-8 and chemokine Gro-α (growth regulated α protein) which attract polymorphonuclear leukocyte inflammatory cells, was found to correlate with measures of disease severity in alcoholic steatohepatitis. Levels of the proinflammatory cytokine precursor, pro-IL-1, are also increased in ALD patients. Inflammasome activation is also proposed to contribute to ALD because expression of its mRNA was demonstrated in the liver [7]. LPS (via TLR4) promotes production of the chemokine CCL20 by Kupffer and hepatic stellate cells which then activates monocytes, dendritic cells, and macrophages to produce proinflammatory cytokines.

Monocyte chemotactic peptide-1 (MCP-1 or CCL2), expressed by hepatocytes and stellate cells in response to inflammation, is also thought to have a role in ALD as it recruits monocytes and macrophages to the sites of injury and inflammation. Levels of MCP-1 were reported to be higher in patients with alcoholic steatohepatitis and its deficiency protects alcohol-fed mice against liver injury through the induction of fatty acid oxidation and inhibition of proinflammatory cytokines. Further work suggests it is responsible for the perpetuation of inflammation in liver tissue and the development of steatosis in alcohol-fed mice [5].

Hepatoprotective and anti-inflammatory factors

Ethanol-induced LPS-stimulated Kupffer cells also produce IL-6 and IL-10 which can attenuate liver injury [7]. Hepatoprotective cytokines such as IL-6 act to reduce liver damage in ALD through the activation of STAT3 (signal transducer and activator of transcription 3) and subsequent induction of hepatoprotective genes and promotion of liver regeneration. Alcohol-fed IL-6 knock-out mice were found to have increased fat accumulation in the liver, lipid peroxidation, mitochondrial DNA damage, and hepatocyte sensitization to TNF-α-induced apoptosis indicative of a protective role. IL-6 levels are elevated in alcoholics. Furthermore, IL-6 treatment prevents alcoholic fatty liver in a rodent disease model. However, its side effects mean it is unsuitable as treatment in humans.

The anti-inflammatory cytokine IL-10 is also associated with ALD via the activation of STAT3 in Kupffer cells, which inhibits inflammation. IL-10 downregulates endogenous TNF-α, and IL-1β released by Kupffer cells during endotoxemia. Levels of these proinflammatory cytokines are increased, and LPS-mediated liver injury is higher, after alcohol feeding IL-10 deficient mice. IL-10 therefore appears to have a protective role in ALD. However, recent work has suggested that IL-10 may also inhibit the hepatoprotective cytokine IL-6, promoting steatosis and inhibiting regeneration, thereby potentiating ALD. Therefore, its contribution to ALD may depend on the balance of proinflammatory and hepatoprotective cytokines being expressed.

IL-22 has also been recently identified as a potential therapeutic as it is suggested to protect against acute and chronic alcoholic liver injury. Similar to IL-6 and IL-10, IL-22 also acts via STAT3 activation leading to upregulation of antiapoptotic genes, antioxidative genes, and downregulation of lipogenic genes in hepatocytes.

Adipokines (cytokines produced by adipose tissue) have also been suggested to have a role in ALD. Adiponectin has been found to have an anti-inflammatory action (apparently via increased fatty acid oxidation) that leads to decreases in liver injury. Chronic alcohol feeding of rats resulted in lowered adiponectin levels and administering adiponectin reduces alcoholic liver steatosis.

Differing responses to acute and chronic alcohol intake

Acute intoxication and chronic alcohol intake have been found to elicit differing immunomodulatory cascades and appear to mediate opposite effects on inflammation via distinct molecular pathways [4]. Studies have shown that acute alcohol exposure is associated with LPS-induced anti-inflammatory effects in monocytic cells in humans both *in vitro* and *in vivo*. This is in contrast to chronic alcohol intake which increases expression of inflammatory cytokines including TNF-α, inflicting liver injury. There is also evidence to suggest that alcohol functionally suppresses cells of the immune system and decreases clearance of bacteria.

Although acute exposure, like chronic intake, causes increased gut permeability to LPS, findings from several research groups support the hypothesis that alcohol intoxication inhibits the inflammatory response. This anti-inflammatory effect may be explained by acute alcohol intake causing cytoskeleton reorganization and redistribution of TLR4, in turn impairing receptor clustering and effectively reducing TLR4-mediated downstream signaling. Acute alcohol intake also interferes with signaling in lipid rafts in monocytes and macrophages as TLR4 is displaced, inhibiting LPS-induced inflammatory signaling.

Murine Kupffer cells show decreased responsiveness to LPS following acute alcohol exposure *in vivo*. This is proposed to involve decreased IRAK expression and reduced NF-κB activity. Similarly, short-term alcohol exposure induces an "LPS hyporesponsive" state in human blood monocytes resulting in suppressed TNF-α production. This response may increase susceptibility to infections similar to that described in patients with septic shock.

Alcohol binge in humans induces TLR tolerance in monocytes and macrophages in which the usual induction of intracellular signaling pathways, stimulating production of proinflammatory cytokines in response to LPS, is diminished. TLR tolerance is mediated by upregulation of negative regulators of TLR signaling and is characterized by a molecular signature including upregulation of NF-κB p50 homodimers, Bcl3,

and IRAK-M. In contrast, prolonged alcohol exposure increases the sensitivity of Kupffer cells to stimulation by LPS, potentiating cytokine-mediated inflammation. Thus, at least in part, explaining apparent differences in the acute and chronic effects of alcohol. Besides the mechanistic distinction between effects, it is notable that chronic alcohol exposure renders the liver more susceptible to injury resulting from cellular changes caused by binge/acute intake.

Fibrosis

Fibrosis is defined by the excessive accumulation of fibrous connective tissue (containing collagens, fibronectin, and hyaluronic acid) in and around damaged tissue. Hepatic fibrosis arises as a "healing" response to persistent and recurrent insult to the liver [8]. Fibrosis may progress to cirrhosis characterized by vascular and architectural distortion and aberrant hepatocyte regeneration [9]. Altered architecture by collagen increases hepatic resistance to blood flow. The progressive build-up of collagen and fibronectin in the extracellular matrix can become irreversible and with progressive fibrosis, the liver loses its ability to detoxify the blood as the number of functional hepatocytes is reduced. The result is decompensated phase of cirrhosis.

Myofibroblast cells are responsible for the majority of the observed deposition of extracellular matrix common to all fibrotic diseases. They also express TIMPs (tissue inhibitors of metalloproteinases) which block matrix degradation and MMPs (matrix metalloproteinases) responsible for matrix remodeling. In the liver, most myofibroblasts are thought to be derived from hepatic stellate cells.

The process of hepatic fibrosis is believed to be primarily driven by inflammatory responses to damaged parenchymal cells. Damaged cells release a variety of factors that recruit inflammatory monocytes and neutrophils to the damage site. These cells can cause further tissue damage. Neutrophil dysfunction with high spontaneous oxidative burst and reduced phagocytosis was recently demonstrated in patients with alcoholic hepatitis and cirrhosis. This was associated with a significantly greater risk of infection, organ failure, and mortality.

Kupffer cells activated in ALD are critical determinants of fibrotic scarring or resolution of injury through the secretion of various factors. Experiments have shown macrophage ablation attenuates fibrosis highlighting their central role. TGF-β (transforming growth factor β) produced by Kupffer cells in ALD has also been postulated to induce early fibrosis and inhibition of this pathway gave reduced liver injury. Evidence suggests TGF-β promotes collagen and TIMP expression, and transition of hepatic stellate cells to myofibroblasts. Conversely, Kupffer cells can induce apoptosis of stellate cells during disease regression. These opposing roles have been proposed to indicate a switch in function in response to the changes in their immunologic microenvironment [9]. NK cells (natural killer T cells) have an important defensive role inhibiting fibrosis: they can induce apoptosis of hepatic stellate cells. However, chronic alcohol intake impairs this function and they appear to be depleted in chronic liver injury suggesting their protective role may be limited to early disease stages.

In ALD, ROS are able to induce the transformation of hepatic stellate cells into myofibroblasts, leading to the excessive production of collagen. Reactive aldehydes derived from lipid peroxidation also stimulate collagen production by hepatic stellate cells. Activation of hepatic stellate cells by LPS directly has also been demonstrated. The activation of MMPs by ROS also results in remodeling of the extracellular matrix. Extracellular matrix fragments also stimulate chemokine/cytokine production by the inflammatory cells further driving fibrosis.

Epigenetic effects

Increasing evidence has established that epigenetic processes (leading to changes in protein expression/activity), particularly protein acetylation and phosphorylation, histone modification (altering gene expression), and DNA methylation are induced by ethanol and also by its metabolites and ROS [10]. These effects are thought to have a vital role in mediating the pathophysiologic responses in ALD. For instance, altered DNA methylation has been linked to liver injury and disease outcome had been demonstrated after short-term alcohol intake while hypomethylation of liver DNA is described following chronic intake.

Recent research has revealed a crucial role for microRNAs (miRNAs) in regulating liver inflammation in ALD [10]. miRNAs are short RNAs that are able to reduce expression of target genes via post-transcriptional mechanisms. miRNAs have been shown to be central mediators of LPS signaling in Kupffer cells,

hepatocytes, and hepatic stellate cells. For example, both miR-155 and miR-21 correlate with LPS signaling after alcohol intake. Induction of miR-155 was also reported in macrophages following acute alcohol exposure and is thought to be directly involved in LPS-induced TNF-α production along with miR-21. Additionally, the increased sensitivity of Kupffer cells from alcohol-fed mice to TLR4/LPS-induced signaling (leading to overproduction of TNF-α), has recently been suggested to be caused by upregulation of miR-155, resulting in increased inflammation [4]. Several studies report dysregulation of both miR-34a and the abundant, liver-specific miR-122 by ethanol. Overexpression of miR-34a induced apoptosis in cultured cells [10]. Roles in regulating lipid metabolism, intestinal permeability, and the cell cycle have been proposed for miR-122 providing molecular mechanisms for pathogenesis.

Other contributing factors

The mechanism of ALD may be further complicated by hepatotoxic comorbid conditions such as obesity which acts synergistically with alcohol to accentuate liver injury. Hepatic iron content is predictive of prognosis in alcoholic steatohepatitis and patients with ALD have elevated hepatic iron uptake, although many alcoholics do have iron overload. However, it is not known how iron may participate in liver injury. Alcohol appears to accelerate the progression of chronic hepatitis C to cirrhosis and also elevates the risk of hepatocellular carcinoma. These effects may be mediated by the immunologic and proinflammatory consequences of alcohol [2].

Conclusions

Excessive alcohol consumption leads to the development of ALD via numerous mechanisms which lead to various pathologic histologies as summarized in Figure 6.3. There is also interplay between these processes which modulates the pathologic development.

Further work is underway to determine the pathway components and investigate the interactions to provide insights into disease mechanisms. A more detailed understanding is important to identify potential therapeutic targets and develop new treatment strategies with minimal detrimental impact.

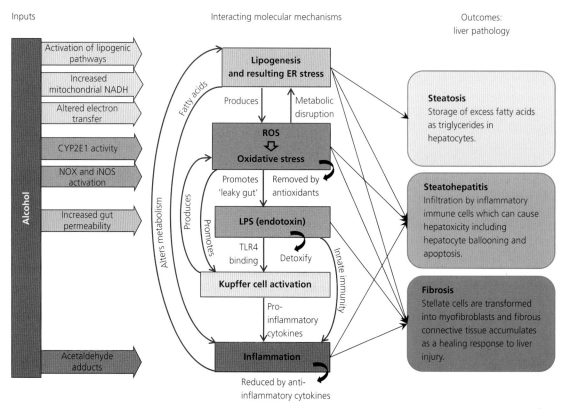

Figure 6.3 Overview of the key interacting pathologic mechanisms contributing to alcoholic liver disease.

References

[1] Setshedi M, Wands JR, Monte SM. Acetaldehyde adducts in alcoholic liver disease. *Oxid Med Cell Longev* 2010; **3**(3): 178–185.

[2] Gramenzi A, Caputo F, Biselli M, et al. Review article: alcoholic liver disease – pathophysiological aspects and risk factors. *Aliment Pharmacol Ther* 2006; **24**(8): 1151–1161.

[3] Syn WK, Teaberry V, Choi SS, Diehl AM. Similarities and differences in the pathogenesis of alcoholic and nonalcoholic steatohepatitis. *Semin Liver Dis* 2009; **29**(2): 200–210.

[4] Shukla SD, Pruett SB, Szabo G, Arteel GE. Binge ethanol and liver: new molecular developments. *Alcohol Clin Exp Res* 2013; **37**(4): 550–557.

[5] Zhu H, Jia Z, Misra H, Li YR. Oxidative stress and redox signaling mechanisms of alcoholic liver disease: updated experimental and clinical evidence. *J Dig Disease* 2012; **13**(3): 133–142.

[6] Jampana SC, Khan R. Pathogenesis of alcoholic hepatitis: role of inflammatory signaling and oxidative stress. *World J Hepatol* 2011; **3**(5): 114–117.

[7] Kawaratani H, Tsujimoto T, Douhara A, et al. The effect of inflammatory cytokines in alcoholic liver disease. *Mediators Inflamm* 2013; **2013**: 495156.

[8] Szabo G, Bala S. Alcoholic liver disease and the gut–liver axis. *World J Gastroenterol* 2010; **16**(11): 1321–1329.

[9] Xu R, Zhang Z, Wang FS. Liver fibrosis: mechanisms of immune-mediated liver injury. *Cell Mol Immunol* 2012; **9**(4): 296–301.

[10] Shukla SD, Lim RW. Epigenetic effects of ethanol on the liver and gastrointestinal system. *Alcohol Res* 2013; **35**(1): 47–55.

CHAPTER 7

Extrahepatic manifestations of alcohol excess

Karl-Heinz Schulz,[1] Sandra van Eckert,[1] and Jens Reimer[2]

[1] *Institute of Medical Psychology and Center for Transplantation Medicine, University Medical Center Hamburg-Eppendorf (UKE), Hamburg, Germany*
[2] *Department of Psychiatry and Psychotherapy, Center for Interdisciplinary Addiction Research, University Medical Center Hamburg-Eppendorf (UKE), Hamburg, Germany*

Alcohol consumption is, depending on the volume and consumption pattern, causally related or linked as a risk factor to a wide variety of diseases. Twenty-five chronic disease and condition codes of the International Classification of Disease 10 (ICD-10) represent diseases for which alcohol is a necessary cause. Accordingly, many of these categories directly carry the term "alcohol" in their name. These diseases and conditions are entirely brought about by alcohol consumption. Furthermore, alcohol is a risk factor in more than 200 other diseases and conditions such as tumors, neuropsychiatric conditions, and cardiovascular and digestive diseases, with a wide dose–response relationship. Therefore, alcohol consumption considerably contributes to the burden of chronic diseases and conditions globally [1]. According to the World Health Organization (WHO), daily consumption of more than 40 g alcohol for men and more than 20 g alcohol for women is associated with an increased risk [2].

In this chapter, extrahepatic manifestations of excess alcohol use are described; therefore hepatic effects are excluded. First, we review effects of alcohol on overarching organ systems such as the central and peripheral nervous systems, the endocrine and the immune systems. We also review the effect of alcohol on carcinogenesis and lipid metabolism. The evidence for the impact of alcohol on different organs including the cardiovascular system, the lungs, the kidney, the gastrointestinal organs, the pancreas, and the skin is summarized. An overview of the impact of alcohol consumption in pregnancy on prenatal development and the fetal alcohol syndrome completes this overview (Figure 7.1).

Overarching systemic effects

Central and peripheral nervous system[1]
Intoxication
Intoxication refers to acute effects of alcohol on the central nervous system (CNS). As alcohol tolerance in humans varies, the following information should be regarded as an approximation. Blood alcohol levels up to 2 parts per thousand result in disinhibition, combativeness, and an enhanced need of conversation. While self-esteem and reaction time increase, perception of pain decreases, and vestibular complaints develop. Alcohol intoxication occurs at a blood alcohol level of 2–3 parts per thousand. The main symptoms comprise speech disturbances, visual impairment, and coordination problems. Nausea, vomiting, amnesia as well as disturbed consciousness and somnolence may also occur. A blood alcohol level of 2.5–5 parts per thousand is regarded as severe alcohol intoxication, which may lead to coma or death.

Effects of long-term alcohol use on the brain
Excessive alcohol consumption leads to extensive brain atrophy (reduction of brain volume and enlargement of the ventricles and sulci). The most susceptible brain structures are the frontal lobes, the limbic system, particularly the hippocampus, and the cerebellum. It is

---

[1] Due to the frequent admission of alcohol intoxicated patients, basic treatment principles for alcohol withdrawal and its complications will be stated.

Alcohol Abuse and Liver Disease, First Edition. Edited by James Neuberger and Andrea DiMartini.
© 2015 John Wiley & Sons, Ltd. Published 2015 by John Wiley & Sons, Ltd.

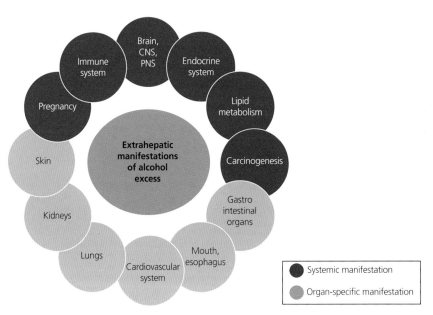

Figure 7.1 An overview of extrahepatic manifestations of alcohol excess. CNS, central nervous system; PNS, peripheral nervous system.

estimated that chronic alcohol consumption induces about 20% loss of neuronal density. Consequently, chronic excessive alcohol consumption is associated with reductions in cognitive functions, such as loss of executive functions, episodic memory, and visuospatial capacities [3]. Furthermore, the development of an addiction involves neuroplastic changes in several brain regions [4].

The brain as a self-regulating organ works to maintain homeostasis even in the face of chronic exposure to alcohol. The sedative effects of alcohol are mediated by gamma-aminobutyric acid type A (GABA-A) receptors, which are downregulated under chronic alcohol influence, whereas N-methyl-D-aspartate (NMDA) receptors are upregulated, as chronic alcohol intake disturbs NMDA receptor functioning. Substance craving seems to be related to several neurotransmitters and hormones, including NMDA, dopamine, GABA, corticotropin-releasing factor (CRF), and norepinephrine, all of which are altered by long-term excessive alcohol use [5].

Epileptic seizure and alcoholic epilepsy
Seizures, often in a tonic–clonic manner, appear within 6–48 hours after alcohol cessation. Although status epilepticus is not common, an epileptic status should be considered in patients with prolonged reduced consciousness during alcohol withdrawal. On the pathophysiologic level, hyperexcitability can be explained by increased NMDA activity, a reduced inhibition through GABA subunits, and increased homocysteine and prolactin. The differential diagnoses include:
- Hypoglycemia;
- Electrolyte disturbances; or
- Meningitis.

Benzodiazepines are the mainstay of treatment using regimens, such as lorazepam 2 mg intravenously [6]. Because the time to reach therapeutic levels exceeds the high-risk period, other antiepileptic drugs are of little benefit in the acute situation [7]. However, antiepileptic drugs may be of benefit if seizures during alcohol withdrawal have occurred despite adequate withdrawal treatment. Long-term antiepileptic drugs are unnecessary in abstinent patients as withdrawal seizures do not recur in abstinent patients [8]. In case of coincidence of alcohol withdrawal and epilepsy, the risk of a future seizure is increased.

Withdrawal symptoms
In subjects physiologically dependent on alcohol, withdrawal symptoms occur on termination or reduction of alcohol consumption. Withdrawal symptoms unmask the compensatory changes induced by chronic exposure

to alcohol, which include downregulation of GABA type A and upregulation of NMDA receptors [9]. If a physiologically dependent subject stops or substantially reduces alcohol intake, the inhibitory effects of alcohol are lost, whereas the adaptive changes persist resulting in overstimulation generating withdrawal symptoms. Common or minor symptoms within the first 72 hours include: apprehension, anxiety, restlessness, tachycardia, insomnia, weakness, irritability, sweating, and gastrointestinal upset. Intermediate symptoms occur between 24 hours to 72 hours, and comprise the above minor symptoms plus:

- Hypertension;
- Illusions;
- Confusion;
- Agitation;
- Disorientation; and
- Fear.

In severe cases, delirium tremens may develop (see Delirium tremens). Benzodiazepines remain the mainstay in prevention of severe withdrawal, seizures, and delirium tremens. Chlordiazepoxide 30 mg three times daily, lorazepam 2 mg three times daily, or oxazepam 15 mg four times daily tapered to zero within 6–7 days can be a useful approach. Medication dosage can vary depending on the severity of withdrawal. Symptom-triggered treatment may reduce the quantity of medication used and the length of withdrawal. Vitamin B substitution helps to prevent Wernicke's encephalopathy [10–12].

Hallucinosis

Alcohol hallucinosis is a psychotic dysfunction comprising (mainly acoustic) hallucinations, anxiety, and delusions, while consciousness and orientation remain intact. The affect is fearful, stressed, and uneasy; some patients show a tendency to violent actions. The progress of hallucinosis is acute and may persist for weeks to months. Recent findings indicate a high risk of rehospitalization and relapse. Treatment includes neuroleptics (haloperidol 5–10 mg/day) and anxiolytic benzodiapines. There seems to be a low risk of a schizophrenia-like course of the illness compared to other drug-induced disorders [13].

Delirium tremens

Delirium tremens is the major representation of alcohol withdrawal and usually appears within 24–72 hours after initiation of withdrawal. As well as the minor and intermediate symptoms described above, the following may occur:

- Hallucinations (often of scenic character or including insects or small animals; in severe cases also with tactile, acoustic, or olfactory character);
- Delusions;
- Seizures;
- Fluctuating levels of disturbed consciousness;
- Cardiac arrhythmias; and
- Circulatory collapse.

Risk factors for the development of delirium tremens comprise:

- Long time lapse since the last consumption of alcohol;
- The presence of medical comorbidity;
- Tachypnea;
- Hypotension;
- Hyperuricemia and
- Hypoalbuminemia.

Again, benzodiazepines are the mainstay of pharmacologic treatment. Diazepam may be chosen because of its more rapid onset, but lorazepam has a shorter half-life and can avoid prolonged sedation, especially in the elderly. Neuroleptic agents may be used as an adjunct if benzodiazepines fail to reduce agitation, thought disorder, or perceptual disturbances. Haloperidol 1–5 mg twice daily may also be a good choice. Older studies describe mortality rates of up to 20% in patients with delirium tremens, though with adequate recognition and treatment the mortality should be as low as 1% [8,11,12].

Wernicke's encephalopathy

Wernicke's encephalopathy (WE) is an acute neuropsychiatric disorder caused by thiamine deficiency leading, amongst other areas of the brain, to damage of the corpora mamillaria, the periaqueductal region, and the tectum. Clinically, WE is characterized by an abrupt onset of confusion, ataxia, and ophthalmoplegia. However, these symptoms may vary.

Mental symptoms can include various confusional states (disorientation, drowsiness, apathy, indifference, incoherence of speech), disorder of memory (mild memory impairment to amnesia), anxiety, fear, coma, and stupor.

Ophthalmoplegia may only represent one of several eye symptoms including nystagmus, lateral rectus palsy, conjugate gaze palsies, papillary abnormalities, retinal hemorrhages, ptosis, scotoma, complete ophthalmoplegia, diplopia, blurred vision, and photophobia.

Ataxia can refer to unsteadiness of gait, dysdiadocho-kinesis, impaired heel–shin testing, past-pointing, and dysarthria.

WE is likely to be underdiagnosed as not all symptoms may be present and, in some cases, none of the classic signs may occur. Substitution of thiamine, preferably intravenously, in doses of 200–500 mg/day until symptoms resolve, is the treatment of choice. For prevention of WE, thiamine may be substituted at doses of 100 mg/day orally in severe alcohol-dependent patients even in the absence of WE symptoms [14,15].

Amnestic syndrome and Korsakoff's syndrome

Korsakoff's syndrome (KS) is a chronic consequence of thiamine deficiency with marked impairment in memory formation. Cardinal KS symptoms comprise permanent anterograde and retrograde amnesia with a focus on episodic memory deficits. The episodic memory is regarded as a long-term memory subcomponent, which gathers features related to specific events, situations, and experiences, and involves encoding, storage, and retrieval in its spatiotemporal context. Additionally, the autonoetic consciousness is impaired (i.e. the ability to travel in one's own memory) and the autobiographic memory and implicit learning are disturbed. Moreover confabulations, namely unintentional and incongruous verbal productions, have been described. Often the patients are not aware of these deficiencies and may be disoriented. Besides KS, patients tend to show characteristics of alcohol-related neurologic illnesses, e.g. oculomotoric disorders, ataxia, or peripheral neuropathy. Thiamine substitution is recommended in patients with WE to prevent KS. Most patients with KS develop long-term impairment some show spontaneous remission [14–16].

Alcoholic polyneuropathy

Alcoholic polyneuropathy progresses slowly showing distal and symmetric sensomotoric symptoms. Superficial sensation is primarily impaired and painful symptoms are the major complaint. Small fiber predominant axonal loss is the characteristic pathologic feature. Alcoholic neuropathy is probably caused by nutritional deficiencies as well as direct neurotoxic effects of ethanol or its metabolites. Treatment comprises a balanced diet and supplementation of all B vitamins. Mild to moderate alcoholic polyneuropathy is associated with a good prognosis within 3–5 years. Painful dysesthesia

can be treated symptomatically using pregabalin, oxcarbazepine, or antidepressants [14,17–19].

Alcoholic myopathy

Chronic alcoholic myopathy occurs in 40–60% of subjects with chronic alcoholism. Ethanol and acetaldehyde are regarded as direct muscle-toxic agents that may inhibit synthesis of contractile and noncontractile muscle proteins. Neurologic examination shows a mild to moderate paresis and atrophy with good reflex. Serum creatine kinase is not elevated. Often, symptoms of alcoholic myopathy are either masked by symptoms of alcoholic polyneuropathy or interpreted as general weakness or malnutrition by patient or physician. With alcohol abstinence, alcoholic myopathy has a good prognosis within 6–12 months [14,20].

Cerebellar degeneration

Excessive alcohol consumption can lead to cerebellar neuronal loss; approximately one-third of all alcohol addicts show signs of a cerebellar dysfunction, more often seen in men. The pathophysiology remains unclear; primary toxic effects of the alcohol, thiamine deficiency, or electrolyte imbalances have all been implicated. Symptoms comprise progressive ataxia of lower limbs (which usually is absent in WE), gait ataxia, and dysarthria. Cerebellar degeneration is often combined with alcoholic polyneuropathy. Ataxia usually improves with alcohol abstinence and a balanced diet. Supplementation of thiamine is recommended [14,19].

Mental disorders

Within the Diagnostic and Statistical Manual of Mental Disorders 5 (DSM-5), alcohol use disorder (AUD) is characterized on the basis of 11 criteria (summarized in NIH publication no 1-7999, November 2013) [21]. The presence of any two of these indicates an AUD. Diagnostic criteria include the domains of physiologic dependence, cravings, and loss of control, and social and behavioral problems related to alcohol use. The severity is defined as mild (2–3 symptoms), moderate (4–5 symptoms), or severe (6 or more symptoms) (for more on diagnosis see Chapter 3).

Subjects with AUD often have additional substance use and further mental disorders. Tobacco smoking in alcohol-dependent persons is increased by a factor of 2–4 compared with the general population, resulting in prevalence rates of 50–80% [22]. In a large US study, the odds ratio for use of any further psychotropic drugs (e.g. sedatives, opioids, amphetamines, cannabis, cocaine) in subjects with AUD was around 7.5 [23]. Nonsubstance use mental comorbidity in alcohol-dependent subjects is prevalent in about 80%, with depression (prevalence 30–60%) and anxiety disorders (prevalence around 20%) found most frequently [24,25].

Endocrine organs

Acute as well as chronic alcohol consumption induces a multitude of dysfunctions in endocrine organs. Nearly every metabolic system is affected by systemic consequences of alcohol use. Effects of chronic use depend on quantity and duration. Alcohol may influence hormone synthesis, storage and release, hormone transport and regulation, and is associated with alteration of blood sugar levels. It may also exacerbate or cause diabetes, impair reproductive function, and interfere with calcium metabolism. Whereas moderate use seems to have some protective effects, e.g. on bone metabolism and on diabetic long-term complications, chronic overconsumption causes dysfunction of:

- the hypothalamic–hypophyseal system (HPA axis);
- the thyroid gland;
- calcium metabolism;
- adrenal function;
- sexual function, hypogonadism, and infertility; and
- carbohydrate metabolism, and late complications in patients with diabetes.

Hypothalamic–pituitary–adrenocortical axis

Chronic alcohol exposure and withdrawal can profoundly disturb the function of the body's neuroendocrine stress response system: the hypothalamic–pituitary–adrenocortical (HPA) axis. During different stages of alcohol misuse and dependence, the HPA axis shows different profiles with different potential consequences for the individual. In high-risk social drinkers there is an enhanced cortisol response to mental stress, amplifying neural reward circuits and increasing positive subjective effects. In the alcohol dependent, an elevated cortisol production but a blunted cortisol response to stress can be found. This can lead to a dysregulation in the reward circuit, to tolerance of rewarding effects, and even cognitive constraints, as cortisol excess has a toxic effect on hippocampal neurons. In acute alcohol withdrawal, cortisol production is markedly elevated with an overactive amygdala, accompanied by anxiety and a higher

motivation to resume drinking. In an abstinent drinker, a low cortisol production and a blunted response to stress induces dysphoria, craving, and further cognitive impairment resulting in a heightened relapse risk. With prolonged abstinence, HPA dynamics usually recover accompanied by a reduction in anxiety and craving [26]. Heavy use of alcohol not only leads to glucocorticoid-mediated dysregulation within the HPA axis, but also changes upstream neural circuits in the prefrontal cortex [27].

Insulin and glucagon

Chronic heavy drinking is associated with hyperglycemia and reduces the responsiveness to insulin thereby causing glucose intolerance. Of patients with alcoholic liver disease, 45–70% are glucose intolerant or are diabetic. Acute as well as chronic alcohol consumption can alter the effectiveness of hypoglycemic medications [28]. The relationship between alcohol use and the risk of diabetes is U-shaped. Nonconsumers and heavy drinkers are at higher risk whereas moderate consumers have a reduced risk according to a meta-analysis [29]. Heavy alcohol consumption promotes the development of obesity, impairs liver function, and leads to pancreatitis, all of which have important roles in the development of type 2 diabetes.

Because chronic overconsumption of alcohol is associated with insufficient dietary intake of glucose it often results in severe hypoglycemia. Acute alcohol consumption furthermore enhances insulin secretion and thereby can also lead to temporary hypoglycemia.

Androgens and estrogens

Reduced testosterone levels in men overconsuming alcohol are brought about by toxic effects to the testes. Testosterone deficiency leads to a "femininization" of male sexual characteristics, for example breast enlargement [30]. In addition, alcohol affects the release of hormones from the hypothalamus and pituitary. These changes can contribute to the impairment of male sexual and reproductive functions. Alcohol also interferes with normal sperm structure and movement by inhibiting the metabolism of vitamin A, which is essential for sperm development [31].

In premenopausal women, chronic heavy drinking can lead to several reproductive disorders, such as cessation of menstruation, irregular menstrual cycles, menstrual cycles without ovulation, early menopause, and increased risk of spontaneous abortions [32].

Calcium and bone metabolism

Chronic heavy drinking can influence vitamin D metabolism, which can lead to an inadequate absorption of dietary calcium. Furthermore, alcohol is directly toxic to bone-forming cells and inhibits their activity. Additionally, chronic heavy drinking can affect bone metabolism by contributing to nutritional deficiencies. All of these factors increase the risk of osteoporosis, which is especially precarious as many falls are related to alcohol use [33].

Growth hormone

Ethanol reduces blood concentrations of growth hormone and furthermore increases cortisol levels, which can lead to muscle atrophy [34].

Immune system

The multiple processes of immunologic response can be seriously disturbed by the modulating effects of alcohol on different components of the immune system [35]. Alcohol-abusing patients are frequently neutropenic and leukopenic; this is mediated by the alcohol-induced suppression of the bone marrow. Chronic alcohol consumption is associated with an increased incidence of bacterial pneumonias. It impairs phagocytosis, superoxide production, and tumor necrosis factor α (TNF-α) production in response to a bacterial challenge in alveolar macrophages. Alcohol exposure of the host also predisposes to pneumonia caused by viral infections. The increased susceptibility to infections after alcohol consumption is not limited to lung infections. *Listeria*-associated meningitis or sepsis is more severe in alcoholics resulting in higher mortality. There is also evidence for ethanol consumption potentiating viral pancreatitis [36]. Several studies demonstrated an association between alcohol consumption and the risk of human immunodeficiency virus (HIV) infection; the incidence of alcohol abuse among HIV-infected individuals is greater than in the general population.

Alcohol abuse is a well-established risk factor for traumatic injuries of all types. Not only does the risk of sustaining an injury increase with the use of alcohol but the severity of trauma-related immune compromise and recovery from trauma-related hospitalization are all negatively affected by alcohol intoxication. Chronic alcohol use was found to be an independent risk factor in the development of sepsis, septic shock, and sepsis-related mortality in critically ill patients [37]. The immunosuppressive cytokine IL-10 is increased in alcoholic patients after surgical interventions [38].

Although alcohol use is associated with impaired immune responses, chronic alcohol use results in an augmentation of macrophage TNF-α production and inflammatory cascade activation. Inflammatory cytokine overproduction and monocyte–macrophage activation in chronic alcohol use are associated with coronary heart disease. Higher endotoxin concentrations in blood, due to a diminished clearance function of the liver and an increased "spill over" from the intestinal mucosa, have been demonstrated, as well as increased levels of proinflammatory (TNF-α, IL-1, IL-6, IL-8) and regulatory cytokines (IL-10, transforming growth factor β; TGF-β).

Beside the nonspecific inflammatory response, the adaptive immune response is altered by alcohol use (Figure 7.2). Reduced lymphocyte proliferation and lymphocyte counts as well as splenic T-cell activation and an increased percentage of effector and/or memory cells have been demonstrated. Furthermore, the presence of circulating autoantibodies to lymphocytes, brain, DNA, serum lipoproteins, and various liver proteins indicate autoimmune processes [35].

Carcinogenesis

A multitude of prospective and case–control studies show a dose-dependent increased risk for carcinomas of the oral cavity, the pharynx, larynx, and the esophagus [39]. Alcohol increases the mucosal permeability, thereby also amplifying the carcinogenic effects of tobacco products.

Cancers of the female breast [40,41] and the colon [42,43] are more frequently detected in drinkers than nondrinkers. Alcohol consumption of ≥4 drinks/day is associated with a fivefold risk for oral and pharyngeal cancer and esophageal carcinoma, a 2.5-fold risk for laryngeal cancer, a 50% increased risk for colorectal and breast cancers, and a 30% increased risk for pancreatic cancer. These estimations are based on a large number of epidemiologic studies. At lower rates of drinking (i.e. ≤1 drink/day) the risk for oral, pharyngeal and cancer of the esophagus is increased by about 20% and 30%. An increase in the risk for breast cancer is seen at more than 3 drinks/week. When combining alcohol consumption and tobacco use the risk for oral and pharyngeal cancers increases drastically [44].

Other cancers such as lung cancer [45] are only marginally associated with alcohol misuse. In prostate

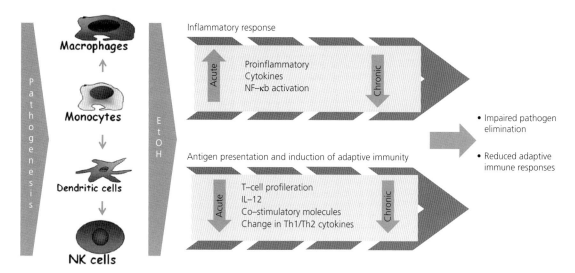

Figure 7.2 Impact of alcohol on innate and adaptive immunity. The response to pathogens of the innate immune system (macrophages, monocytes, dendritic cells, and natural killer cells) is moderated. Acute alcohol exposure inhibits inflammatory responses, while chronic alcohol use augments it. The induction of adaptive immune responses is impaired: both acute and chronic alcohol use inhibits cytokine production and T-cell proliferation. These changes result in impaired pathogen elimination. (Source: Szabo and Mandrekar 2009 [35]. Reproduced with permisison of Research Society on Alcoholism)

cancer there are conflicting findings. While Rohrmann et al. [46] did not find an association between alcohol use and prostate cancer, several systematic reviews [47–49] came to the conclusion that, whereas moderate alcohol consumption does not influence prostate cancer risk, heavy consumption of more than 7 drinks/day may be associated with an excess risk.

The total amount and duration of alcohol consumption are more important than the type of alcoholic beverage consumed. One of the main mechanisms by which alcohol can promote cancerogenesis is mediated by acetaldehyde. Ethanol may also stimulate carcinogenesis by inhibiting DNA methylation and by interacting with retinoid metabolism [50]. Several other mechanisms are summarized in Box 7.1. The effect of alcohol is modulated by polymorphisms in genes encoding enzymes for ethanol metabolism (e.g. alcohol dehydrogenases, aldehyde dehydrogenases, and cytochrome P450 2E1), folate metabolism, and DNA repair (Box 7.1) [51].

Lipid metabolism

Alcohol use leads to alterations in all lipid fractions regarding their concentration in serum or plasma, their structure, and their composition. Increased high-density lipoprotein

Box 7.1 Carcinogenic mechanisms in extrahepatic tumors. (Source: adapted from Boffetta and Hashibe 2006 [51]. Reproduced with permission of Elsevier)

Strong evidence
- DNA damage by acetaldehyde
- Increase in estrogen concentration

Moderate evidence
- Solvent for other carcinogens (e.g. for tobacco carcinogens)
- Production of reactive oxygen and nitrogen species
- Changes in folate metabolism

Weak evidence
- DNA damage by ethanol
- Nutritional deficiencies
- Reduced immune surveillance
- Carcinogenicity of constituents other than ethanol

(HDL) levels represent the best-known consequence of moderate alcohol use. Cardioprotective effects of alcohol can probably be in large part ascribed to this phenomenon.

While alcohol induces an increase in triglyceride-rich lipid molecules, alcohol restriction leads to a decrease in the triglyceride level. Alcohol-induced hypertriglyceridemia is associated with an increase in very low density lipoproteins, chylomicrons, intermediate density lipoproteins, impaired lipolysis, and increased free fatty acid fluxes from adipose tissue to the liver [52]. In extreme cases, massive increases of triglycerides can cause an acute pancreatitis. Furthermore, alcohol and a diet rich in calories represent the main cause of symptomatic hyperuricemia.

Specific organ systems

Cardiovascular system
Hypertension
Increased blood pressure is significantly associated with high ethanol consumption as shown in epidemiologic, preclinical, and clinical studies. Several possible mechanisms have been proposed (Box 7.2 and Figure 7.3) [53,54]. Hypertension usually improves on withdrawal, and treatment is to that of a nonalcoholic patient.

Box 7.2 Basic pathophysiologic mechanisms underlying ethanol-induced hypertension. (Source: adapted from Husain et al. 2014 [53]; Marchi et al. 2014 [54])

Endocrine and neural mechanisms
- Increased cortisol levels
- Stimulation of the renin–angiotensin–aldosterone system
- Increase in activity of the central and sympathetic nervous systems

Myogenic mechanism
- Stimulation of the endothelium to release vasoconstrictors
- An increase of intracellular Ca^{2+} in vascular smooth muscle and enhanced vascular reactivity to vasoconstrictor agents
- Impairment of the vascular relaxation

Oxidative stress
- Increase in generation of reactive oxygen species
- Reduction of antioxidant systems
- Loss of relaxation caused by inflammation and oxidative injury of the endothelium leading to inhibition of endothelium-dependent nitric oxide production

Cardiomyopathy
Heavy alcohol consumption is associated with cardiomyopathy and reduced myocardial contractility, cardiac arrhythmias, and hemorrhagic stroke [55–57], whereas light to moderate alcohol consumption is associated with a reduced risk of multiple cardiovascular outcomes [58,59]. This could be due to a reduction in clotting factors (fibrinogen, factor VII, von Willebrand factor) in chronic alcohol users and a reduced thrombocyte function. However, a hypofibrinolytic state caused by elevated plasminogen activator inhibitor (PAI-1) levels can also be seen. Cardiomyopathy usually refers to a dilated cardiomyopathy and presents with symptoms and signs of heart failure; the diagnosis is made by chocardiography. Treatment consists of absolute alcohol abstinence and symptomatic control.

Oral cavity and esophagus
In the oral cavity alcohol abuse causes mucosal changes, periodontitis as well as early and distinct caries. Bacteria accumulate on the dental enamel and create a sticky, acid plaque. Within this plaque, bacteria transform food residue into acids that attack and ultimately destroy the dental hard tissues. Micronutrient deficiencies and malnutrition can intensify the destructive effect of plaque. Heavy alcohol consumers lose their teeth on average two to three times more frequently than people who rarely consume alcohol.

Alcohol abuse also has an adverse effect on the esophagus, causing a reduced pressure in the lower esophageal section which, in turn, results in a reflux of acid gastric juices and heartburn. There is a higher risk of developing reflux esophagitis which could trigger considerable pain, cause frequent nausea, and ultimately damage the esophagus.

Gastrointestinal tract
Overconsumption of alcohol leads to an increased production of hydrochloric acid and digestive enzymes, can damage the stomach, and leads to chronic gastritis or enteritis. This, in turn, results in an impaired digestion with a diminished ability to absorb nutrients.

Alcohol and its by-products attack the intestinal wall. As a result, digestion becomes sluggish and intestinal contents remains longer inside the body. Chronic alcohol abuse also frequently leads to diarrhea, malnutrition, weight loss, and a reduction in the surface of the small intestines (atrophy). The main reason for the

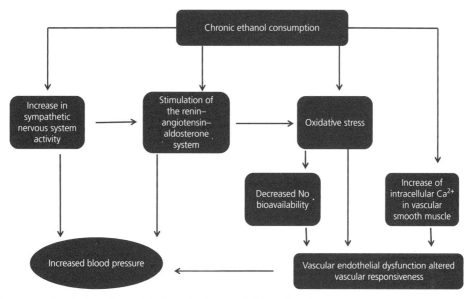

Figure 7.3 Summary of the basic pathophysiologic mechanisms underlying ethanol-induced hypertension. (Source: adapted from Marchi et al. 2014 [54])

malnutrition and weight loss is the reduced supply of nutrients. Chronic alcoholics receive some 50% of their daily caloric intake from ethanol, and alcoholic beverages lack the essential nutrients. The diarrhea is the result of the malabsorption of nutrients through the digestive tract, an increased secretion of water and electrolytes, and a bacterial overgrowth in the small intestines.

In addition, the utilization of nutrients can become disrupted, specifically the absorption of monosaccharides, such as glucose, certain amino acids, and water-soluble vitamins, as folic acid, vitamin B1 and B12. Of particular concern is the resulting folic acid deficiency which, in turn, causes further problems in nutrient uptake [60].

Pancreas

There is an exponential dose–response relationship between alcohol consumption and pancreatitis with a threshold of 4 drinks/day (50 g alcohol) leading to pancreatitis [61]. Via toxic metabolites of alcohol and oxidative stress, pancreatic acinar cells are predisposed to autodigestive damage. Trigger factors such as endotoxins initiate pancreatic inflammation and necrosis. Pancreatic stellate cells are activated and secrete excessive amounts of extracellular matrix proteins leading to the development of pancreatic fibrosis (Figure 7.4) [62]. Other causes of pancreatitis must be excluded (such as

stones, other toxins, drugs, and some infections). Treatment is primarily symptomatic and with abstinence.

The lungs

Alcohol enters the airway passages both, by bronchial circulation and direct inhalation. Chronic alcohol consumption results in dysfunctional ciliary clearance which leads to difficulty in clearing inhaled particles such as pollutants, bacteria, and viruses. This results in persistent massive exposure which, in turn, leads to enhanced injury. Furthermore, alcohol exposure weakens the epithelial barrier function and the repair responses to wound healing [63].

The increased susceptibility to lung injury and infections in the context of chronic alcohol use is largely caused by oxidative stress, which leads to tissue injury and barrier dysfunction, phospholipid peroxidation, DNA oxidation, fibronectin production, apoptosis, and dysregulation of cellular zinc transport and immune function [64].

In the otherwise healthy heavy alcohol consumer, there is no clinical evidence of alveolar dysfunction. However, the chronic alcohol consumption does predispose to an enhanced reaction from a "second hit", such as lung injury or sepsis. Alveolar functions that are impaired due to alcohol exposure include impaired surfactant production and barrier dysfunction [65].

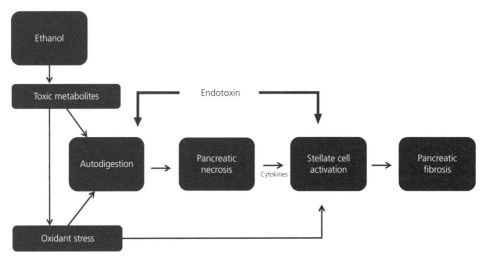

Figure 7.4 Pathogenesis of alcoholic pancreatitis. (Source: Apte et al. 2009 [61]. Reproduced with permission of Journal of Gastroenterology and Hepatology Foundation and Blackwell Publishing Asia Pte Ltd.)

Heavy alcohol consumption is well recognized as a significant risk factor for serious pulmonary infections. The mechanisms by which alcohol abuse increases the risk of pneumonia include an increased risk of aspiration of gastric acid and/or microbes from the upper part of the throat (i.e. oropharyngeal flora), decreased mucous-facilitated clearance of bacterial pathogens from the upper airway, and impaired pulmonary host defenses.

A history of chronic alcohol use is associated with an increased occurrence and severity of the acute respiratory distress syndrome (ARDS) in critically ill patients. Particularly in combination with nicotine, chronic alcohol abuse was determined as a significant comorbid variable, almost tripling the incidence of ARDS [60].

The kidneys
Excessive alcohol consumption can have profoundly negative effects on the kidneys and their function of maintaining the body's fluid, electrolyte, and acid–base balance. Alcohol increases the basal metabolic rate of the renal tubules and also selectively increases renal perfusion thus resulting in an escalated diuresis, causing much more frequent micturition and even leading, at times, to massive dehydration, indirect renal damage, and the formation of renal calculi. Alcoholism is associated with a higher risk of postinfectious glomerulonephritis, acute kidney injury, and kidney graft failure [60]. There is no robust evidence for a direct relation

between chronic alcohol use and chronic renal disease; however, the hypertensive effect of alcohol could indirectly lead to an increased risk of chronic renal diseases.

Alcohol and the skin
The effects of alcohol and its metabolites on the skin may serve as important indication for the diagnosis of chronic alcohol use. Flush, alcoholic facies, palmar erythema, and even spider nevi are well-recognized signs. These acute or chronic vascular alterations are caused by alcohol and its metabolites and seem to be mediated by the central nervous system, as in tetraplegics alcohol does not induce these changes. Less well-recognized effects are the appearance of fat deposits on the trunk, loss of body hair, and other signs (Table 7.1) [66]. In addition to the direct effects of alcohol on the skin, alcohol may also exacerbate dermatoses. Indirect effects of alcohol producing skin symptoms can arise from hepatotoxicity, gastrointestinal disturbances including changes in vitamin metabolism, and damage to the peripheral nervous system. Suppression of the immune system may lead to increased susceptibility to mycotic or bacterial infections.

Alcohol abuse is also frequently linked to changes in social behavior with increased risk taking and unsafe sexual practices (e.g. abandoning protective measures). This leads indirectly to an increase in sexually transmitted infections [67].

Table 7.1 Dermatologic manifestations of alcohol. (Source: adapted from Liu et al. 2010 [66]. Reproduced with permission of Elsevier)

Specific dermatologic manifestations		
Vascular changes	Urticaria	Black hairy tongue
Spider telangiectasia	Nail changes	Glossitis
Palmar erythema	Terry's nails	Leukoplakia
Corkscrew sclera vessels	Red lunulae	Parotid swelling
Caput medusa	Koilonychia	Hyperpigmentation
Plethoric facies	Clubbing	Lichenoid dermatitis
Flushing	Skin cancer	Oral changes
Unilateral nevoid telangiectasia	Jaundice	Pruritus
Exacerbations of skin disease		
Psoriasis	Rosacea	Discoid eczema

Alcohol consumption and pregnancy

Alcohol consumption in pregnancy has serious lifelong consequences for the affected child, and results in a broad spectrum of damages. Alcohol represents the most common and most significant toxic substance in relation to prenatal development. Ethanol and its by-products (especially acetaldehyde) pass the placental barrier with the potential of causing direct organic and functional developmental disorders of the fetus. Alcohol and acetaldehyde are toxins that can have an adverse effect on mitosis with the central nervous system being particularly vulnerable.

The term fetal alcohol spectrum disorders (FASD) is in itself not a clinical diagnosis but rather describes the full range of disabilities that may result from prenatal exposure to alcohol:

- *Fetal alcohol syndrome (FAS):* the child experiences stunted growth and learning difficulties. The child has distinctive facial features and structural abnormalities as a consequence of prenatal exposure to alcohol.
- *Partial FAS:* the child shows some though not all features of FAS.
- *Alcohol-related neurodevelopmental disorders (ARND):* this refers to the child with learning and behavioral difficulties related to alcohol exposure.
- *Alcohol-related birth defects (ARBD):* refers to physical and cognitive deficits (e.g. abnormal organ development, notably of the heart and kidneys), due to the alcohol consumption by the mother during pregnancy. Currently, FAS is the only expression of prenatal alcohol exposure defined by the International Statistical Classification of Diseases and Related Health Problems with assigned ICD-10 diagnoses.

Alcohol crosses the placental barrier and can stunt fetal growth or weight, create distinctive morphologic changes of the face, damage neurons and brain structures resulting in mental retardation and other psychologic or behavioral problems. Consumption of alcohol during pregnancy can cause both minor and major physical abnormalities. The main effect of FAS is a permanent damage of the central nervous system and especially of the brain [68]. Developing brain cells and cell structures can become malformed or have their development interrupted by prenatal alcohol exposure. This, in turn, can create an array of primary cognitive and functional disabilities including poor memory, attention deficits, impulsive behavior, and poor cause–effect reasoning as well as secondary disabilities (e.g. predispositions to mental health problems and drug addiction).

Genetic studies have identified a continuum of long-lasting molecular effects that are both, time- and dosage-specific with even moderate amounts of alcohol being able to cause significant alterations [69]. Organic brain damage caused by the mother's prenatal alcohol consumption is irreversible and cannot be cured by therapeutic measures.

According to the Centers for Disease Control and Prevention (CDC), a diagnosis of FAS requires that all criteria in Table 7.2 must be fully met [68].

Breastfed infants of alcohol-consuming mothers stand a higher risk of developing sleep disorders and of slower mobility development. In addition, alcohol-containing breast milk affects the sucking reflex of the child who drinks much less than usual, thus achieving lower body weight and slower weight gain. Alcohol intake of the mother inhibits the milk ejection reflex causing a temporary decrease in milk yield [70].

Conclusions

Although the liver is considered the major organ affected by excessive alcohol consumption, all organs can be affected. Many of the effects of alcohol and its metabolites are a consequence of direct metabolic

Table 7.2 Criteria of the fetal alcohol syndrome. (Source: Centers for Disease Control and Prevention)

Growth deficiency	Confirmed prenatal or postnatal height or weight, or both, at or below the 10th percentile, documented at any one point in time (adjusted for age, sex, gestational age, and race or ethnicity).
Facial dysmorphia	Based on racial norms, individual exhibits all three characteristic facial features (smooth philtrum, thin vermillion border, small palpebral fissures)
Central nervous system abnormalities	Clinically significant structural, neurologic, or functional impairment
Maternal alcohol exposure	Confirmed or unknown prenatal alcohol exposure

effects, other factors such as dietary deficiency, comorbid conditions and other toxins, such as tobacco and illicit drugs, must be considered. Full assessment of the patient must evaluate not only the impact of alcohol on the liver, but on all body systems.

References

[1] Shield KD, Parry C, Rehm J. Chronic diseases and conditions related to alcohol use. *Alcohol Res* 2013; **35**:155–173.

[2] World Health Organization (WHO). *International guide for monitoring alcohol consumption and related harm.* Department of Mental Health and Substance Dependence, World Health Organization, Geneva; 2000 http://apps.who.int/iris/handle/10665/66529#sthash.zvuAdEaw.dpuf (accessed 4 December 2014).

[3] Bernardin F, Maheut-Bosser A, Paille F. Cognitive impairments in alcohol-dependent subjects. *Front Psychiatry* 2014; **16**(5): 78.

[4] Koob GF, Volkow ND. Neurocircuitry of addiction. *Neuropsychopharmacology* 2010; **35**: 217–238.

[5] Tabakoff B, Hoffman PL. The neurobiology of alcohol consumption and alcoholism: an integrative history. *Pharmacol Biochem Behav* 2013; **113**: 20–37.

[6] D'Onofrio G, Rathley NK, Ulrich AS, Fish SS, Freedland ES. Lorazepam for the prevention of recurrent seizures related to alcohol. *N Engl J Med* 1999; **340**: 915–919.

[7] Minozzi S, Amato L, Vecchi S, Davoli M. Anticonvulsants for alcohol withdrawal. *Cochrane Database Syst Rev* 2010; **3**: CD005064.

[8] Welch KA. Neurological complications of alcohol and misuse of drugs. *Pract Neurol* 2011; **11**: 206–219.

[9] Hughes JR. Alcohol withdrawal seizures. *Epilepsy Behav* 2009; **15**: 92–97.

[10] Kattimani S, Bharadwaj B. Clinical management of alcohol withdrawal: a systematic review. *Ind Psychiatry J* 2013; **22**: 100–108.

[11] Lutz UC, Batra A. Diagnostics and therapy of alcohol withdrawal syndrome: focus on delirium tremens and withdrawal seizure [in German]. *Psychiat Praxis* 2010; **37**: 271–278.

[12] McKeon A, Frye MA, Delanty N. The alcohol withdrawal syndrome. *J Neurol Neurosurg Psychiatry* 2008; **79**: 854–862.

[13] Soyka M. Alcohol-induced psychotic disorders: a diagnostic entity of its own? [in German]. *Nervenarzt* 2014; **85**: 1093–1098.

[14] Gass A, Singer OC. Hirnorganische Erkrankungen und peripheres Nervensystem. In: Singer, Manfred V, Batra A, Mann K, eds. *Alkohol und Tabak: Grundlagen und Folgeerkrankungen.* Thieme, Stuttgart; 2011.

[15] Isenberg-Grzeda E, Kutner HE, Nicolson SE. Wernicke–Korsakoff syndrome: under recognized and under-treated. *Psychosomatics* 2012; **53**: 507–516.

[16] Brion M, Pitel AL, Beaunieux H, Maurage P. Revisiting the continuum hypothesis: toward an in-depth exploration of executive functions in Korsakoff syndrome. *Front Human Neurosci* 2014; **8**: 498.

[17] Chopra K, Tiwari V. Alcoholic neuropathy: possible mechanisms and future treatment possibilities. *Br J Clin Pharmacol* 2011; **73**: 348–362.

[18] Koike H, Sobue G. Alcoholic neuropathy. *Curr Opin Neurol* 2006; **19**: 481–486.

[19] Uhl A, Bachmayer S, Kobrna U, et al. *Handbuch: Alkohol – Österreich: Zahlen, Daten, Fakten, Trends 2009,* 3rd edn. BMGFJ, Wien; 2009.

[20] Wijna JW, Wielders JPM, Lips P, et al. Is vitamin D deficiency a confounder in alcoholic skeletal muscle myopathy? *Alcohol Clin Exp Res* 2013; **37**: E209–E215.

[21] Dawson DA, Goldstein RB, Grant BF. Differences in the profiles of DSM-IV and DSM-5 alcohol use disorders: implications for clinicians. *Alcohol Clin Exp Res* 2013; **37**(Suppl 1):E305–E313.

[22] Romberger DJ, Grant K. Alcohol consumption and smoking status: the role of smoking cessation. *Biomed Pharmacother* 2004; **58**: 77–83.

[23] Stinson FS, Grant BF, Dawson DA, et al. Comorbidity between DSM-IV alcohol and specific drug use disorders in the United States: results from the National Epidemiologic Survey on Alcohol and Related Conditions. *Drug Alcohol Depend* 2005; **80**: 105–116.

[24] Kessler RC, Crum RM, Warner LA, et al. Lifetime co-occurence of DSM-III-R alcohol abuse and dependence with other psychiatric disorders in the National Comorbidity Survey. *Arch Gen Psychiatry* 1997; **54**: 313–321.

[25] Regier DA, Farmer ME, Rae DS, et al. Comorbidity of mental disorders with alcohol and other drug abuse: results from the Epidemiologic Catchment Area (ECA) Study. *JAMA* 1990; **264**: 2511–2518.

[26] Stephens MA, Wand G. Stress and the HPA axis: role of glucocorticoids in alcohol dependence. *Alcohol Res* 2012; **34**: 468–483.

[27] Lu YL, Richardson HN. Alcohol, stress hormones, and the prefrontal cortex: a proposed pathway to the dark side of addiction. *Neuroscience* 2014; **277C**: 139–151.

[28] Bi Y, Wang T, Xu M, et al. Advanced research on risk factors of type 2 diabetes. *Diabetes Metab Res Rev* 2012; **28**(Suppl 2): 32–39.

[29] Koppes LL, Dekker JM, Hendriks HF, Bouter LM, Heine RJ. Moderate alcohol consumption lowers the risk of type 2 diabetes: a meta-analysis of prospective observational studies. *Diabetes Care* 2005; **28**: 719–725.

[30] Emanuele MA, Emanuele N. Alcohol and the male reproductive system. *Alcohol Res Health* 2001; **25**: 282–287.

[31] Muthusami KR, Chinnaswamy P. Effect of chronic alcoholism on male fertility hormones and semen quality. *Fertil Steril* 2005; **84**: 919–924.

[32] Sharma R, Biedenharn KR, Fedor JM, Agarwal A. Lifestyle factors and reproductive health: taking control of your fertility. *Reprod Biol Endocrinol* 2013; **11**: 66.

[33] Berg KM, Kunins HV, Jackson JL, et al. Association between alcohol consumption and both osteoporotic fracture and bone density. *Am J Med* 2008; **121**: 406e18.

[34] Bianco A, Thomas E, Pomara F, et al. Alcohol consumption and hormonal alterations related to muscle hypertrophy: a review. *Nutr Metab* 2014; **11**: 26.

[35] Szabo G, Mandrekar P. A recent perspective on alcohol, immunity, and host defense. *Alcohol Clin Exp Res* 2009; **33**: 220–232.

[36] Jerrells TR, Vidlak D, Strachota JM. Alcoholic pancreatitis: mechanisms of viral infections as cofactors in the development of acute and chronic pancreatitis and fibrosis. *J Leukoc Biol* 2007; **81**: 430–439.

[37] O'Brien JM Jr, Lu B, Ali NA, et al. Alcohol dependence is independently associated with sepsis, septic shock, and hospital mortality among adult intensive care unit patients. *Crit CareMed* 2007; **35**: 345–350.

[38] Sander M, von Heymann C, Neumann T, et al. Increased interleukin-10 and cortisol in long-term alcoholics after cardiopulmonary bypass: a hint to the increased postoperative infection rate? *Alcohol Clin Exp Res* 2005; **29**: 1677–1684.

[39] Baan R, Straif K, Grosse Y, et al; WHO International Agency for Research on Cancer Monograph Working Group. Carcinogenicity of alcoholic beverages. *Lancet Oncol* 2007; **8**: 292–293.

[40] Collaborative Group on Hormonal Factors in Breast Cancer. Alcohol, tobacco and breast cancer: collaborative reanalysis of individual data from 53 epidemiological studies, including 58,515 women with breast cancer and 95,067 women without the disease. *Br J Cancer* 2002; **87**: 1234–1245.

[41] Seitz HK, Pelucchi C, Bagnardi V, La Vecchia C. Epidemiology and pathophysiology of alcohol and breast cancer: update 2012. *Alcohol Alcohol* 2012; **47**: 204–212.

[42] Cho E, Smith-Warner SA, Ritz J, et al. Alcohol intake and colorectal cancer: a pooled analysis of 8 cohort studies. *Ann Intern Med* 2004; **140**: 603–613.

[43] Oyesanmi O, Snyder D, Sullivan N, et al. Alcohol consumption and cancer risk: understanding possible causal mechanisms for breast and colorectal cancers. *Evid Rep Technol Assess* 2010; **197**: 1–151.

[44] Pelucchi C, Tramacere I, Boffetta P, Negri E, La Vecchia C. Alcohol consumption and cancer risk. *Nutr Cancer* 2011; **63**: 983–990.

[45] Freudenheim JL, Ritz J, Smith-Warner SA, et al. Alcohol consumption and risk of lung cancer: a pooled analysis of cohort studies. *Am J Clin Nutr* 2005; **82**: 657–667.

[46] Rohrmann S, Linseisen J, Key TJ, et al. Alcohol consumption and the risk for prostate cancer in the European Prospective Investigation into Cancer and Nutrition. *Cancer Epidemiol Biomarkers Prev* 2008; **17**: 1282–1287.

[47] Dennis LK, Hayes RB. Alcohol and prostate cancer. *Epidemiol Rev* 2001; **23**: 110–114.

[48] Middleton Fillmore K, Chikritzhs T, Stockwell T, Bostrom A, Pascal R. Alcohol use and prostate cancer: a meta-analysis. *Mol Nutr Food Res* 2009; **53**: 240–255.

[49] Rizos Ch, Papassava M, Golias Ch, Charalabopoulos K. Alcohol consumption and prostate cancer: a mini review. *Exp Oncol* 2010; **32**: 66–70.

[50] Seitz HK, Stickel F. Molecular mechanisms of alcohol-mediated carcinogenesis. *Nat Rev Cancer* 2007; **7**: 599–612.

[51] Boffetta P, Hashibe M. Alcohol and cancer. *Lancet Oncol* 2006; **7**: 149–156.

[52] Klop B, do Rego AT, Cabezas MC. Alcohol and plasma triglycerides. *Curr Opin Lipidol* 2013; **24**: 321–326.

[53] Husain K, Ansari RA, Ferder L. Alcohol-induced hypertension: mechanism and prevention. *World J Cardiol* 2014; **26**: 245–252.

[54] Marchi KC, Muniz JJ, Tirapelli CR. Hypertension and chronic ethanol consumption: what do we know after a century of study? *World J Cardiol* 2014; **6**: 283–294.

[55] Movva R, Figueredo VM. Alcohol and the heart: to abstain or not to abstain? *Int J Cardiol* 2013; **164**: 267–276.

[56] Higashiyama A, Okamura T, Watanabe M, et al. Alcohol consumption and cardiovascular disease incidence in men with and without hypertension: the Suita study. *Hypertens Res* 2014; **36**: 58–64.

[57] Patra J, Taylor B, Irving H, et al. Alcohol consumption and the risk of morbidity and mortality for different stroke types: a systematic review and meta-analysis. *BMC Public Health* 2010; **10**: 258.

[58] Ronksley PE, Brien SE, Turner BJ, Mukamal KJ, Ghali WA. Association of alcohol consumption with selected cardiovascular disease outcomes: a systematic review and meta-analysis. *BMJ* 2011; **22**; 342:d671.

[59] Bergmann MM, Rehm J, Klipstein-Grobusch K, et al. The association of pattern of lifetime alcohol use and cause of death in the European Prospective Investigation into Cancer and Nutrition (EPIC) study. *Int J Epidemiol* 2013; **42**: 1772–1790.

[60] Singer MV, Batra A, Mann K, eds. *Alkohol und Tabak. Grundlagen und Folgeerkrankungen*. Georg Thieme Verlag, Stuttgart; 2011.

[61] Apte M, Pirola R, Wilson J. New insights into alcoholic pancreatitis and pancreatic cancer. *J Gastroenterol Hepatol* 2009; **24**(Suppl 3): S51–S56.

[62] Irving HM, Samokhvalov AV, Rehm J. Alcohol as a risk factor for pancreatitis: a systematic review and meta-analysis. *JOP* 2009; **10**: 387–392.

[63] Wyatt TA, Sisson JH. Alcohol, the upper airway, and mucociliary dysfunction in the conducting airways. In: Guidot DM, Mehta AJ, eds. *Alcohol Use Disorders and the Lung: A Clinical and Pathophysiological Approach*. Springer, New York; 2014, 49–62.

[64] Yeligar SM, Liang Y, Brown LAS. Alcohol-mediated oxidative stress in the airway: the unique role of thiol depletion. In: Guidot DM, Mehta AJ, eds. *Alcohol Use Disorders and the Lung: A Clinical and Pathophysiological Approach*. Springer, New York; 2014, 103–114.

[65] Molina SA, Koval M. Alcohol and the alveolar epithelium. In: Guidot DM, Mehta AJ, eds. *Alcohol Use Disorders and the Lung: A Clinical and Pathophysiological Approach*. Springer, New York; 2014, 83–101.

[66] Liu S, Lien M, Fenske N. The effects of alcohol and drug abuse on the skin. *Clin Dermatol* 2010; **28**: 391–399.

[67] Rehm, J. The risks associated with alcohol use and alcoholism. *Alcohol Res Health* 2011; **34**: 135–143.

[68] USA National Task Force on FAS/FAE. *Fetal Alcohol Syndrome: Guidelines for Referral and Diagnosis*. Centers for Disease Control and Prevention, Atlanta, GA; 2004.

[69] Laufer BI, Mantha K, Kleiber ML, et al. Long-lasting alterations to DNA methylation and ncRNAs could underlie the effects of fetal alcohol exposure in mice. *Dis Model Mech* 2013; **6**: 977–992.

[70] Haastrup M, Pottegård A, Damkier P. Alcohol and breastfeeding. *Basic Clin Pharmacol Toxicol* 2014; **114**: 168–173.

CHAPTER 8

Patterns of alcohol-associated liver damage

Peter Hayes and Michael Williams

Department of Gastroenterology, Royal Infirmary of Edinburgh, Edinburgh, UK

KEY POINTS

- Alcohol excess can cause various patterns of liver injury, including steatosis, hepatitis, and cirrhosis.

- Steatosis is almost universal in heavy drinkers but generally asymptomatic and reversible with abstinence.

- Alcoholic hepatitis occurs in less than one-third of heavy drinkers and severe cases carry a high short-term mortality.

- Alcoholic cirrhosis occurs in 10–20% and is associated with portal hypertension and liver failure.

- Hepatocellular cancer develops in patients with alcoholic cirrhosis with an incidence of 1–2% per year.

- All of the patterns of liver injury seen with alcohol can also be associated with nonalcoholic fatty liver disease.

Alcoholic liver disease (ALD) develops in patients consuming excessive quantities of alcohol. However, only a minority of heavy drinkers develop symptomatic liver disease. This is not explained simply by the amount or duration of alcohol consumed, and suggests that other factors are important in determining an individual's response to alcohol [1]. In order to understand this further, it is important to understand the ways in which alcohol can damage the liver.

Chronic alcohol excess is associated with a range of different patterns of liver damage, including simple steatosis, alcoholic hepatitis, fibrosis, and cirrhosis [2]. Although these patterns are defined histologically, they are often associated with discrete clinical syndromes which can help to distinguish the different stages of ALD. The key features of each of these is summarized in Table 8.1.

Although ALD is often viewed as a spectrum, there is not necessarily a stepwise progression through all of the stages. Patients can have varying degrees of the different elements, as shown in Figure 8.1.

Alcoholic steatosis

Fatty liver is the most common manifestation of ALD and is seen in the majority of heavy drinkers. Fatty liver is estimated to occur in at least 90% of those regularly consuming >60 g/day of alcohol, but also occurs in a proportion of those drinking less than this [3]. It reflects a pathologic accumulation of lipids (predominantly triglycerides) within hepatocytes. The build-up of fat is likely to be multifactorial, as alcohol has been shown to increase fatty acid synthesis, increase mobilization of fatty acids from adipose tissue, reduce fatty acid oxidation, and impair very low density lipoprotein export [4]. It is not currently clear which of these effects is most important in the development of steatosis.

Alcohol Abuse and Liver Disease, First Edition. Edited by James Neuberger and Andrea DiMartini.

Table 8.1 Patterns of alcohol-related liver damage.

	Steatosis	Alcoholic hepatitis	Cirrhosis
Key histologic features	Fat droplets in hepatocytes	Ballooning Mallory's hyaline Neutrophil infiltration Pericellular fibrosis	Thick bands of fibrosis Nodule formation
Key clinical features	Asymptomatic	Asymptomatic Jaundice Tender hepatomegaly Fever	Asymptomatic Ascites Jaundice Ascites Encephalopathy
Proportion of heavy drinkers affected	90–95%	10–35%	10–20%
Reversible	Usually	Often	No

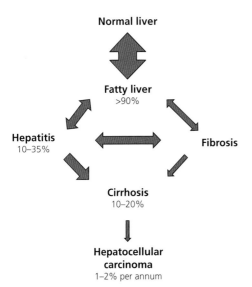

Figure 8.1 Relationship between patterns of liver damage in alcoholic liver disease. The different patterns of liver damage seen in individual patients is likely to reflect the interplay between the amount and pattern of alcohol consumed, and both genetic and environmental factors.

Pathology

Macroscopically, the liver is often large and pale with a greasy appearance. Microscopically, although the lipid is usually dissolved during preparation of routine histologic sections, the empty vacuoles left behind can be clearly seen. If there is diagnostic uncertainty, special lipid stains such as Sudan dyes can demonstrate fat more conclusively. Alcohol-related fatty liver is typically macrovesicular, with a single large fat droplet in the

hepatocyte which displaces the nucleus, as shown in Figure 8.2. Alcohol can also produce a microvesicular steatosis, with multiple smaller lipid droplets within the hepatocyte. Fat tends to accumulate preferentially in the centrilobular hepatocytes, but can be diffusely distributed in severe steatosis.

Clinical presentation

The vast majority of cases of steatosis are asymptomatic, and are discovered as a result of abnormal liver biochemistry or imaging. However, it may be associated with some nonspecific upper abdominal symptoms as a consequence of hepatomegaly, such as right upper quadrant discomfort and nausea. Hepatomegaly may be detected on routine clinical examination.

Differential diagnosis

The main alternative causes of steatosis are shown in Table 8.2. In particular, nonalcoholic fatty liver is commonly seen in association with features of the metabolic syndrome (obesity, type 2 diabetes, hypertension, hyperlipidemia). Medications associated with fatty liver include methotrexate, glucocorticoids, amiodarone, and tamoxifen. Fatty liver therefore requires careful evaluation of the patient prior to attributing it solely to alcohol.

Investigations

Many patients will have deranged liver biochemistry. The most common abnormality is an elevated gamma glutamyltransferase (GGT), although the correlation between GGT and degree of steatosis is poor. Patients

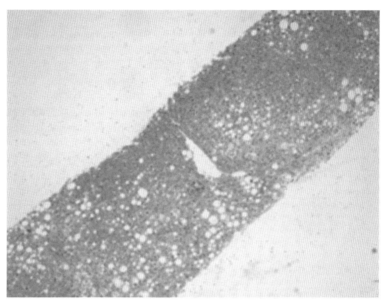

Figure 8.2 Steatosis. Hepatocytes show typical large vacuoles seen in macrovesicular steatosis. *(See insert for color representation of the figure)*

Table 8.2 Differential diagnosis of alcoholic liver disease.

Steatosis	Alcoholic hepatitis	Cirrhosis
NAFLD	NAFLD	NAFLD
Drug-induced	Drug-induced	Chronic viral hepatitis B or C
Hepatitis C		Hereditary hemochromatosis
genotype 3		Autoimmune hepatitis
Malnutrition		Primary biliary cirrhosis
		Primary sclerosing cholangitis
		Alfa-1-antitrypsin deficiency
		Wilson's disease

NAFLD, nonalcoholic fatty liver disease.

may also have mild increases in serum aspartate transaminase (AST) and alanine transaminase (ALT), with AST generally higher than ALT. This is thought to be a result of deficiency of pyridoxal-6-phosphate, a cofactor necessary for the enzymatic activity of ALT, in patients with chronic alcohol excess.

Liver fat typically causes a bright appearance of the liver on ultrasound caused by increased echogenicity. It has been suggested that magnetic resonance imaging (MRI) may be able to quantify liver fat more reliably to aid in noninvasive evaluation of steatosis but this requires further validation.

Natural history

Steatosis can develop rapidly and has been demonstrated within as little as 8 days of excess alcohol consumption, and is potentially completely reversible with abstinence. Complete resolution of fatty change has been shown on both liver biopsy and imaging within 4–6 weeks of stopping drinking. No specific interventions other than abstinence have been shown to be beneficial in fatty liver.

Only a minority of patients with alcoholic steatosis will progress to develop other patterns of injury. However, ongoing consumption of alcohol is associated with a risk of developing cirrhosis. Approximately 10–20% of patients with fatty liver (without evidence of alcoholic hepatitis) who continue to drink will develop advanced fibrosis or cirrhosis, especially those with a mixed macro- and microvesicular pattern of steatosis and perivenular fibrosis. Other factors that predict progression to cirrhosis include a pattern of daily drinking rather than periodic binges, female gender, and coexisting liver diseases such as viral hepatitis and nonalcoholic fatty liver disease (NAFLD).

Alcoholic hepatitis

A proportion of heavy drinkers will develop hepatocellular damage and inflammation, or alcoholic hepatitis. Although there is a lack of robust data on prevalence, it is estimated that between 10 and 35% of heavy drinkers will develop alcoholic hepatitis.

Pathology

Microscopically, alcoholic hepatitis is characterized by several features [5]. Hepatocytes lose osmotic control and isolated cells will undergo swelling and necrosis, known as ballooning degeneration. The cytoplasm of these cells often has a pale granular appearance, or may be broken up into cobweb-like strands. Damage to the hepatocyte cytoskeleton results in tangled clumps of intermediate filaments which are visible as eosinophilic cytoplasmic inclusions, called Mallory bodies or Mallory's hyaline. Although Mallory bodies are characteristic of alcoholic hepatitis, they are not pathognomonic and may also be seen in cholestatic syndromes and NAFLD. There is also an acute inflammatory infiltrate which is composed predominantly of neutrophils, densest around areas of ballooned hepatocytes and those containing Mallory bodies. These features are shown in Figure 8.3.

Alcoholic hepatitis is also associated with pericellular fibrosis, which produces a lattice-like "chicken wire" appearance as it surrounds individual hepatocytes and small clusters.

Clinical presentation

Some patients with a histologic diagnosis of alcoholic hepatitis may be asymptomatic. However, severe alcoholic hepatitis can present as an acute illness with rapid onset of jaundice, accompanied by malaise, anorexia, upper abdominal pain, tender hepatomegaly, fever, and leukocytosis. Patients may have an audible bruit over the liver. It can be associated with transient portal hypertension. Alcoholic hepatitis may progress to hepatic failure and alcoholic hepatitis carries a significant short-term mortality. Up to 40% of patients with severe alcoholic hepatitis will die within 6 months [6].

Differential diagnosis

Nonalcoholic steatohepatitis (NASH) associated with the metabolic syndrome and drug-induced liver injury can produce identical histologic changes.

The clinical presentation of alcoholic hepatitis with an acute inflammatory response can also be diagnostically challenging. Although fever and tachycardia can both be manifestations of alcoholic hepatitis, these also occur with sepsis and alcohol withdrawal, and these conditions should be actively sought and treated.

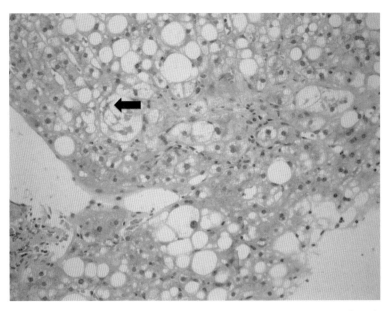

Figure 8.3 Alcoholic hepatitis. The arrow shows a hepatocyte undergoing ballooning degeneration with evidence of Mallory's hyaline accumulation. *(See insert for color representation of the figure)*

Investigations

In contrast to other forms of hepatocellular injury, serum ALT and AST are only mildly raised. Even in severe alcoholic hepatitis, the serum AST is usually less than 300 IU/L, and the ALT even lower. Higher values should prompt consideration of alternative diagnoses, such as acute viral hepatitis, acetaminophen toxicity, or ischemic hepatitis. The AST : ALT ratio is often greater than 2 in alcoholic hepatitis, in contrast to these other conditions in which AST : ALT is typically less than 1.

Patients with severe alcoholic hepatitis have significantly raised bilirubin levels and prolonged prothrombin times. The extent of these abnormalities can help to predict prognosis, and are the basis of several prognostic scoring systems for alcoholic hepatitis such as the Maddrey discriminant function, Lille Score, and Glasgow Alcoholic Hepatitis Score.

Ultrasound and other imaging modalities are unable to distinguish simple fatty change from inflammation. The clinical syndrome of severe alcoholic hepatitis as described is usually sufficient for diagnosis. However, in atypical cases, a liver biopsy may be necessary to confirm the diagnosis, and to exclude other coexistent causes of liver injury.

Natural history

Severe alcoholic hepatitis is associated with a high short-term risk of death from acute liver failure, sepsis, or renal failure. If patients survive, alcoholic hepatitis usually resolves with abstinence within 6 weeks to 3 months. Ballooned hepatocytes and Mallory bodies disappear and areas of necrosis are converted to scar. However, alcoholic hepatitis is often viewed as a major risk for development of fibrosis. With ongoing alcohol consumption, alcoholic hepatitis can progress to cirrhosis within months to years and it is associated with a much higher rate of cirrhosis than fatty liver alone. Approximately 70% of patients with alcoholic hepatitis will subsequently develop cirrhosis.

Alcoholic hepatitis can coexist with cirrhosis. In approximately 50% of cases of alcoholic hepatitis, there is already underlying cirrhosis.

Alcoholic cirrhosis

Alcohol excess can also be associated with progressive fibrosis, characterized by the abnormal accumulation of collagen-rich extracellular matrix. This typically begins in a pericentral distribution with perivenular sclerosis, extending into the sinusoids and encircling individual hepatocytes in a "chicken wire" pattern. The fibrosis eventually forms bridges between adjacent central veins, and between central and portal areas, leading to the formation of nodules. The end result is cirrhosis, when the liver architecture is disrupted with multiple nodules separated by bands of fibrous scar, as shown in Figure 8.4. The increased resistance to flow in the portal vein associated with increased splanchnic blood flow leads to portal hypertension, which is responsible for ascites, varices, and encephalopathy.

Fibrosis is considered to be the wound-healing response to liver injury, and is closely associated with inflammation. Episodes of alcoholic hepatitis may trigger or accelerate the development of cirrhosis. However, it is thought that fibrosis can also occur in the absence of any inflammation and may be a direct consequence of steatosis in a minority of patients. Certainly, a significant proportion of patients with alcoholic cirrhosis will not have had any preceding clinical episodes of alcoholic hepatitis.

Alcoholic liver disease is typically associated with a micronodular or Laënnec's cirrhosis, with most nodules measuring less than 3 mm in diameter. Following abstinence, this frequently transforms to a macronodular cirrhosis. Although steatosis is very common in heavy drinkers, there is often loss of much of the fat from the liver as cirrhosis develops, even with ongoing alcohol consumption. Macroscopically, the liver tends to become shrunken with an irregular surface.

Although technically a histologic diagnosis, cirrhosis is usually diagnosed on the basis of a combination of clinical signs, biochemical findings, and imaging.

Clinical presentation

The presentation of alcohol-related cirrhosis is similar to that of cirrhosis of other causes. Cirrhosis can be asymptomatic in compensated patients. Physical signs that should raise suspicions of cirrhosis include spider nevi, palmar erythema, gynecomastia, and loss of body hair. Patients may have palpable hepatomegaly or splenomegaly. Decompensation is signified by the development of ascites or edema, variceal bleeding, hepatic encephalopathy, or jaundice.

Ascites is the accumulation of fluid in the peritoneal cavity. This presents as abdominal distension, often with associated discomfort, early satiety, and breathlessness as a result of the raised abdominal pressure. It can be demonstrated clinically by the finding of shifting dullness, or a

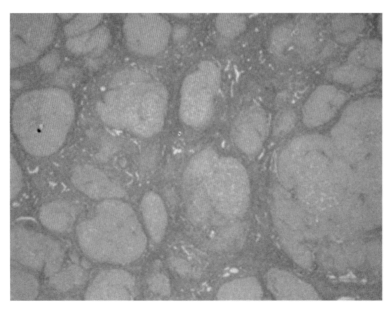

Figure 8.4 Cirrhosis. The liver architecture is disrupted with nodules separated by thick fibrous septa. *(See insert for color representation of the figure)*

fluid thrill. Ascites is treated by dietary salt restriction, diuretic therapy, or by insertion of a drain (paracentesis).

Ascites can become infected despite an absence of any obvious source, resulting in spontaneous bacterial peritonitis (SBP). This can present in a very nonspecific manner with few if any localizing signs. SBP is associated with a risk of renal failure and carries a significant mortality. As a result, SBP should be considered in any hospitalized patient with ascites.

Gastroesophageal varices are enlarged tortuous blood vessels typically found in the distal esophagus and stomach, and are present in approximately 50% of patients with cirrhosis. These can bleed spontaneously, which carries a short-term mortality of 10–20%. Screening endoscopies to assess for varices are therefore recommended for all cirrhotic patients. Prophylactic treatment with nonselective beta-blockers or band ligation reduces the risk of bleeding.

Hepatic encephalopathy refers to varying degrees of altered consciousness that can arise from cirrhosis. In its mildest form, this can cause sleep disturbance, irritability, and forgetfulness. However, it can also result in lethargy, confusion, and depressed conscious level to the point of coma. It is frequently precipitated by constipation, dehydration or diuretic therapy, infection, gastrointestinal bleeding or drugs, including sedatives or opiates.

Rapid onset of jaundice is often caused by superimposed alcoholic hepatitis; however, a gradual rise in bilirubin is seen as a result of liver failure in advanced cirrhosis.

Differential diagnosis

Cirrhosis can arise as a result of numerous other etiologies, listed in Table 8.2. As discussed in the section on alcoholic hepatitis, NAFLD is histologically indistinguishable from ALD, and this remains true when the patient is cirrhotic.

Hereditary hemochromatosis (HH) should also be considered as a differential diagnosis. However, patients with alcoholic cirrhosis also frequently have a raised serum ferritin level, and evidence of secondary iron overload on liver biopsy. Furthermore, both HH and alcohol can be associated with cardiomyopathy, pancreatic damage leading to insulin resistance, and testicular atrophy. Testing for mutations in the HH gene (*HFE*) can be helpful in distinguishing the two conditions.

Investigations

A low platelet count (thrombocytopenia) is suggestive of cirrhosis, as a consequence of splenic sequestration of platelets. This may be associated with anemia or leukopenia. Additionally, patients may have a raised bilirubin, low albumin, and prolonged prothrombin time.

Cirrhosis may be evident on imaging, as a small shrunken liver with an irregular contour and heterogeneity of the parenchyma. Right lobe atrophy and hypertrophy of the caudate and left lobes are also suggestive of cirrhosis. Portal hypertension as a consequence of cirrhosis may also be suspected on abdominal imaging if there is evidence of splenomegaly or intra-abdominal varices.

Elastography is an ultrasound-based technique for assessing liver stiffness. This is commonly used in the form of FibroScan to quantify fibrosis and to diagnose cirrhosis. Serum fibrosis markers are also useful diagnostically and have a reasonable accuracy in the diagnosis of cirrhosis, although are less useful in distinguishing between the varying degrees of fibrosis.

Natural history

The natural history of alcohol-related cirrhosis is heavily dependent on whether the patient continues to drink alcohol or not. Although abstinence from alcohol will not result in complete reversal of the architectural changes within the liver, it can result in histologic improvements and reduces the risk of decompensation. Patients with compensated cirrhosis who abstain from alcohol have a 5-year survival of over 90%. With continuing alcohol consumption, this drops to less than 70%. Episodes of decompensation predict a worse prognosis, and ongoing alcohol use in this setting carries a 5-year survival of less than 30%. Following the development of ascites, the median survival is less than 2 years. Encephalopathy is associated with the worst prognosis, with the majority of patients dying within a year.

Several prognostic scores can be used to predict survival. The Child–Turcotte–Pugh score combines biochemical parameters (bilirubin, albumin, and prothrombin time) with the development of clinical complications (ascites and encephalopathy). The Model for End-stage Liver Disease (MELD) score is based on bilirubin, international normalized ratio for prothrombin time (INR), and creatinine. Prognosis is also dependent on nutritional status and comorbid conditions such as chronic viral hepatitis.

Hepatocellular carcinoma

Alcohol is well-recognized as an etiologic factor in a number of cancers, including those of the oropharynx, larynx, esophagus, and possibly breast and colon.

Patients with alcoholic cirrhosis are also at risk of developing primary liver cancer, or hepatocellular carcinoma (HCC) [7]. The incidence of HCC in alcoholic cirrhosis is approximately 1–2% per year, which is lower than that associated with cirrhosis due to chronic viral hepatitis or hemochromatosis. HCC can develop even after many years of abstinence, and should be considered as a cause of sudden decompensation. HCC has been reported to occur in noncirrhotic livers, although this is very uncommon. Men are at higher risk of developing HCC than women, and the incidence increases with age.

Clinical presentation

HCC is often clinically silent in its early stages. In more advanced disease, it can present with right hypochondrial pain, anorexia, and weight loss. Alternatively, HCC can present with an episode of decompensation of underlying cirrhosis, such as worsening ascites or a variceal bleed. An enlarged liver may be palpable on examination, and there may be an audible arterial bruit on auscultation.

Investigations

A focal liver lesion may be visible on ultrasound, but this modality is unable to distinguish HCC from other solid liver lesions. Cross-sectional imaging with computed tomography (CT) and MRI is required to define the lesion further. HCC typically demonstrate early arterial enhancement with rapid washout during the portal venous phase. CT and MRI are quite accurate at diagnosing lesions greater than 2 cm diameter, but it can be difficult to confidently classify lesions less than 2 cm.

Alfa-fetoprotein (AFP) is an alfa1-globulin expressed during fetal development which is normally present at only very low levels in adult serum. As it can be elevated in HCC, it is used as a screening test (along with ultrasound scans) for HCC in cirrhotic patients. However, it should be noted that not all HCCs produce AFP. Furthermore, elevated AFP levels may be seen in cirrhotic patients without HCC, especially those with chronic viral hepatitis. Nevertheless, a progressively rising AFP is strongly suggestive of underlying HCC.

Natural history

The prognosis of HCC is generally poor because of its late presentation. Disease may be staged according to the Barcelona Clinic Liver Cancer (BCLC) classification which takes into account both tumor burden and underlying liver function.

Early stage disease may be curable by liver transplantation, resection, or possibly radiofrequency ablation. More advanced disease may be treated by transarterial chemoembolization (TACE) or sorafenib as palliative treatments. Patients with advanced liver disease may not be suitable for any active treatment and may be managed with symptom control alone.

Current recommendations are for screening with ultrasound every 6 months in alcoholic cirrhotic patients [8]. The use of AFP as a screening test is more controversial because of concerns over its specificity and sensitivity but is still widely practiced, and serial changes may be valuable in triggering further imaging.

Distinction from nonalcoholic fatty liver disease

NAFLD can produce histologically indistinguishable changes for all of the stages of ALD. In patients with features of the metabolic syndrome who consume alcohol, it can therefore be challenging to identify the relative contributions of the two processes. The distinction between the two conditions therefore has to be made on clinical grounds, and has traditionally been made using a threshold of 21 units of alcohol per week for men and 14 units for women. However, it is likely that some patients will have potential contributions from both processes. Indeed, obesity has been shown to be a risk factor for the development of cirrhosis in alcoholic liver disease.

Determinants of injury pattern

The clinical pattern of liver damage for any individual can be affected by the amount and pattern of alcohol consumption, as well as a range of genetic and nongenetic factors. Ethnicity, gender, nutrition, and comorbidities have all been shown to influence the pattern of liver damage seen. A number of genes have been proposed, including those involved in alcohol and lipid metabolism, oxidative stress, and immune response [9].

However, many of the suggested genes have conflicting or poor quality evidence. The most robust association has been shown for variation in the gene coding for patatin-like phospholipase encoding 3 (PNPLA3). The PNPLA3 rs738409 GG genotype was significantly more frequent in both alcoholic cirrhotics and noncirrhotic alcoholics with elevated liver enzymes than in alcoholics without liver damage.

Conclusions

In summary, alcohol can result in a range of different liver injury patterns, including steatosis, alcoholic hepatitis, cirrhosis, and hepatocellular cancer. All patients with evidence of any form of ALD should be advised to abstain completely from alcohol, as even fatty liver is associated with a risk of progression to cirrhosis. Patients with the more severe forms of alcohol-related liver damage may require additional therapies. Even in patients who drink alcohol heavily, other causes of liver disease should be considered according to the presentation.

References

[1] Gramenzi A, Caputo F, Biselli M, et al. Review article: alcoholic liver disease – pathophysiological aspects and risk factors. *Aliment Pharmacol Ther* 2006; **24**(8): 1151–1161.

[2] Adachi M, Brenner DA. Clinical syndromes of alcoholic liver disease. *Dig Dis* 2005; **23**(3–4): 255–263.

[3] O'Shea RS, Dasarathy S, McCullough AJ. Alcoholic liver disease. *Hepatology* 2010; **51**(1): 307–328.

[4] Gao B, Bataller R. Alcoholic liver disease: pathogenesis and new therapeutic targets. *Gastroenterology* 2011; **141**(5): 1572–1585.

[5] Alcoholic liver disease: morphological manifestations: review by an international group. *Lancet* 1981; **1**(8222): 707–711.

[6] Lucey MR, Mathurin P, Morgan TR. Alcoholic hepatitis. *N Engl J Med* 2009; **360**(26): 2758–2769.

[7] Morgan TR, Mandayam S, Jamal MM. Alcohol and hepatocellular carcinoma. *Gastroenterology* 2004; **127**(5 Suppl 1): S87–S96.

[8] Bruix J, Sherman M. Management of hepatocellular carcinoma: an update. *Hepatology* 2011; **53**(3): 1020–1022.

[9] Stickel F, Hampe J. Genetic determinants of alcoholic liver disease. *Gut* 2012; **61**(1): 150–159.

CHAPTER 9

Cofactors and alcohol-related liver disease

John G. O'Grady

Institute of Liver Studies, King's College Hospital, London, UK

KEY POINTS

- Excess weight and diabetes mellitus increase the risk of fibrosis and cirrhosis developing in regular alcohol consumers.

- There is considerable overlap in the phenotype of alcohol and nonalcohol-related live disease and the designation of cause may simply reflect the history of alcohol consumption.

- Alcohol increases the risk of cirrhosis in homozygous and compound heterozygous *HFE* gene mutations.

- Iron deposition increases disease progression in high alcohol consumers.

- Alcohol is the strongest environmental influence on disease progression in patients with hepatitis C.

- Previous or active alcohol consumption decreases the response to interferon-based regimens.

- Alfa-1 antitrypsin phenotype PiMZ is significantly over-represented in patients with alcohol-related cirrhosis and counseling about alcohol consumption is warranted.

Introduction

There is a poor correlation between the quantity of alcohol consumed and the risk of developing severe liver injury. The recognized risk factors are discussed in Chapter 5 and in this chapter attention turns to coexisting conditions that may have a role in reducing the threshold for the development of fibrosis and cirrhosis. This phenomenon is sometimes referred to as the "two hit" theory. The cofactors may cluster and, for example, there is considerable overlap with the comorbidities recognized with nonalcohol-related fatty liver disease and the attribution of the disease may be based on the history of alcohol consumption rather than a diagnostic phenotype. Similarly, alcohol, chronic hepatitis, and iron accumulation can interact to promote disease progression. The second observed effect of cofactors is to alter the trajectory of the disease, both by promoting progression of fibrosis and the time to clinical decompensation once cirrhosis has developed.

Body weight, obesity, and diabetes mellitus

Increased body weight in alcohol consumers heightens the risk of developing cirrhosis [1]. The mechanisms that have been postulated include:
- Upregulation of the microsomal cytochrome CYP2E1;
- Enhanced delivery of free fatty acids;
- Generation of reactive oxygen species;
- Lipid peroxidation;

- Endotoxin-induced Kupffer cell activation;
- Production of interleukin 1β; and
- Adiponectin resistance.

A study of 1604 patients with a history of excessive alcohol consumption included 608 with cirrhosis of which 411 were proven on liver biopsy [2]. The four variables that correlated with the development of cirrhosis were:

- Age;
- Female sex;
- Total duration of alcohol abuse; and
- Being overweight for at least 10 years.

The definition of overweight was a body mass index (BMI) >24 (kg/m²) in females and >26 (kg/m²) in males and the lowest weight during the 10-year period was used to classify the patients. This definition was satisfied in 172 patients accounting for 60% of the cirrhotic patients and 35% of the others. After adjustment for the other variables, the calculated increased risk of developing cirrhosis when overweight was 2.2-fold higher. An association with being overweight and risk of developing acute alcoholic hepatitis was also established in this cohort. In a different cohort the risk of developing cirrhosis was doubled in patients with a BMI of 29 (kg/m²) compared with those whose BMI was 21 (kg/m²).

Higher weight acting as a surrogate marker for higher alcohol consumption does not appear to explain this association. However, there is a relationship between being overweight and having a poor diet and this in turn is a well-recognized correlate with an increased risk of developing severe liver disease. Mechanistically, it was hypothesized that increased presentation of free fatty acids to the liver enhanced the risk of liver injury in overweight individuals. However, it was also considered that the simple step of developing steatosis may represent the entry point in the disease process.

The data on the link between diabetes mellitus and more advanced alcohol-related liver disease are limited. Early studies may be unreliable before the strong link between diabetes mellitus and nonalcoholic-related fatty liver disease was appreciated and the more recent literature is dominated by the latter condition. The incidence of diabetes mellitus is high in patients with alcohol-related cirrhosis but is unclear the extent to which this is cause or effect. The incidence of diabetes mellitus doubles with a weekly alcohol consumption in excess of 270 g. Higher glycemia levels were demonstrated in patients with alcohol-related liver disease and

more severe fibrosis. Up to 20% of those with end-stage liver disease have diabetes mellitus but this is the most likely of the observations to be a consequence of the liver disease.

Abstinence from alcohol has the potential to fairly rapidly improve this risk profile. The degree of steatosis reduces more predictably with the interventions than with nonalcohol-related liver disease. The reduced caloric intake usually leads to weight loss and altered behavioral patterns result in improved nutritional status. Glycemic control also improves but it is less clear whether interventions to increase insulin sensitivity are as relevant as with the nonalcoholic variant of fatty liver disease. Exercise is recommended on general grounds rather than on an evidence base.

Iron

Alcohol and iron act synergistically to cause liver injury [3,4]. Alcohol consumption increases serum iron and this effect is reversed within periods of abstinence as short as 6 weeks. The iron is deposited in the hepatocytes initially but also in macrophages as disease progresses. Postulated mechanisms include:

- Iron release as a consequence of cellular injury;
- *HFE* mutations;
- Dysregulation of hepcidin;
- Release of proinflammatory cytokines; and
- Upregulation of alfa-smooth muscle and procollagen.

There is clear evidence that alcohol consumption increases the severity of disease in patients with the C282Y homozygous state and associated predisposition to genetic hemochromatosis [5]. This was calculated as a fourfold increase with two drinks per day and a ninefold increase when the alcohol consumption was 60 g/day or greater. C282Y/H63D compound heterozygosity patients with disease penetrance were twice as likely to be heavy consumers of alcohol than C282Y homozygotes with similar patterns of disease. There are few data available on heterozygotes for either mutation although a study of first-degree relatives of C282Y heterozygotes failed to identify an excess of clinical liver disease. In a study of patients with alcohol-related liver disease, iron deposition was identified as a significant determinant of disease progression along with age, female sex, BMI, and glucose intolerance [6]. The role of iron depletion is well established in the management but there is little evidence that it alters the rate of progression in disease predominantly attributable to alcohol.

Hepatitis C

Alcohol is the most conspicuous environmental risk factor for the development of cirrhosis in patients with hepatitis C infection. It has a role from the point of infection through to the terminal stages of the disease.

- The prospects of spontaneously clearing the virus are reduced by half in alcohol consumers.
- Patients who consume alcohol have higher hepatitis C viral loads which fall within months of reducing alcohol consumption.
- Severe liver disease rates are two- to threefold higher in patients who consume alcohol.
- The interval between the time of acquisition of the virus and the development of cirrhosis is reduced by about 10 years.
- Once cirrhosis has developed the pace of decompensation is accelerated.

A seminal study of fibrosis progression in 2235 patients with hepatitis C identified three risk factors for developing cirrhosis:

1 Age greater than 40 years;
2 Alcohol consumption of 50 g/day or higher; and
3 Male sex.

The most rapid progression to cirrhosis was 13 years compared to 42 years in nonalcohol-consuming women who were aged less than 40 years at the time of acquisition of hepatitis C [7]. However, the negative impact of alcohol has been detected at alcohol consumption rates of 20 g/day or higher. There appears to be no safe level of alcohol consumption in patients with hepatitis. The mechanisms are poorly understood but are considered to include:

- Increased hepatitis C virus replication;
- Higher occurrence of quasispecies;
- Immune impairment;
- Impaired dendritic cell function;
- Mitochondrial dysfunction;
- Proteasome activity and generation of reactive oxygen species; and
- High rates of apoptosis.

Active and previous alcohol consumption decreased the likelihood of responding to interferon-based antiviral therapy. It was unclear if this was a direct effect or a risk factor for reduced adherence to the challenging interferon-based therapies. This consideration is now less important as the direct acting antiviral drugs are likely to rapidly replace interferon-based regimens.

Alfa-1 antitrypsin phenotype

Alfa-1 antitrypsin is a proteolytic enzyme and an acute phase protein. There are two clinically relevant genetic mutations with the normal phenotype termed M and the abnormalities designated as S and Z. Homozygous or compound heterozygous abnormalities are classically considered to be required to be associated with clinical disease, although this expresses variable penetration.

There is accumulating evidence that the PiMZ phenotype acts as a cofactor with alcohol to increase the rate of fibrosis progression and increase the overall risk of developing cirrhosis. This phenotype is over-represented by a factor of 5 in patients with alcohol-related cirrhosis and was found in 10% of potential candidates for liver transplantation. However, the observation is not unique to alcohol and the rate of detection in transplant candidates in the setting of nonalcohol-related fatty liver disease was 17% [8]. The mechanism of action for the acceleration of disease progression appears to be accumulation of misfold alfa-1 antitrypsin aggregates in hepatocytes. A study of liver tissue confirmed a small, but independent, aggravating effect on fibrosis in alcohol-related liver disease in patients with PiMZ phenotype.

There is no effective treatment for alfa-1 antitrypsin related liver disease but it does not recur after liver transplantation. However, counseling patients who are identified as having the PiMZ phenotype about their alcohol consumption seems prudent although it is not widespread practice. Respiratory physicians are more proactive in counseling against smoking because of the risk of chronic obstructive airways disease in PiMZ individuals.

Cofactors and liver histology

Liver histology is the most informative way of assessing the impact of cofactors. The pattern of cirrhosis is characteristic of alcohol-related liver disease except in patients with hepatitis C virus infection when the appearances associated with chronic hepatitis dominate with significant portal tract infiltration. Additional information achieved from the biopsy includes:

- Semi-quantitative assessment of steatosis;
- Distribution and intensity of iron accumulation; and
- Detection of alfa-1 antitrypsin globules in PiMZ phenotypes.

Serial liver biopsies give the most accurate information on the rate of progression of fibrosis and insight into the relevance of cofactors. This approach translated into definitions of slow, intermediate, and fast fibrosers in hepatitis C virus infected patients.

References

[1] Powell EE, Jonsson JR, Clouston AD. Steatosis: co-factor in other liver diseases. *Hepatology* 2005; **42**: 5–13.

[2] Naveau S, Giraud V, Borotto E, et al. Excess weight risk factor for liver disease. *Hepatology* 1997; **25**: 108–111.

[3] Siddique A, Kowdley KV. Review article: the iron overload syndromes. *Aliment Pharmacol Ther* 2012; **35**: 876–893.

[4] Purohit V, Russo D, Salin M. Role of iron in alcoholic liver disease: introduction and summary of the symposium. *Alcohol* 2003; **30**: 93–97.

[5] Fletcher LA, Dixon JL, Purdie DM, Powell LW, Crawford DHG. Excess alcohol greatly increases the prevalence of cirrhosis in hereditary hemochromatosis. *Gastroenterology* 2002; **122**: 281–289.

[6] Raynard B, Balian A, Fallik D, et al. Risk factors for fibrosis in alcohol-induced liver disease. *Hepatology* 2003; **35**: 635–638.

[7] Poynard T, Bedossa P, Opolon P. Natural history of liver fibrosis progression with chronic hepatitis C. *Lancet* 1997; **348**: 825–832.

[8] Cacciottolo TM, Gelson WTH, Maguire G, Davies SE, Griffiths WJH. Pi*Z heterozygous alpha-1 antitrypsin states accelerate parenchymal but not biliary cirrhosis. *Eur J Gastroenterol Hepatol* 2014; **26**: 412–417.

CHAPTER 10

Impact of alcohol and liver disease on prescribing

Richard Parker[1,2] and Amanda Smith[2]

[1] Centre for Liver Research and Biomedical Research Unit, University of Birmingham, Birmingham, UK
[2] University Hospitals Birmingham NHS Foundation Trust, Birmingham, UK

KEY POINTS

- It should be a priority to help patients reduce or stop hazardous drinking.

- Most drugs that are commonly used in the field of hepatology are safe in the context of cirrhosis.

- Many drugs are metabolized by the liver and may accumulate in liver disease.

- Avoid nephrotoxic drugs whenever possible.

- Avoid drugs that may affect conscious status if possible.

- A general priniciple of prescribing in hazardous alcohol use and/or liver disease is to start with low doses of drugs and carefully titrate dosage upwards if necessary.

Hepatic drug metabolism

The liver is the main site of drug metabolism. The liver predominantly converts lipid-soluble drugs to water-soluble hydrophilic metabolites so that they may be excreted via the kidneys. Some inactive prodrugs may be converted to active forms through hepatic metabolism. Three pathways or phases of drug metabolism exist in the liver:

- *Phase I:* reactions catalyzed by the cytochrome P450 enzyme superfamily, in the endoplasmic reticulum of hepatocytes.
- *Phase II:* enzymatic reactions found in both endoplasmic reticulum and cytoplasm of hepatocytes (e.g. gluconoryl transferases).
- *Phase III:* nonenzymatic reactions, transport of drugs across membranes into bile.

Effect of liver disease on the metabolism of drugs

Chronic liver disease can affect hepatic drug metabolism in several ways [1]. Differing patterns of liver injury cause different effects on hepatic drug metabolism (Table 10.1). Parenchymal liver injury will reduce cytochrome P450-dependent drug metabolism, although significant hepatic reserve may allow normal or near-normal metabolism to continue until very end-stage disease. Typically, phase II reactions are less affected. Cholestatic disease will adversely affect mechanisms of biliary drug excretion. Portal hypertension with systemic shunting of portal blood will decrease hepatic drug extraction and first pass hepatic metabolism leading to increased systemic levels of a drug. All of these phenomena may occur simultaneously and individual patients should be carefully assessed for

---

Alcohol Abuse and Liver Disease, First Edition. Edited by James Neuberger and Andrea DiMartini.
© 2015 John Wiley & Sons, Ltd. Published 2015 by John Wiley & Sons, Ltd.

Table 10.1 Mechanisms of hepatic drug metabolism and consequences of liver disease.

	Function	Signs of impairment	Consequences of impairment
Cytochrome P450-dependent mechanisms	Lipid-soluble drugs made water soluble	Low albumin Increased prothrombin time or international normalized ratio	Reduced metabolic capability when reduced hepatic mass
Biliary excretion via specific transporter	Excretion of drugs via bile and bowel	Raised bilirubin, alkaline phosphatase	Cholestasis reduced excretion of drugs
Hepatic uptake		Ascites, varices, hepatic encephalopathy	Reduced first pass hepatic metabolism

potential effects before prescribing. Decreased serum albumin concentration and increased bilirubin concentration may increase the free fraction of drugs that are highly protein bound.

Metabolism of alcohol

Alcohol is metabolized to acetaldehyde, a toxic compound that is normally quickly converted to acetate. Acetate is transported in the blood and converted to carbon dioxide, fatty acids, and water. In health, alcohol is metabolized principally by alcohol dehydrogenase (ADH). ADH is found predominantly in hepatocytes but is also present in smaller concentrations in the stomach. Two other enzyme systems also metabolize alcohol: the microsomal ethanol oxidizing system (MEOS) and catalase. Of the two MEOS is of more physiologic significance, particularly at higher concentrations and in chronic alcohol use, as it is an inducible enzyme system. MEOS involves the cytochrome P450 enzyme system, particularly CYP2E1. Metabolism of alcohol through this pathway produces free radicals and oxidative stress, contributing to the development of hepatic inflammation and damage. Acetaldehyde, a common product of all of these enzymatic pathways, is cleared through acetaldehyde dehydrogenase (ALDH) in mitochondria.

Effect of alcohol on metabolism of drugs

Chronic alcohol use can affect metabolism of drugs through several mechanisms. Alcohol induces the cytochrome P450 enzyme system [2], responsible for

metabolism of many classes of drugs. Pharmacodynamic effects may be exacerbated, for example benzodiazepines causing greater sedation. Alcohol can also alter gastric motility and thus absorption of drugs. Additionally, reports of drug interactions with alcohol are common although definitive evidence of harmful interactions is often lacking. It is therefore difficult to make recommendations but caution should be used in prescribing for patients who drink hazardously. Alcohol may increase the risk the hepatotoxicity of many drugs. Some commonly used medications with good evidence of interactions with alcohol are summarized in Table 10.2.

Specific prescribing problems: hepatology

The overriding principle in the treatment of alcoholic liver disease (ALD) is to achieve and maintain abstinence. Drugs that may be used to support abstinence are discussed (see Drugs used for treatment of alcohol abuse); otherwise there are few specific therapies for ALD. Prednisolone or pentoxifylline may be used in the treatment of severe alcoholic hepatitis in the context of recent hazardous alcohol use [4].

General management of chronic liver disease may involve the use of drugs to control the complications of portal hypertension – ascites, varices, and hepatic encephalopathy. Noncardioselective beta-blockers for primary and secondary prophylaxis of variceal bleeding are used safely in the context of chronic liver disease. Alcohol use may exacerbate the hypotensive effect of beta-blockade, although there are reports that it may attenuate the hemodynamic effects of propranolol. There has been interest in the use of

Table 10.2 Interaction of alcohol with commonly used medications [3].

Drug	Interaction with alcohol
Drugs causing sedation and/or psychomotor impairment	Possible greater effect with alcohol
Aspirin	Greater risk GI bleeding
Metronidazole	Disulfiram-like reaction
Interferons	Reduced efficacy with heavier alcohol use
Nicotine	Some evidence of increased tachycardic effect of alcohol with nicotine patches
NSAIDs	Increased risk of gastrointestinal bleeding, especially with greater alcohol consumption
Paracetamol	Hepatotoxicity potentiated in the context of chronic alcohol abuse
Phenytoin	Lower serum concentration in heavy drinking; higher doses may be required to maintain effective levels
Acitretin	Increased formation of metabolite etretinate
Tacrolimus	Skin flushing with topical tacrolimus and alcohol
Doxycycline	Reduced serum levels in chronic alcoholism
Vitamin A	Potential for increased liver injury and interactions with metabolism of vitamin A
Warfarin	Appears safe with mild–moderate alcohol consumption

GI, gastrointestinal, NSAID, nonsteroidal anti-inflammatory drug.

Table 10.3 Summary table of drugs used in hepatology.

Drug	Indication	Known interaction with alcohol	Known consequence of liver disease
Noncardioselective beta-blockers	Primary and secondary prophylaxis of variceal bleeding	Potential enhanced hypotensive effect	Safely used in cirrhotic liver disease
Spironolactone	Treatment of ascites or hepatic hydrothorax	Additional diuresis, disorder electrolytes, etc.	Safely used in cirrhotic liver disease
Furosemide	Treatment of ascites or hepatic hydrothorax	Additional diuresis, disordered electrolytes	Safely used in cirrhotic liver disease
Neomycin	Treatment of hepatic encephalopathy		Safely used in cirrhotic liver disease
Rifaximin	Treatment of hepatic encephalopathy	Dizziness	Safely used in cirrhotic liver disease

beta-blockers to prevent seizures in alcohol withdrawal although this is not established and not recommended for routine practice. Alcohol may interact with the treatment of ascites with diuretics (spironolactone or furosemide), causing excessive diuresis, disordered serum electrolytes, or hypotension. Nonabsorbable antibiotics such as neomycin and rifaximin have been used in the treatment of hepatic encephalopathy. Neomycin has no known interactions with alcohol, but rifaximin and alcohol can cause marked dizziness (Table 10.3).

It is not uncommon for patients with other chronic liver diseases to consume dangerous amounts of alcohol. Antiviral treatment for hepatitis B or C can be problematic in the presence of alcohol use, which may reduce the efficacy of interferon-based regimens [5]. Again, the safest option is to address alcohol use and this should be a priority. Alcohol use after liver transplantation for ALD is common, although hazardous use is unusual. Tacrolimus, a calcineurin inhibitor, has been reported to cause facial flushing or skin irritation if alcohol is used, but this only seems to be in the context of topical tacrolimus.

Specific drug interactions: psychiatry

Antidepressants

Many antidepressants are extensively metabolized by the liver, and should be used with caution in liver disease (Table 10.4). As a general principle, the lowest possible dose should be used to start treatment, and the dosage titrated according to response. It should also be remembered that some antidepressants can cause liver injury, in particular tricyclics. Many antidepressants are metabolized by CYP2D6, and it should be borne in mind that poor metabolizers may have increased plasma levels, which may be exacerbated further by liver disease.

Selective serotonin reuptake inhibitors

All selective serotonin reuptake inhibitors (SSRIs) are significantly metabolized by the liver, and many have long half-lives which are increased in liver impairment, leading to accumulation and the potential for toxicity. Many also are highly protein bound. They are less sedating than tricyclic antidepressants. The choice of drug will depend on the extent of disease, as some are contraindicated in severe liver impairment, and other factors such as drug interactions or side effect profile. They should be used with caution in liver impairment, and treatment should be commenced with a low dose, and the patient monitored closely.

Fluoxetine and its active metabolite both have particularly long half-lives, which are considerably increased in alcoholic cirrhosis. Citalopram and escitalopram can increase the QT interval, so need to be used with caution with other drugs that can also have this effect, particularly bearing in mind accumulation in liver impairment.

Tricyclic antidepressants

Tricyclics are more sedating than SSRIs, which may be exacerbated if patients are still drinking. The sedating and constipating effects of tricyclics can be an issue in encephalopathy. Imipramine, lofepramine, and nortriptyline are less sedating, but lofepramine in particular has been associated with drug-induced liver injury, and imipramine may be more constipating. Tricyclics are metabolized by the liver, and all should be used with caution in liver disease, and commenced at low doses; they should be avoided in decompensated cirrhosis because of limited safety data. Tricyclics may lower the seizure threshold, so should be used with caution in alcohol withdrawal.

Mirtazapine

Mirtazapine is metabolized by the liver with a variable elimination half-life (20–40 hours) which is increased in liver impairment. It is approximately 85% plasma protein bound. Mirtazapine should be used with caution in liver impairment, and should be commenced with a low dose. The CNS depressant effects of alcohol may be increased, so mirtazapine may not be appropriate if the patient is still drinking. Drug-induced liver injury has

Table 10.4 Summary table of drugs used in psychiatry.

Drug	Indication	Known interaction with alcohol	Known consequence of liver disease
SSRIs	Antidepressant		Liver metabolized – may accumulate in liver disease
Tricyclics	Antidepressant	Increased sedative effects	Liver metabolized – may accumulate in liver disease Constipation and sedation may cause problems in encephalopathy. Avoid in decompensated cirrhosis
Mirtazapine	Antidepressant	Increased sedative effects	Liver metabolized – may accumulate in liver disease
SNRIs	Antidepressant		Liver metabolized – may accumulate in liver disease Avoid duloxetine
MAOIs	Antidepressant		Contraindicated in liver disease
Benzodiazepines	Anxiolytic	Increased sedative effects	Liver metabolized – may accumulate in liver disease
Buspirone	Anxiolytic	Increased sedative effects	Liver metabolized – may accumulate in liver disease Contraindicated in severe liver disease

MAOI, monamine oxidase inhibitor; SNRI, serotonin–norepinephrine reuptake inhibitor; SSRI, selective serotonin reuptake inhibitor.

been reported. Mirtazapine can commonly cause weight gain, which is often an issue in alcoholic patients particularly those without end-stage liver disease.

Serotonin and noradrenaline reuptake inhibitors

The clearance of duloxetine is greatly reduced and the area under the curve substantially increased in liver impairment, so it is not recommended. Venlafaxine is extensively metabolized by the liver, and accumulation may occur in impairment, although there is considerable inter-patient variability. A low starting dose should be used.

Monoamine oxidase inhibitors

Monoamine oxidase inhibitors (MAOIs) are generally considered to be contraindicated in liver disease [6].

Anxiolytics
Benzodiazepines

Benzodiazepines are metabolized by the liver, and may accumulate in impairment. They are widely used in alcohol withdrawal, but should be used with caution when there is also liver impairment, as accumulation can lead to coma. They should be used with caution, and in low doses. Drugs such as lorazepam or oxazepam may be preferable, as they have a shorter half-life and are inactivated by hepatic glucuronidation alone, which is less affected by liver impairment than oxidation, but they should still be used with caution, and commenced at low doses. Lorazepam may also be given intravenously or intramuscularly, although caution is required with intramuscular injection in patients with deranged blood clotting. Benzodiazepines may be reversed with flumazenil which may make benzodiazepines a more attractive option than nonreversible agents. The sedative effects of alcohol are enhanced by benzodiazepines, which may be synergistic rather than just additive [7].

Buspirone

Buspirone is extensively metabolized by CYP3A4 in the liver, and is highly protein bound. The clearance is markedly decreased in cirrhosis, and it should be used with caution; accumulation may increase the incidence of side effects such as drowsiness and confusion, which can cause problems in patients at risk of encephalopathy. Buspirone is contraindicated in severe liver impairment.

Drugs used for treatment of alcohol abuse

In patients with ALD, drugs as an adjunct to counseling are recommended to decrease the likelihood of relapse to alcohol use in those who achieve abstinence [4].

Naltrexone is an opioid antagonist, which blocks the effects of opioids by competitive binding at opioid receptors. Clinical studies have shown the efficacy of naltrexone in reducing alcohol consumption in alcohol dependence. Metabolism takes place in both hepatic and extrahepatic sites, with evidence of enterohepatic cycling. Excretion is via the kidneys and to some extent via the gut. Studies in patients with cirrhosis show a slower rate of production of the active metabolite, 6-beta-naltrexol, and consequently higher circulating levels of naltrexone. Acamprosate and disulfiram, also used for treatment of alcoholism, have few data to guide their use in cirrhosis. Baclofen has been shown to be safe in patients with cirrhosis, although further trial evidence is required before routine use of baclofen can be recommended [8].

Other commonly used drugs

Analgesia
Nonsteroidal anti-inflammatory drugs

There are a number of risks associated with the use of nonsteroidal anti-inflammatory drugs (NSAIDs) in liver impairment which usually outweigh the benefits, and their use should be avoided. NSAIDs can cause gastrointestinal irritation and hemorrhage, and it is possible that they increase the risk of bleeding in patients with cirrhosis with portal hypertension and varices. It should also be borne in mind that many patients with liver impairment also have impaired clotting. Prostaglandin inhibition by NSAIDs can decrease glomerular filtration rate and increase sodium retention, worsening ascites and increasing risk of hepatorenal syndrome. Most NSAIDs are metabolized by the liver, so metabolism may be impaired in liver disease, leading to accumulation. Most are also highly protein bound. In addition, NSAIDs can rarely cause hepatotoxicity.

Opioids

Opioids may be used with caution in compensated cirrhosis, although it can be difficult to predict their pharmacokinetics. They are metabolized by the liver and are all likely to accumulate in liver impairment; plasma levels may also be higher than predicted if portosystemic shunts are present, because of a reduction in first pass metabolism. There may also be decreased elimination of morphine and codeine in cholestasis. Long-acting preparations should be avoided, and treatment initiated at low dosage. Generally, treatment should be initiated with a weak opioid. Constipation and sedation are common side effects of opioids, which may be problematic in patients with encephalopathy. Consideration should be given to concomitant prescribing of laxatives to prevent constipation. If possible, naloxone should be available to reverse the opioid if necessary.

Weak opioids

Codeine may be a less suitable choice, as it is more constipating, and depends on liver metabolism to be converted to morphine, so it may be less effective in cirrhosis. Tramadol is less constipating and associated with less respiratory depression, but may lower the seizure threshold so should be used with caution in alcoholics. The analgesic effect of dihydrocodeine is largely due to the parent compound, so it may be more effective than codeine in cirrhosis, but it may still accumulate, so low doses should be used.

Strong opioids

Strong opioids should be used with extreme caution in cirrhosis, and preferably only used after discussion with a liver unit. Pethidine (meperidine) should be avoided, as there is likely to be accumulation of the toxic metabolite norpethidine, which may increase the risk of toxicity, for example seizures and/or hallucinations. Most opioids are likely to accumulate in liver impairment. Where portosystemic shunts are present there may be higher than expected plasma concentrations of opioids with high first pass metabolism following oral administration (e.g. morphine), so very low doses should be used, and titrated as appropriate.

Paracetamol/acetaminophen

Chronic hazardous alcohol use induces enzymes that metabolize paracetamol to its toxic metabolite, thus increasing the potential toxicity. Indeed, chronic alcohol use is common in accidental paracetamol overdose. This susceptibility appears reversible if abstinence is achieved. In the absence of established liver disease, newly abstinent alcoholics including those with alcoholic hepatitis and hepatitis C virus infection showed only minor changes in liver function tests when given paracetamol

[9]. A reduced dose of paracetamol is advised in patients with chronic liver disease, especially those with advanced disease who may have other risk factors for toxicity, for example sarcopenia.

Cardiovascular drugs

As hazardous alcohol intake is associated with increased risk of cardiovascular disease, commonly used cardiovascular medications may be indicated.

Aspirin

Aspirin for the secondary prevention of coronary artery disease and ischemic stroke may be indicated in patients with a background of hazardous drinking. Aspirin is associated with gastrointestinal bleeding which may be potentiated by alcohol consumption particularly at higher levels of intake. There are few data regarding other antiplatelet drugs such as clopidogrel or dipyridamole; these should be used with caution. Of note, proton-pump inhibitors (PPIs) have been linked with an increased risk of spontaneous bacterial peritonitis, thus gastroprotection with PPIs may be inadvisable.

Warfarin

Mild to moderate alcohol use appears safe with warfarin and other coumarins, although the half-life of warfarin is lower in alcoholics. In liver disease the anticoagulant effect of warfarin may be difficult to predict and thus preclude effective anticoagulation.

Statins

Dyslipidemia is common in liver disease, particularly nonalcoholic fatty liver disease (NAFLD). Statins are effective to reduce cardiovascular risk, but there may be reluctance to use these drugs in view of possible hepatotoxicity. However, serious side effects are rare and statins may generally be used safely with appropriate monitoring. Hydrophilic statins – atorvastatin, rosuvastatin, fluvastatin, and pravastatin – may be associated with a lower risk of side effects in liver impairment (Table 10.5).

Monitoring therapy in liver disease

Monitoring liver function can be undertaken in most cases by performing liver function tests (LFTs) before and during treatment. LFTs should include bilirubin, albumin, and alanine transaminase (ALT) or aspartate

Table 10.5 Summary table of other commonly used drugs.

Drug	Indication	Known interaction with alcohol	Known consequence of liver disease
NSAIDs	Analgesia		Risk of GI bleeding, increased sodium retention, worsening ascites and increasing risk of hepatorenal syndrome
Opioids	Analgesia	Tramadol may lower seizure threshold.	Difficult to predict their pharmacokinetics.
		Increased sedation	Side effects may be problematic in patients with encephalopathy
Paracetamol/acetaminophen	Analgesia	Greater risk of toxicity	Reduced dose of paracetamol is advised in chronic liver disease
Aspirin	Secondary prevention of cardiovascular disease	Potentiates risk of GI bleeding	Potentiates risk of GI bleeding
Warfarin	Anticoagulation	Appears safe with alcohol mild to moderate alcohol use	Difficult to predict clinical effects
Statins	Dyslipidemia		Side effects rare

GI, gastrointestinal; NSAID, nonsteroidal anti-inflammatory drug.

transaminase (AST). Unexpected fluctuations in LFTs should prompt cessation or at least review of new drugs. Nevertheless, regular blood testing may not be completely effective in preventing liver injury; ensuring that patients are aware of potential side effects and are instructed to report them promptly may be of more value [10]. In advanced liver disease, clinical condition is also important, for example a new drug may cause deterioration in hepatic encephalopathy. Again, good communication between clinicians, patients, and their family and carers can detect early changes.

Conclusions

The liver is the major site for drug metabolism and abnormalities in liver function have significant effects on drug metabolism. This is mediated through both biochemical and structural disturbances. Hazardous alcohol intake, even in the absence of significant liver disease, will also change the pharmacokinetics of many drugs. Prescribers therefore need to be aware of the potential for harm when either of these conditions are present. To complicate matters further, alcohol abuse and significant liver disease may often present together. It is important that those who drink hazardous amounts of alcohol are given assistance to reduce or stop drinking. This may be supported with drug treatment.

Hepatologists and gastroenterologists are accustomed to treating patients with cirrhosis, and most drugs in this field have direct evidence from trials including such patients. However, active alcohol abuse complicates this and some drugs, for example antiviral therapy, may not be suitable for active drinkers. Outside of hepatology, there is far less experience with liver disease. Some risks are theoretical without clear data. In the absence of observed interactions with liver disease or alcohol, great caution must be exercised and a mantra of "start low, go slow" adopted when a particular drug is indicated.

References

[1] Veerbeeck RK. Pharmacokinetics and dosage adjustment in patients with hepatic dysfunction. *Eur J Clin Pharmacol* 2008; **64**(12): 1147–1161.

[2] Pirmohamed M. Prescribing in liver disease. *Medicine* 2011; **39**(9): 541–544.

[3] Baxter K, Preston CL, eds. *Stockley's Drug Interactions*, 10th edn. Pharmaceutical Press, 2013. Accessed online March–April 2014.

[4] O'Shea RS, Dasarathy S, Mccullough AJ. Alcoholic liver disease. *Hepatology* 2010; **51**(1): 307–328.

[5] Tabone M, Sidoli L, Laudi C, et al. Alcohol abstinence does not offset the strong negative effect of lifetime alcohol consumption on the outcome of interferon therapy. *J Viral Hepat* 2002; **9**(4): 288–294.

[6] Timmer CJ, Sitsen JM, Delbressine LP. Clinical pharmacokinetics of mirtazapine. *Clin Pharmacokinet* 2000; **38**(6): 461–474.

[7] Tanaka E, Misawa S. Pharmacokinetic interactions between alcohol ingestion and single doses of benzodiazepines, and tricyclic and tetracyclic antidepressants: an update. *J Clin Pharm Ther* 1998; **23**: 331–336.

[8] Liu J, Wang LN. Baclofen for alcohol withdrawal. *Cochrane Database Syst Rev* 2013; **2**: CD008502.

[9] Dart RC, Green JL, Kuffner EK, et al. The effects of paracetamol (acetaminophen) on hepatic tests in patients who chronically abuse alcohol: a randomized study. *Aliment Pharmacol Ther* 2010; **32**(3): 478–486.

[10] Senior JR. Monitoring for hepatotoxicty: what is the predictive value of liver "function" tests? *Clin Pharmacol Ther* 2009; **85**(3): 331–334.

CHAPTER 11

Psychiatric examination of liver transplant patients with alcohol use disorders

Robert M. Weinrieb[1] and Omair Abbasi[2]

[1] Department of Psychiatry, University of Pennsylvania Health System, Perelman School of Medicine, Philadelphia, PA, USA
[2] Department of Psychiatry and Human Behavior, Thomas Jefferson University Hospitals, Sidney Kimmel School of Medicine, Philadelphia, PA, USA

KEY POINTS

- Every patient with a history of addiction being assessed for liver transplant needs assessment by a mental health professional with addictions expertise.

- The pretransplant evaluation is a judgment of the suitability of the candidate for transplantation not a therapeutic intervention.

- Those assessing the transplant candidate must be aware of the common myths held by the transplant candidate.

- Risk factors for relapse include a shorter duration of sobriety, a family history of alcoholism, and poorer social support.

- A robust rehabilitation is important in supporting sobriety.

- The interview should be structured and include an alcohol history, treatment history, psychosocial functioning, comorbid psychiatric and substance use disorders.

- Subsequent collateral interviews should be with the family, spouse, or partner and supported by other screening methods.

- Strctural assessment tools (such as High Risk Alcohol Relapse Scale, Transplant Evaluation Rating scale, and the Stanford Integrated Psychsocial Assessment for Transplantation have been used with good effect.

Introduction

Despite the fact that liver transplantation for decompensated alcoholic liver disease affords patients the best chance of long-term survival, only a fraction of patients who could be eligible for a liver transplant are referred for formal transplant evaluation. More specifically, 90–95% of patients with decompensated alcoholic liver disease are not referred for transplant evaluation; thus, approximately 12 000 die each year [1]. When compared with the figure of nearly 1200 with end-stage alcoholic liver disease who will be transplanted in a given year, we must conclude that the patients we evaluate are a select and fortunate group indeed. We can speculate about the reasons for this disparity, but the goal of this chapter is to give transplant care providers some understanding and guidance regarding the assessment of alcohol intake in patients with liver disease. The psychiatric assessment of an alcoholic patient in the setting of a liver transplant evaluation has specific goals that may be different from most interviews of alcoholic patients. While the focus of this chapter is primarily on the psychiatric interview in the liver transplant candidate, the same approach to and content of assessment applies to patients at any stage of their alcoholic liver disease.

It has been suggested that a psychiatrist or mental health professional with addictions expertise interview

---

Alcohol Abuse and Liver Disease, First Edition. Edited by James Neuberger and Andrea DiMartini.
© 2015 John Wiley & Sons, Ltd. Published 2015 by John Wiley & Sons, Ltd.

every patient with a history of addictions in need of a liver transplant [2]. However, before we discuss the psychiatric interview from the perspective of the examiner, it may be helpful to understand the process through the eyes of the patient. In our experience, if interviewed sensitively, most patients being evaluated for liver transplant as a result of alcoholic liver disease will acknowledge that they drank too much and that they have "learned their lesson." Many will say with sincerity, "After what I've been through, I will never drink again." Patients have also said that before they were sick enough to be considered for a liver transplant, their gastroenterologist told them to "cut back on their drinking," as opposed to "Stop drinking or you will die." Whether these physicians actually told alcohol-dependent patients to control their drinking or that is the message their patients heard, it nonetheless resulted in a reduction of their alcohol consumption for a period of time, but eventually many would return to their previous level of consumption, if not more. Although some patients may have perfunctorily completed a court stipulated sentence to attend Alcoholics Anonymous (AA) meetings for a driving under the influence (DUI) conviction, many have never had formal alcoholism treatment or attended an AA meeting by the time they present with symptoms of liver disease or for a liver transplant evaluation [3]. Consequently, it has been observed that many transplant candidates lack the intrinsic motivation to take a hard look at their alcoholism and begin the work that is needed, not just to remain abstinent from alcohol for the rest of their lives, but to accept and recover from their addiction [4]. In addition, our group and others have found even after transplant listing when the alcoholic patient's confidentiality from the transplant team is assured, as many as 25% will endorse drinking alcohol while on the waiting list [3,5]. This demonstrates the difficulty in maintaining abstinence even when confronted with a life-threatening illness and underscores the need for ongoing monitoring.

The patient's perspective

DiMartini and Dew have written, "The pretransplant evaluation is not a therapeutic interaction but a judgment of the suitability of the individual for solid organ transplantation" [5]. Whether the referring transplant teams explained this to their patients, most understand that the psychiatric interview is likely to have a significant role in their transplant eligibility. Not surprisingly, this may result in patients' minimizing or obfuscating the severity of their addiction. In addition, patients may be reluctant to vocalize questions or admit to critical feelings about the psychiatric interview out of fear that these disclosures may adversely implicate them or render them ineligible for transplant. In our experience, many patients arrive at the psychiatric interview with a host of erroneous preconceived notions, therefore we illustrate some common examples of misconceptions or "myths" patients often have about the psychiatric interview, and describe how liver specialists can interpret and address them. By identifying and addressing some of these misleading notions, it is hoped that hepatologists can facilitate a more open and trusting relationship with the consulting psychiatrist or mental health professional who conducts the pretransplant psychiatric evaluation.

Myth 1: "You're the last one I have to see to 'pass the test' so I can get my liver"

This misconception can lead to the patient's view of the psychiatrist as someone who will make a final and unilateral decision to either let the patient live or die. This must be addressed at the start of the interview to allow patients to feel comfortable enough to open up and be honest about their problems. Our group has found that when we introduce ourselves to a new patient, it is important to let the patient know our role on the transplant team (i.e. that we are consultants to the team and one voice among the many team members who decide upon listing as a group). We also explain that our job is to learn about their strengths and limitations so that we can develop a comprehensive treatment plan that may facilitate transplant listing rather than block their path to transplant. Patients should be told that everything discussed will be shared with the transplant team, and that their permission is sought to discuss their case with their referring provider and to speak to a family member or significant other. If the patient is too ill or cognitively impaired to retain the information and instructions from the psychiatrist or liver specialist, it can be helpful if they designate an individual with whom they are close who can communicate regularly with the key transplant team members. This can minimize confusion amongst multiple caregivers who may understandably want to be involved in the patient's care.

Myth 2: "I feel badly that someone died so I can live"

Patients do not always understand the process of donation, and some may believe that their donor's lives were lost because they needed an organ, and others may feel guilty that someone died so that they can benefit from their death. Patients are relieved to hear that deceased organ donors would not have survived regardless of donation, and because the donor and their families chose to give the "gift of life," it can be a source of comfort to the donor's family to know that their tragic loss will not be in vain.

Myth 3: "There are so many others who deserve a liver more than I do, and besides, I am probably not going to get a liver anyway"

It is not uncommon for patients with addictions to feel less worthy of receiving a transplant than patients without a history of addiction. This can be an opportunity to explore the guilt and shame that many addicted patients carry that leads to their feeling ambivalent about transplantation. Of course most want to live, but because they may not feel "equal" to their nonaddicted peers, they can lose hope about their chances of being selected for the waiting list or being transplanted. Patients who are made aware of this ambivalence are eager to discuss it when it is raised, and it can be useful for them to hear that their feelings of inferiority are very common in the early phases of addiction recovery, whether or not they have liver disease. The mental health professional or liver specialist can use this explanation to emphasize how this underscores the importance of engaging in formal counseling for their addictions where these issues can be addressed.

Myth 4: "You're saying I'm an alcoholic, but I'll bet you think that because you never took a drink in your life"

This is a classic transference reaction toward the psychiatrist or liver specialist and is based upon the patients' worries that they are being judged or will not be accepted or helped by the doctor. Again, this is best approached in a nondefensive, nonjudgmental fashion by the interviewer. Patients with addictions are very sensitive to feeling that their care providers are judging them, whether it is true or not. We recommend that the interviewer try to reassure patients by explaining to them that they agree that their problems are unique to them and although the doctor can never know *exactly* what it feels like to be them, they can still help and care for them. It can be emphasized that therapy is most fulfilling when viewed as a partnership in which patients help the doctor appreciate their problems through mutual understanding, honesty, and respect.

Myth 5: "I'm depressed, but I have to live with it because my doctors told me I can't take any medicine for depression; it's not good for my liver"

In general, it is important for the mental health professional to diagnose accurately and recommend appropriate treatment to patients with comorbid mental illnesses. Depression and anxiety disorders are common in patients with alcohol use disorders, and if untreated can lead to relapse. Reassure patients that most medications used to treat depression or other mental health disorders, if carefully monitored, are safe to take even in patients with cirrhosis. A word of caution is advised about the risk of spontaneous bleeding associated with the use of selective serotonin reuptake inhibitors (SSRIs) in patients at risk for bleeding [6]. Physicians treating depression or anxiety in patients with liver disease should nonetheless not be deterred from the appropriate use of SSRIs in this population. If the risk of bleeding seems too great to use an SSRI, then serotonin–norepinephrine reuptake inhibitors (SNRIs) like venlafaxine or non-SSRIs such as bupropion may be safer. Most antidepressants are just as safe for patients with cirrhosis as many of the other nonpsychiatric drugs they take, especially if started at a low dose and increased slowly [7].

Myth 6: "I don't need rehab, I am strong willed and I know I will never drink again"

While this may be true for some, approximately half of all patients who receive a liver transplant as a result of alcohol overuse will return to some drinking as long as 5 years post-transplantation [8]. Although most transplant recipients who drink do so infrequently and lightly, approximately 20% of those who "slip" (i.e. sample alcohol) will relapse and drink heavily relatively soon after transplant and develop significant health problems [9]. In a meta-analysis by Dew et al. [10], it was determined that relapse to drinking was associated with short sobriety (<6 months), a family history of alcoholism, and having a poorer social support system. Knowing these primary risk factors for relapse is especially important for the examiner to probe.

Merely describing the validity of this information or the nuances of which post-transplant predictors of drinking apply most closely to the patient does not seem particularly persuasive to those patients who are proud of being strong willed and feel insulted that they are not being trusted to never drink again. They may also feel offended that they are being required to attend rehabilitation and may feel as if this demeans their own success in abstinence. In these situations, it can be useful to explain that this process is not about whether the transplant team (or their liver doctor) lacks trust in them, it is that the disease of alcoholism can express itself in the form of a relapse, even in the most well-intentioned patient. Therefore, if patients reject the opportunity to learn new tools and coping skills, they subject themselves to an increased risk of drinking. Without a good rehabilitation program, patients will often resort to passive coping, which has been shown to be far less effective in maintaining sobriety than active coping mechanisms such as attending AA meetings and engaging in an open and honest dialog about their alcoholism with a professional [11].

Referral for alcoholism treatment requires the examiner to have an understanding of the types of programs that may be available to patients. Alcoholism treatment options are typically inpatient, outpatient, or residential (see Chapter 18). Inpatient rehabilitation programs in the United States may last up to 30 days and are typically staffed by a psychiatrists, nurses, and therapists. Usually, patients who need to be in such a controlled environment do so because of co-occurring mental illness. If actively drinking, patients may also be admitted to an inpatient detoxification program for a safe, monitored, detoxification only and then referred for outpatient aftercare. Outpatient treatment is typically delivered via an Intensive Outpatient Program (IOP) in the United States. IOPs in the United States accept a variety of insurance plans and patients attend 3–5 days per week for up to 16 weeks.

In the United Kingdom, Community Alcohol Teams (CATs) provide a wide range of support services including home-based and community detoxification programs, counseling, and group work. Most CATs are managed by the National Health Service (NHS) and often have a multidisciplinary staff team including link workers, health care workers, and social workers. Some CATs will accept self-referrals although others only deal with clients referred by GPs or other professionals. Day programs in the United Kingdom provide a structured, full-time program for clients and can last from 6 weeks to 9 months. Some residential services also take clients on a nonresidential basis and offer day programs.

In all of these programs, the most common form of addiction treatment used employs the "Minnesota Model," a 12-step program that relies heavily on group participation. With alcohol use disorders, relapse is common; thus, directing patients to rehabilitation that provides therapeutic tools and allows patients to take responsibility for their recovery will improve their potential for success in sobriety. This should not be viewed differently from if they were told that learning to manage their diabetes or hypertension is necessary in order to regain hepatic health or to be considered for a liver transplant.

The significance of putting information concerning patients' perspectives, fears, and myths at the start of the chapter was meant to emphasize the fact that patients who are misinformed about the transplant process or the role of the psychiatrist on the team are less likely to disclose aspects of their history that they perceive as potential barriers to their transplant eligibility. If these misconceptions are anticipated, recognized, and addressed by the interviewer early in the interview process, patients may be more relaxed through the psychiatric interview and provide a more honest account of their lives and the severity of their problems.

In the following section, we discuss the role of the psychiatrist or mental health professional conducting psychiatric evaluations of liver transplant patients with alcohol use disorders and the unique perspectives that are inherent to this process.

The psychiatrist's perspective

The psychiatric assessment of alcohol use disorders can often seem like a difficult task. The very process of undergoing a liver transplant evaluation for alcohol-related cirrhosis is predicated on the fact that the patient has lost control of their alcohol consumption. In light of this, patients often feel guilty and ashamed about being in their condition and are understandably defensive about discussing the consequences of their drinking. It is important to remember that patients often realize the destruction that alcohol has caused in their lives, but may fear having to undertake the task of reinforcing their new-found sobriety and the potential failure that may arise from attempting to maintain it. Therefore, when obtaining a history from a patient, one should keep in mind that contradictory statements are not necessarily an attempt at manipulation, but may reflect the patient's own internal struggle in creating a meaningful dialog about his or her alcohol use. In some instances, the psychiatrist may be the first individual to ask the patient to narrate and quantify their alcohol use, and in so doing, their recollection may be inconsistent. In addition, there may also be indecision on the part of the patient to be candid out of concern that their history may exclude them from liver transplant or further treatment. Thus, methods for interviewing that can allow for a more honest narrative of the patient's alcohol history can improve the ability to identify treatment targets.

The patient interview

After introductions are made and the purpose of the interview has been explained, it is vitally important for the interviewer to start the examination by asking the patient how he or she physically feels that day. If the patient is feeling poorly, the interviewer should enquire whether this is a recent change in their condition. If the patient reports a change in their condition, enquire whether they have informed their doctors. Psychiatrists should know how to recognize the symptoms of hepatic encephalopathy (HE), and its varying degrees of severity. More severely encephalopathic patients may appear intoxicated, with slurred speech, somnolence, and an ataxic gait. This can occur in those patients who avoid taking lactulose for the trip to the transplant assessment center. Patients can present with more subtle signs of HE, such as prolonged latency of speech or problems with word finding. The psychiatrist should be aware that if their patient has HE, their self-report may be inaccurate and they may even be somewhat suggestible. An example with the potential for serious consequences for the patient is when they erroneously endorse recent drinking after being asked when their last drink was despite long-term sobriety. Postponing the psychiatric interview and seeking appropriate medical treatment when the patient is physically unstable is prudent and necessary in these instances.

Similarly, the transplant interview may have to be conducted while the patient is acutely hospitalized and displays cognitive limitations secondary to HE and/or medications (i.e. opiates, benzodiazepines, anticholinergics). Ambiguous statements made by the patient can be identified and clarified later either through review of records, reinterviewing the patient when they are more cogent, or through collateral interview. More detail regarding the collateral interview is discussed later in the chapter.

Structure of the psychiatric interview

It should be noted that there is no singular method that is universally effective in assessing alcohol intake. Rather, it is a combination of strategies that allows for the physician to make as accurate an assessment as possible of the patient's drinking habits. This process begins by interviewing the patient alone, then again with their family member, spouse, or partner. In addition to interviewing, the use of screening measures and laboratory testing can aid in confirming reported abstinence (see Chapter 13).

It is the authors' recommendation that the assessment for alcoholic intake be part of an overall psychosocial evaluation rather than its own singular encounter with the patient. Presenting it in this manner provides benefits in two ways:

1 It allows for the interviewer to establish rapport with the patient; and
2 It facilitates the gathering of multiple psychosocial data points that are necessary for an accurate and comprehensive evaluation.

As described in Myth 1, the evaluation should be introduced to the patient as a means of deriving information that can be used to obtain the best possible outcomes in the treatment of his or her liver disease. In other words, preface the interview by stating that the mental health professional's role is not to block the patient's access to transplant, but to do the best to develop a treatment plan tailored to the individual patient's needs. The patient's openness can facilitate eventual placement on the transplant waiting list, with the ultimate goal of total abstinence both before and after the transplant.

All aspects of the psychiatric interview should be included: chief complaint, history of the present illness, past psychiatric history, past medical and surgical history, a current review of symptoms, medications, allergies, family history, developmental history and, finally, the addiction history. In the following paragraphs, we primarily emphasize the alcohol intake assessment.

Alcohol use history

In longitudinal observational studies, alcohol misuse usually presents in one or more of three primary patterns.

1 The individual who begins abusing alcohol but maintains a steady pattern of the quantity and frequency of alcohol consumption for most of his or her life.

2 The patient who begins drinking socially or moderately but, as they get older, their drinking escalates and becomes out of control. These patients may have experienced alcohol withdrawal symptoms and/or alcohol withdrawal seizures.

3 Episodic, heavy exacerbations in drinking (binges) with periods of sobriety lasting days to months in the interim [12].

Individuals with alcohol use disorders have also been classified in the literature as type A (for the Roman god Apollo) or type B (for the Roman god Bacchus) in Babor's classification [13]. Type B describes those who start drinking heavily early in life, usually in their teens or early twenties. They rapidly develop marked tolerance to alcohol and have strong family histories of alcoholism in their first degree relatives. Type A alcoholics tend to develop alcohol problems later in life, usually in response to psychosocial stressors such as a death in the family or loss of a job. Of the two types, type B is considered the more severe form of alcoholism with heavier genetic influence (see Chapter 3).

Beginning the interview

The interview can begin in reverse chronologic order to allow for the patient to establish historical drinking patterns and become comfortable speaking about his or her alcohol use. A good starting statement may be, "Tell me when alcohol started to play a role in your life." Having the patient begin with his or her first recollection of drinking will set the stage to create a narrative of how the addiction progressed. Early drinking age (prior to 18 years old) may indicate the patient used drinking as a tool for coping with stressful life circumstances in lieu of learning healthier coping strategies that would have normally developed in his or her formative years. This is of concern as the patient may turn to alcohol to cope

with stress or anxiety, which he or she will inevitably face during medical treatment for liver disease.

After establishing an age at which the patient began drinking, the next step is to ask the patient about the first time he or she felt that drinking affected him or her negatively. In some cases, the patient may respond by stating he or she never thought it was a problem until the doctor informed him or her about the recent liver disease diagnosis. The patient may report having been able to maintain work and social responsibilities in the setting of excessive alcohol intake. Asking the above questions allows the interviewer to gauge the level of insight and motivation the patient has in regards to the alcohol misuse. When faced with a patient with limited insight, the CAGE questionnaire may prove to be helpful – CAGE is an acronym for asking patients if they ever felt they needed to "**C**ut down" their intake; if they've ever become **A**ngry when others question their alcohol intake; if they've ever felt **G**uilty about their drinking; or if they have ever needed an "**E**ye opener" to reduce withdrawal symptoms at the start of their day [14]. Additional questions about withdrawal symptoms (tremors), delirium tremens (DTs), or a history of seizures may provide some additional information as to the intensity of problematic drinking patients have experienced. Surprisingly, patients may respond affirmatively to several of these questions yet not believe they have a "drinking problem." Minimizing the adverse consequences of their drinking is common, so the interviewer can take this opportunity to ask the patient if it is acceptable to invite their significant other in to talk. This is invaluable because patients' partners often see problems in them that they do not.

Quantity and frequency of intake

Many patients feel more comfortable providing quantitative information about their alcohol consumption after they have been asked about the psychosocial consequences of their drinking. Intake of alcohol should be described by quantity and frequency of use. This may be assessed in three domains:

1 The variability in frequency and amount of consumption during the lifespan (was the patient a binge drinker or someone who drank several drinks on a daily basis?);

2 The maximum amount they were able to consume in a sitting; and

3 The current level of consumption.

This should include asking about when was the last time they had "even a sip" to drink. To aid in this process, the examiner may use additional tools such as the Alcohol Time Line Follow Back (TLFB) [15]. The TLFB is a retrospective measure of alcohol use that is used to provide improved recall of quantity and frequency of drinking. Studies show that it has excellent reliability and validity for recall of up to 3 months. The TLFB uses an event calendar on which specific anchor points (e.g. holidays, birthdays, special occasions) are identified that assist in the patient's recall of events. The type and amount of alcohol consumed is noted on the calendar for each day of the recall period. Consumption should be measured in specific amounts (i.e. number of drinks and type of drink consumed). Dividing intake into amounts consumed per type of beverage (beer, wine, liquor) has been shown to result in a higher reported intake [16]. In the United States, a standard drink is ~14 g for a 12-oz beer, 8 oz of wine or 1 oz of hard liquor; however, in the United Kingdom, a standard drink is referred to as a "unit" and is 10 mL (~7.9 g) of EToH [17]. Remember to quantify the size of a can of beer (12, 16, 22, or 40 oz in the United States), or if it was beer with a high alcohol content per volume (malt liquor). If patients have difficulty quantifying their drinking, suggesting an amount may be useful. If the interviewer begins with a large amount, patients may feel more comfortable admitting to heavier use. For example, "When was the heaviest drinking period of your life?" "At your heaviest, could you drink a case of beer per day" (there are 24 12-oz beers in a case in the United States) or "How many 12 packs of beer do you think you could drink in a day?" The patient will either be able to answer this question with a number or he or she may balk at the large amount proposed. If the latter occurs, follow up by asking the patient "Well, how long would a 12-pack (or bottle of wine or fifth of a gallon of liquor ~750 mL) last then?" This tactic may aid the patient in being able to more easily quantify his or her intake or at least place it on a comparable scale. A follow-up question may be, "Was there ever a time in the past when you could finish off 12–18 beers in a single sitting?" This allows the patient to more easily admit to excessive drinking in the past since he or she may feel that his or her most recent intake was much lower.

This may be a good time to ask patients if anyone ever suggested they "cut down" on their drinking?

Frequently, they did so because they were told to by their physicians, and once they did cut back for a period of time, nearly all will have returned to their previous level of consumption. In the mind of the alcoholic, this will translate to "Yes, I did cut down for a period of time and because I was able to do that, I don't have a drinking problem." Patients with liver disease must never be advised to simply "cut down." The very nature of alcohol dependence is the inability to control the substance. Physicians must not be ambiguous; the key to recovery is total abstinence. Patients need to hear that if they do not stop drinking now, they may very well die in the very near future. When the physician provides a stern and dire warning, it may be the only way to get past a patient's deeply entrenched denial. Nevertheless, education alone, even if it contains information about a life-threatening condition, is rarely sufficient to permanently stop alcohol consumption. Most patients require a formal addiction treatment program (see Chapter 18).

Patients will sometimes admit to drinking nonalcoholic beer or wine, or ask permission to do so. Addiction specialists should probe patients' motivations for drinking these beverages and explain to them that they do contain alcohol (0.05% per bottle of nonalcoholic beer). Patients should be advised not to drink them and that consuming them may lead them to relapse.

Treatment history

Once a timeline for alcohol intake has been established, it is important to identify whether the patient was able to achieve periods of sobriety. For a given period of sobriety, it is important to follow up with what led the patient to seek sobriety – threat of impending divorce, job loss, health issues, prison sentence, etc. How did the patient achieve sobriety? Did the patient quit "cold turkey" or was he or she involved in a formal inpatient or outpatient program? Did he or she attend AA meetings? If he or she did attend any form of treatment, was it court ordered or volitional, and was the patient able to complete the program he or she started? If the patient left the program prior to completing it, what was the reason? Specific dates for treatment should be recorded along with duration of sobriety after each treatment. Any history of psychiatric care, whether it was inpatient, outpatient, or medication prescribed by the family doctor, should also be noted.

Psychosocial functioning

A psychosocial history is integral to the alcohol intake assessment and may provide clues to the accuracy of the patient's self-report of his or her alcohol use. Certain jobs (e.g. bartender, restaurant owner) may lend to a higher propensity to drink in the workplace. Reviewing past relationships may also aid in identifying problematic drinking. Divorces, separations, and estrangement from family members may signal ways in which alcohol use interfered with patients' social obligations. Because poorer social support has been shown to be a predictor of relapse [10], patients who live alone, especially those who live in isolated areas, should raise concern. If patients do not live alone, the interviewer should ask about whether their current support person drinks alcohol and how they truly feel about that. In a recent psychiatric interview, a patient said that he felt very vulnerable when going to pick up his wife when she was drinking at the bar they used to drink in together. Patients must have clear strategies to stay sober in situations where they are with actively drinking family members. It may be helpful for patients to explain to their host that they will join the family for the meal, but will not come early or linger long after the meal because that is when they feel most at risk to drink. In the United Kingdom, because the pub is such a significant part of a community's culture and is so integral to people's social networks, many patients will need to develop alternatives for sober socializing. Legal history can also prove valuable; in one study by Bajaj et al. [18], of 76 liver disease patients, 22% were found to have a DUI upon review of records from the state Department of Transportation, which the patient did not report. What is more, 61% of the DUIs found occurred during the period of time for which the patients had claimed sobriety on pretransplant interview.

In addition to the above challenges, the majority of alcoholics with liver disease have quit drinking without professional treatment on their own prior to the psychiatric interview because they were too ill to keep drinking or had been told to stop by their doctors. This can result in patients' minimizing their drinking history and the effects that alcohol has played in their lives. Motivational enhancement therapy (MET) was developed as a therapeutic strategy to measure patients' motivation to accept their addiction and make changes toward lasting recovery [19]. Four distinct phases describing the degree to which patients view their alcoholism have been defined and can be measured by the Stages of Change questionnaire: the *pre-contemplation* phase is when a patient has not given much, if any thought to having an addiction problem at all; the *contemplation* phase is when patients recognize that a problem does exist, but they have not taken steps toward meaningful change; the *action* phase is when patients actively seek help for their problem, and the *maintenance* phase is when patients have reached stable sobriety and have developed methods to maintain their sobriety by attending self-help groups or another form of aftercare. A study that compared the motivational stages of change in alcoholic liver transplant candidates to a matched control group of alcoholics without liver disease found that significantly more patients in the liver transplant candidate group did not acknowledge that alcoholism was a problem for them and that they did not see the need to make changes in their lives to maintain sobriety [4]. Because liver transplant patients so often report having achieved abstinence from alcohol on their own and typically refuse formal alcoholism treatment because they feel they have "moved past it," it should be explained to them that alcohol dependence is a lifelong disease with remissions and relapses. While it is warranted to congratulate patients on their newly earned sobriety, it is even more important for them to understand how and why they must create a safety net of support they can rely upon if they find themselves craving a drink or in a social situation in which everyone is drinking and they think to themselves "One will not hurt, things are different now." They should understand that recovering from alcohol-related liver injury or transplanting their liver would not change their brain's response to losing control of their alcohol consumption. As AA teaches, "One drink is too many and 100 are not enough."

Comorbid psychiatric and substance use disorders

The psychiatric interviewer must also probe into the existence of comorbid psychiatric and substance use disorders, including nicotine dependence. Studies show that 80–95% of alcoholics smoke [20], and those with untreated anxiety and depressive disorders are even less likely to quit smoking successfully [21,22]. Given that smoking and ongoing untreated psychiatric illness can be associated with a greater risk of alcohol relapse, the implications for seeking appropriate treatment is crucial. Similarly, untreated substance use disorders, such as marijuana or opiates, can also lead to higher rates of alcohol relapse.

Collateral interview

In addition to interviewing the patient, inviting a collateral to the interview is vital to obtaining an accurate history and confirming consumption patterns and dates of last use. Meeting a family member or friend who is familiar with the patient or resides with the patient can be very informative when evaluating the patient's psychosocial support network. It cannot be overemphasized how helpful family members are in pointing out a more accurate account of how harmful the effects of the patient's drinking was to them, and to the family.

Use of laboratory testing

The veracity of evaluating alcohol intake and current sobriety by patient self-report is controversial. A meta-analysis by Dew et al. [10] demonstrated that studies relying on self-reports of alcohol use after transplantation are just as likely to identify alcohol use as studies using other methods. By contrast, Hempel et al. [23] published a study in which 35% of patients had a positive serum biomarker of recent alcohol use (methanol), compared with only 3% who were identified by standard serum blood alcohol levels or verbal reports. For interested readers, DiMartini and Dew [24] published an editorial response to the Hempel paper in which they provided an excellent review of methods to monitor alcohol use in transplant patients. They suggest that the optimal therapeutic approach to garner the greatest likelihood of patient candor is to conduct regular interviews and random biologic measures by a team not connected to the transplant team. The highest yield would come from a combination of those two methods and the report from an independent caregiver.

Specific biologic tests for recent alcohol use such as blood ethanol levels, breathalyzer testing, methanol levels, carbohydrate-deficient transferase (CDT), gamma-glutamyl transferase (GGT), ethyl glucuronide (EtG), and ethyl sulfate (EtS), or combinations of these tests, can be useful. More details regarding these and other specific tests are described in Chapter 13.

Use of structured assessment tools

While various structured assessment tools that can aid in the evaluation of transplant candidates with psychiatric or addiction histories exist and are in use in some programs, we did not addressed them in detail here because the older instruments, such as the High Risk Alcohol Relapse (HRAR) scale [25] and Transplant Evaluation Rating Scale (TERS) [26] do not have convincing data suggesting that they are more effective at predicting poor psychosocial outcomes in liver transplant patients than a thorough psychiatric interview. The most recently studied instrument is the Stanford Integrated Psychosocial Assessment for Transplantation (SIPAT) [27]. The SIPAT is a comprehensive screening instrument that can be administered by psychiatrists, psychologists, and social workers to assess psychosocial history and functioning to predict adverse post-transplant outcomes. Maldonado et al. [27] found that SIPAT scores were predictive of transplant psychosocial outcomes and had excellent inter-rater reliability. The SIPAT can take 30–45 minutes to administer, and although preliminary results are promising, these results were based on the use of retrospective chart reviews and linked to patients' subsequent post-transplant outcomes. The investigators are currently conducting a prospective study evaluating the ability of the SIPAT to predict medical outcomes.

Conclusions

The objective of this chapter is to provide liver specialists and mental health professionals with a framework for conducting or interpreting the psychiatric assessment of patients with alcoholic liver disease. Although much of this chapter is focused on patients being considered for liver transplantation, the information provided is applicable to patients with any stage of alcohol-related liver disease. A thorough and nuanced psychiatric examination can provide transplant teams with information describing the existence and severity of risk factors that may lead to adverse medical and psychosocial outcomes, such as poor adherence to medical care, relapse to drinking, drug use, smoking, and/or depressive or anxiety disorders.

Additionally, the psychiatric evaluation of the alcoholic liver transplant patient can provide the most useful data if patients are interviewed repeatedly over time, with collateral information and random toxicology screens. Given the complexity of these patients and the limited number of skilled examiners available, the repeated interview process may not be feasible for some transplant programs. Future development of assessment tools specifically designed for the evaluation of patients with alcoholic liver disease and transplant candidates with addictions may facilitate objective data gathering.

References

[1] Kotlyar DS, Burke A, Campbell M, Weinrieb RM. A critical review of candidacy for orthotopic liver transplantation in alcoholic liver disease. *Am J Gastroenterol* 2008; **103**: 734–743.

[2] Lucey MR. Liver transplantation in patients with alcoholic liver disease. *Liver Transpl* 2011; **17**: 751–759.

[3] Weinrieb RM, Van Horn DH, Lynch KG, Lucey MR. A randomized, controlled study of treatment for alcohol dependence in patients awaiting liver transplantation. *Liver Transpl* 2011; **17**(5): 539–547.

[4] Weinrieb RM, Van Horn DH, McLellan AT, et al. Drinking behavior and motivation for treatment among alcohol dependent liver transplant candidates. *J Addict Dis* 2001; **20**(2): 101–115.

[5] DiMartini AF, Dew MA. Monitoring alcohol use on the liver transplant wait list: therapeutic and practical issues. *Liver Transpl* 2012; **18**: 1267–1269.

[6] Weinrieb R, Auriacombe J, Lynch KG, Lewis KD. Selective serontonin re-uptake inhibitors and the risk of bleeding. *Expert Opin Drug Saf* 2007; **4**(2): 337–344.

[7] Surman OS, Cosimi AB, DiMartini A. Psychiatric care of patients undergoing organ transplantation. *Transplantation* 2009; **87**(12): 1753–1761.

[8] DiMartini A, Dew MA, Day N, et al. Trajectories of alcohol consumption following liver transplantation. *Am J Transplant* 2010; **10**(10): 2305–2312.

[9] DiMartini A, Day N, Dew MA, et al. Alcohol consumption patterns and predictors of use following liver transplantation for alcoholic liver disease. *Liver Transpl* 2006; **12**(5): 813–820.

[10] Dew MA, DiMartini AF, Steel J, et al. Meta-analysis of risk for relapse to substance use after transplantation of the liver or other solid organs. *Liver Transpl* 2008; **14**(2): 159–172.

[11] Moos RH, Moos BS. Rates and predictors of relapse after natural and treated remission from alcohol use disorders. *Addiction* 2006; **101**(2): 212–222.

[12] Vaillant GE. *The Natural History of Alcoholism, Revisited.* Harvard University Press, Cambridge, MA; 1995.

[13] Tam TW, Mulia N, Schmidt LA. Applicability of type A/B alcohol dependence in the general population. *Drug Alcohol Depend* 2014; **138**: 169–176.

[14] Ewing JA. Detecting alcoholism: the CAGE questionnaire. *JAMA* 1984; **252**: 1905–1907.

[15] Sobell LC, Brown J, Leoa GI, Sobell MB. The reliability of the Alcohol Timeline Followback when administered by telephone and by computer. *Drug Alcohol Depend* 1996; **42**(1): 49–54.

[16] Feunekes GI, van't Veer P, van Staveren WA, Kok FJ. Alcohol intake assessment: the sober facts. *Am J Epidemiol* 1999; **150**(1): 105–112.

[17] Calculator for equivalent values of unit drinks. http://www.cleavebooks.co.uk/scol/ccalcoh1.htm (accessed 6 December 2014).

[18] Bajaj JS, Saeian K, Hafeezullah M, et al. Failure to fully disclose during pretransplant psychological evaluation in alcoholic liver disease: a driving under the influence corroboration study. *Liver Transpl* 2008; **14**: 1632–1636.

[19] Miller W, Zweben A, DiClemente C. Motivational enhancement therapy manual. In Mattson ME, ed. *Project Match Monograph Series*, Vol. **2**, DHHS No. 92–1894, Rockville, MD; 1992, 1–121.

[20] Patten CA, Martin JE, Owen, N. Can psychiatric and chemical dependency treatment units be smoke free? *J Subst Abuse Treat* 1996; **13**(2): 107–118.

[21] Cinciripini PM, Wetter DW, Fouladi RT, et al. The effects of depressed mood on smoking cessation: mediation by postcessation self-efficacy. *J Consult Clin Psychol* 2003; **71**(2): 292–301.

[22] Ziedonis D, Hitsman B, Beckham JC, et al. Tobacco use and cessation in psychiatric disorders: National Institute of Mental Health report. *Nicotine Tob Res* 2008; **10**(12): 1691–1715.

[23] Hempel JM, Greif-Higer G, Kaufmann T, Beutel ME. Detection of alcohol consumption in patients with alcoholic liver cirrhosis during the evaluation process for liver transplantation. *Liver Transpl* 2012; **18**(11): 1310–1315.

[24] DiMartini AF, Dew MA. Monitoring alcohol use on the liver transplant wait list: therapeutic and practical issues [Editorial]. *Liver Transpl* 2012; **18**(11): 1267–1269.

[25] De Gottardi A, Spahr L, Gelez P, et al. A simple score for predicting alcohol relapse after liver transplantation results from 387 patients over 15 years. *Arch Intern Med* 2007; **167**: 1183–1188.

[26] Twillman RK, Manetto C, Wellisch DK, Wolcott DL. The transplant evaluation rating scale a revision of the psychosocial levels system for evaluating organ transplant candidates. *Psychosomatics* 1993; **34**(2): 144–153.

[27] Maldonado JR, Dubois HC, David EE, et al. The Stanford Integrated Psychosocial Assessment for Transplantation (SIPAT): a new tool for the psychosocial evaluation of pretransplant candidates. *Psychosomatics* 2012; **53**: 123–132.

CHAPTER 12

Abnormal liver tests in the context of alcohol excess

James Ferguson

Liver Unit, Queen Elizabeth Hospital Birmingham, Birmingham, UK

KEY POINTS

- Abnormal liver function test results are common in asymptomatic individuals and often no cause is found.
- Despite the term liver function test, this does not actually measure liver function.
- Gamma-glutamyl transpetidase activity can be raised secondary to alcohol excess but can also be high as a result of other causes.
- An aspartate aminotransferase : alanine aminotransferase ratio of greater than 2 : 1 can suggest liver disease secondary to alcohol.
- Plasma bilirubin is raised in alcoholic hepatitis and can be very high in severe cases.
- Clinical history is more useful than laboratory findings in detecting individuals drinking alcohol to excess.

Liver function tests

This broad term describes a group of tests used in clinical practice to identify liver disease, understand the cause of jaundice, to follow the course of an illness longitudinally, and detect toxicity secondary to medications. Despite the name, a number of these tests do not measure liver function and can be affected by a number of factors outside the liver. The tests usually include:

- *Transaminases:* aspartate aminotransferase (AST), alanine aminotransferase (ALT) increased secondary to damage to hepatocytes;
- *Bilirubin:* a measure of hepatic transport;
- *Alkaline phosphatase* (ALP): increased in biliary obstruction;
- *Gamma-glutamyl transpeptidase* (GGT): increased in biliary obstruction and alcohol excess; and

- *Albumin:* a major protein synthesized by the liver. A low albumin is a feature of advanced liver disease.

As with all tests, defining what is normal is difficult. Values in well people are not distributed normally and can be affected by age, sex, ethnicity, and body mass. Therefore a healthy person may have an abnormal liver test result. Furthermore, although liver tests do accurately reflect severe disease they may not reveal mild or moderate abnormalities. It is well described that patients with steatosis or hepatitis C may have normal liver test results.

Transaminases (ALT and AST)

Both ALT and AST are widely used in the diagnosis of liver disease. ALT is found within the liver but despite being widely distributed within the rest of the human

---

Alcohol Abuse and Liver Disease, First Edition. Edited by James Neuberger and Andrea DiMartini.

© 2015 John Wiley & Sons, Ltd. Published 2015 by John Wiley & Sons, Ltd.

body it is specific for liver disease because of its low activity in other organs. AST is present in large amounts in the liver and heart and to a lesser extent in the pancreas, brain, skeletal muscle, and red blood cells. Both enzymes are normally present within the serum. Serum AST may also be derived from mitochondria (mAST) and high levels of mAST may be seen in liver damage from alcohol.

Acute liver injury irrespective of the cause leads to a rise in transaminases. Very high concentrations (200-fold or more) are seen in paracetemol poisoning, shock, and severe hypoxia. The ratio of AST : ALT can also give helpful clues to the etiology of liver disease. An AST : ALT ratio of greater than 2 : 1 can suggest alcoholic liver disease, whereas a ratio of less than 1 is more typical of nonalcoholic fatty liver disease or viral hepatitis.

Bilirubin

Bilirubin is derived from heme. The majority (75%) of heme comes from the breakdown of mature red blood cells. Initially, bilirubin is unconjugated and insoluble in water. It is transported in the blood bound to albumin. It then enters the liver where it is metabolized and excreted in a water-soluble form in the bile. Normal serum contains bilirubin that is almost entirely unconjugated. Men tend to have higher concentrations than women.

A common cause of an isolated raised bilirubin (unconjugated) is the benign condition Gilbert's syndrome, usually diagnosed on the basis of the demonstration of a raised unconjugated serum bilirubin in the absence of hemolysis as shown by normal reticulocyte count and haptoglobin: Gilbert's syndrome may be confirmed by genetic testing showing increased TATA repeats. Increased hemolysis may be seen in association with alcohol excess as well as many other causes.

Jaundice is said to be clinically recognizable with serum bilirubin levels exceeding 35 µmol/L but in practice this is less simple. In those with established liver disease, the degree of elevation of serum bilirubin due to hemolysis is usually greater than normally seen.

The causes of a raised bilirubin are numerous but can be broadly broken down into the following groups:
- Unconjugated:
  ○ Increased bilirubin production;
  ○ Failure of bilirubin transport.

- Conjugated:
  ○ Failure of bilirubin transport;
  ○ Hepatocellular damage;
  ○ Biliary obstruction.

Alkaline phosphatase

ALP is normally present in the serum with the majority coming from liver, bone, and small intestine. During pregnancy (from week 8 onwards) the placenta produces ALP and by term concentrations may reach two times normal. Increased activity due to disease is predominantly caused by either liver or bone disease. Biliary obstruction leads to the increased production of ALP irrespective of the site of obstruction. In bone disease the increase is secondary to osteoblastic activity in diseases such as Paget's, metastases, and osteomalacia. Classically, ALP has been used in liver disease to differentiate acute hepatitis from biliary obstruction in cases of jaundice.

Gamma-glutamyl transpeptidase

GGT is present in the serum and widely distributed in the body. Within the liver it is found in the hepatocytes and biliary epithelium. In the clinical setting it is used to detect biliary disease and alcohol excess. In the context of biliary disease it gives no indication of the site of biliary obstruction.

Increased GGT activity is often used to detect the abuse of alcohol. However, it is important to note that GGT does not rise in one-third of heavy drinkers and raised activity can be secondary to many other causes. It can increase in relation to liver disease, the administration of certain drugs, and extrahepatic diseases such as pneumonia and pancreatitis. GGT activity is also raised in men, the obese, and the elderly. Where brought about by alcohol excess, levels of GGT usually normalize with alcohol cessation within 3 months unless there is underlying liver disease.

Albumin

Albumin is the major protein synthesized by the liver. Nutrition, liver function, and hormonal changes impact on its production. Its two main functions are maintaining colloid pressure and carrying substances in the blood such as hormones and drugs.

A low albumin is a feature of advanced chronic liver disease. This is related to a reduced rate of albumin synthesis by the injured liver. Of note, a reduced albumin is associated with a poor prognosis in patients with cirrhosis.

Patterns of liver function tests in alcoholic liver disease

Alcohol excess

Serum GGT activity is a widely used marker of alcohol abuse. Its use can supplement the alcohol history but it is not a specific test for alcohol excess. GGT activity can be increased for other reasons than alcohol excess including certain drugs, hyperlipidemia, and as a normal variant in the healthy population.

Consistent heavy drinking leads to a raised GGT whereas a single episode of heavy alcohol intake does not increase GGT activity. An increase of two- to four-fold in GGT is often observed in heavy alcohol users but it can rise to 20 times the upper limit of normal. Serum activity can take 1–2 months to fall after abstinence commences.

Some papers have reported the effect of combining several measurements to improve the diagnostic accuracy of laboratory tests to diagnosis individuals drinking to excess. These models have combined GGT, ALP, and erythrocyte macrocytosis. Although they have demonstrated an improved accuracy over one single test they are relatively insensitive in screening well individuals. Clinical history is more useful than laboratory findings in detecting individuals drinking alcohol to excess [1].

Alcoholic steatosis

The presence of fat within the liver (steatosis) is the most common form of liver disease related to alcohol. Patients may present with a tender, enlarged liver but it is most commonly asymptomatic. It is often associated with a raised GGT and an AST : ALT ratio of >2 : 1. Tests of synthetic function (albumin, prothrombin time) are normal. Steatosis will usually resolve within months of abstinence and the associated abnormalities in liver tests should return to normal.

Alcoholic hepatitis

Alcoholic hepatitis is serious condition and carries a substantial mortality, 40% in its severe form [2]. Most patients will have drunk heavily for some time and not uncommonly the patient will have stopped drinking prior to the onset of symptoms. It presents with jaundice, weight loss, and signs of liver failure. A fever is common and can be associated with a raised neutrophil count. The plasma bilirubin is raised and can be higher than 500 mmol/L (29 mg/dL) in very severe cases. Aminotransferases are only moderately raised and rarely more than four times the upper limit of normal [3]. Alkaline phosphatase is only moderately elevated. Plasma albumin is often low, reflecting poor synthesis function and in some cases poor nutrition. Lastly, a coagulopathy is common, representing synthetic failure and demonstrated by a raised prothrombin time.

Cirrhosis of the liver secondary to alcohol excess

Cirrhosis occurs in the context of long-term alcohol excess. It is characterized by the replacement of healthy liver tissue by scar tissue and regenerative nodules. This change in architecture leads to changes in function. In its early stages patients may be asymptomatic and liver test results may be normal [4]. As the disease progresses tests can indicate signs of impaired liver function including a raised bilirubin, prothrombin time, and a decreased plasma albumin.

The most effective treatment is abstinence and impaired liver function can improve even in advanced cases of liver cirrhosis.

Liver function tests in asymptomatic individuals

Liver function tests are common tests and can indicate serious disease. However, many individuals with abnormal liver tests will not have a particular disease process. In a study examining liver function tests in a UK primary care setting, 40% of patients who underwent testing had abnormalities found in one or more analyate [5]. GGT was the most frequently found abnormal test. Despite extensive investigation with history, blood tests, and imaging, no cause could be found in 45% of individuals.

References

[1] Skinner HA, Holt S, Sheu WJ, Israel Y. Clinical versus laboratory detection of alcohol abuse: the alcohol clinical index. *BMJ* 1986; **292**: 1703–1708.

[2] Lucey M, Mathurin P, Morgan T. Alcoholic hepatitis. *N Engl J Med* 2009; **360**: 2758–2769.

[3] Furlop M, Katz S, Lawrence C. Extreme hyperbilirubinaemia. *JAMA* 1971; **127**: 254–258.

[4] Walsh K, Alexander G. Alcoholic liver disease. *Postgrad Med J* 2000; **76**: 280–286.

[5] Armstrong M, Houlihan D, Bentham L, et al. Presence and severity of non-alcoholic fatty liver disease in a large prospective primary care cohort. *J Hepatol* 2012; **56**(1): 234–240.

CHAPTER 13

Biochemical determination of alcohol consumption

Friedrich Martin Wurst*,[1,2] Natasha Thon*,[3] Wolfgang Weinmann,[4] Michel Yegles,[5] Jessica Wong,[6] and Ulrich W. Preuss[6,7]

[1] Paracelsus Medical University (PMU), Salzburg, Austria

[2] Centre for Interdisciplinary Addiction Research, University of Hamburg, Germany

[3] Department for Psychiatry and Psychotherapy II, Christian–Doppler Hospital, Paracelsus Medical University (PMU), Salzburg, Austria

[4] Institute of Forensic Medicine, University of Berne, Switzerland

[5] Laboratoire National de Santé, Division de Toxicologie, Centre Universitaire Luxembourg, Luxembourg

[6] Kreiskrankenhaus Prignitz, Perleberg, Germany

[7] Department of Psychiatry, Psychotherapy and Psychosomatic Medicine, University of Halle, Germany

KEY POINTS

- Indirect serum markers of alcohol consumption include gamma-glutamyl transpeptidase (GGT), red cell mean corpuscular volume, and carbohydrate deficiency transferrin (CDT). These are influenced by age, gender, other toxins, and non-alcohol-related diseases, or a combination of these.

- Combinations of markers such as the Antilla Index using CDT and GGT allow detection of regular and longer term (days, weeks) alcohol consumption.

- Ethanol metabolites, such as ethyl glucuronide (EtG), phosphatidylethanol (PEth), and fatty acid ethyl esters in blood, serum, and hair, are being used increasingly as markers of recent alcohol use.

- Urinary levels of EtG are most useful for assessing recent ethanol intake, and PEth and ethyl glucuronide in hair for longer term ethanol consumption.

Introduction

Alcohol use disorders (AUD) are among the top ten of the most common diseases worldwide. AUD are common, expensive in their course, and often under diagnosed. According to the WHO Global Status Report on Alcohol, approximately 4% of deaths worldwide are attributable to alcohol – more deaths than caused by HIV, violence, or tuberculosis. To facilitate early diagnosis and therapy of alcohol-related disorders and prevent secondary complications, questionnaires like the Alcohol Use Disorders Identification Test (AUDIT) and biomarkers are useful.

Both indirect and direct state markers are routinely used to detect alcohol. The indirect state markers such as gamma-glutamyl transpeptidase (GGT), mean corpuscular volume (MCV), and carbohydrate deficiency transferrin (CDT) are influenced by age, gender, various substances, and non-alcohol-related illnesses, and do not cover the entire timeline for alcohol consumption.

*Both the authors have contributed equally.

Ethanol metabolites have gained interest in recent decades as they are metabolites of alcohol that become positive in the presence of alcohol. As biomarkers with high sensitivity and specificity covering the complementary timeline, they are routinely applied and contribute to new perspectives in prevention, interdisciplinary cooperation, diagnosis, and therapy of alcohol-related disorders [1].

Traditional biomarkers for alcohol consumption

Many clinical–chemical parameters show pathologic changes as evidence of the biochemical burden of ethanol metabolism. Evidence of long-term alcohol consumption can be obtained from these state markers, especially when using a combination of several individual indicators.

Gamma-glutamyl transferase

A well-known, inexpensive, and widely used biomarker is the membrane bound glycoprotein enzyme GGT which occurs ubiquitously in the organism, but mainly in liver, pancreas, and renal proximal tubules. GGT detectable in serum arises mainly from the liver so that an increase in serum enzyme activity would be a sensitive indicator for hepatobiliary disease. Chronic alcohol consumption induces an increase in enzyme synthesis and, through direct activation of the enzyme from membrane binding, leads to increased levels of GGT in serum which indicates chronic alcoholic hepatitis [2]. To exceed normal values (4–18 U/L in women and 6–28 U/L in men) requires chronic, daily alcohol intake over at least 4–6 weeks while this does not occur in a short-term, higher alcohol burden [3].

The sensitivity of GGT varies, according to age, gender, and body weight, from 35% to 85% [4]. Contrarily, in young adults less than 30 years, even when they are alcohol dependent, the sensitivity of the markers is very low. Other studies have reported that GGT levels can also be increased by various other causes, such as obesity (BMI >35), the effects of medication and teratogens, adiposities, diabetes, cholestatic or inflammatory liver diseases [4]. Accordingly, the specificity of 63–85% is not satisfactory and using GGT as the sole

indicator of chronic alcohol use and current liver disease is not practical [2].

Mean corpuscular erythrocyte volume

Measurement of the MCV is common in standard investigations; an increase occurs in 4% of the general population and in 40–60% of patients with alcohol misuse [4]. A marked dose-dependent relationship between MCV and the intensity of alcohol consumption has been reported. Increase in MCV is to be expected in long-term alcohol consumption and the values normalize slowly during abstinence over a period of 2–4 months. Compared with GGT, the sensitivity of MCV in screening for alcohol misuse, at least in men, is inferior. In interpreting MCV values, other causes such as vitamin B_{12} or folic deficiency, non-alcoholic liver diseases, reticulocytosis, and hematologic diseases should be considered.

The mechanism responsible for an increase in MCV is unclear. Direct hematotoxic damage or interaction of ethanol and its metabolites, especially acetaldehyde, with the erythrocyte membrane, have been suggested [2].

Carbohydrate deficient transferrin

The most important iron transport molecule in humans is transferrin. Its synthesis and glycolization occur in hepatocytes. Isoforms of CDT can be differentiated by measurement of isoelectric points (pI), where values depend on the load of bound iron ions and number of sialin acid residuals in carbohydrate chains [3]. Stibler and Kjellin found abnormal isoforms with much increased pI-values over 5.65 in the serum of alcohol-dependent patients, and traced this back to low levels of bound sialin acid residuals. In subsequent investigations, all abnormal isoforms were included as CDT and all isoforms are increased in those with chronic alcohol intake [3].

The underlying pathogenetic mechanism for CDT formation is not fully understood but may be related to inhibition of intracellular transmission of carbohydrates to transferring its toxic effects from ethanol or acetyldehyde as well as the effect of ethanol on the activities of membrane-bound sialine transferases and plasma sialidases in hepatocytes [3].

In earlier studies, there was no consensus on the correlation between CDT concentrations in serum and the amount of alcohol consumed; however, an increase in CDT with daily consumption of 60–80 g alcohol over 7 days has been reported in some but not all studies [3].

The clinical usefulness of CDT as a biomarker varies depending on gender, BMI, age, nicotine abuse, and anorexia. CDT is a more sensitive indicator for alcohol-related diseases in men than women. Among the various conventional alcohol markers, CDT is currently considered the most useful and significant indicator [4]. Information on sensitivity and specificity varies, because no methodical standardization exists. Furthermore, the heterogeneity of test populations concerning age, gender, alcohol consumption, duration of abstinence before serum extraction as well as current liver diseases makes the comparison with other traditional markers difficult. In selected clinical patient groups, various test methods with specificity of 90–100% and high sensitivity (50–90%) were reported [3].

Most patients with liver diseases have only marginally raised CDT levels so that the specificity, especially in comparison with other markers, is high and usually >90%. Thus, CDT could be used for detection of chronic alcohol consumption and changes in drinking patterns in these patients. With a half-life of 14 days and normalization of CDT values with abstinence, evidence of drinking relapses in the post-acute phase after alcohol withdrawal treatment can be obtained [3].

Serum transaminases

Increases in levels of aspartate aminotransferase (AST) and alanine aminotransferase (ALT) in serum are nonspecific markers of hepatocellular damage. While AST is produced in many cells including hepatocytes and both skeletal and cardiac muscle cells, ALT is a liver-specific enzyme. Thus, an increase in ALT strongly indicates liver diseases (fatty degeneration, tumors, metastases, cirrhosis, cholangitis). By contrast, measurements of AST must differentiate between the alcohol sensitive, mitochondrial (m-AST) and the cytoplasmic isoform (c-AST). An increased m-AST : c-AST ratio strongly suggests alcohol-related liver damage. Increased AST values are found in 39–47% of alcohol-dependent patients [2]. Thus, measurements of the De Ritis quotient (AST : ALT) increase the alcohol

specificity of both markers – a ratio > 1 strongly suggests an alcohol-related etiology [3].

In summary, the sensitivity and specificity of both enzymes as indicators for alcohol misuse are considered variable so that an interpretation of an increased serum activity is mainly meaningful in the context of other liver values (bilirubin, alkaline phosphatase, GGT).

Combination of individual markers

Combinations of markers may be helpful. The more frequently used combinations comprise CDT, GGT, MCV, and AST.

Gamma-glutamyl transferase and carbohydrate deficient transferrin

Some studies showed that the combined use of GGT and CDT resulted in higher sensitivity and specificity compared to use of either one alone [3]. Sillanaukee et al. [5] reported a sensitivity of 75% and specificity of 93% for γ-CDT. γ-CDT is estimated using the formula [γ-CDT = 0.8 ln(GGT)+1.3 ln (CDT)], the Antilla Index.

Values for γ-CDT correlate to current levels of consumption, regardless of whether a heavily alcohol-dependent individual or an occasional drinker was tested. γ-CDT can thus be used to monitor abstinence, though in continuing abstinence the values normalize within 2–3 weeks.

Alc-index

Brinkmann et al. [6] developed the Alc-index to differentiate between alcohol-dependent patients and non-drinkers by combining methanol, aceton/isopropanol, GGT, and CDT in a logistic regression formula. The basic principle for the investigations was the hypothesis that each of these alcohol markers shows overlap in values in the collective with none or low alcohol consumption and alcoholics. From the results, an Alc-index of 1.7 as cutoff was defined with a specificity of 100% and a sensitivity of 90% to differentiate between alcohol-dependent and nonalcohol-dependent individuals. The advantage of this index is the single cutoff point instead of four individual markers, and drawing false conclusions based on raised values of an isolated marker is prevented.

> **Key points**
>
> - Traditional biomarkers have various limitations besides clear advantages such as practicability and cost efficiency.
>
> - A combination (such as the Antilla Index) of various laboratory parameters (such as CDT and GGT) allows sufficient inference on regular, even longer term (days, weeks) alcohol consumption.
>
> - The diagnostic sensitivity of individual parameters, such as AST or ALT, is low, the specificity is moderately high, with the exception of CDT which shows moderate sensitivity and high specificity to differentiate between alcohol-dependent individuals and control persons.
>
> - The strengths of these traditional markers in routine practice lies in their practicability and, with the exception of CDT, cost-effectiveness.
>
> - Normalization of CDT occurs only after weeks or months of abstinence so that inference of current or short-term recent alcohol consumption can be made.

Ethanol metabolites

Ethanol metabolites are formed in the presence of alcohol, are minor pathways of ethanol elimination, and cover different time frames of detection. Routinely measured ethanol metabolites are as follow:
- Ethyl glucuronide (EtG) in serum, urine, and hair;
- Ethyl sulfate (EtS) in urine and serum;
- Phosphatidylethanol (PEth) in whole blood; and
- Fatty acid ethyl ester (FAEE) especially in hair.

The abovementioned ethanol metabolites are detectable in serum for hours, in urine for up to 7 days, in whole blood over 2 weeks, and in hair over months [7–9].

Blood and urine analysis
Ethyl glucuronide

EtG is a phase II metabolite of ethanol and has a molecular weight of 222 g/mol. It is metabolized by the UDP-glucuronosyl transferase. Whereas EtG is not of relevance for alcohol elimination as it is less than 0.1%, it is a useful biomarker, detectable during or after the ingestion of ethanol. EtG is nonvolatile, water-soluble, stable in storage and can, depending on the amount consumed and the duration of consumption, still be detectable in the body long after completion of alcohol elimination. EtG can be detected in urine up to 90 hours following ingestion [10]. There is no difference between the elimination rate in the healthy population and heavy alcohol consumers at the beginning of detoxification treatment.

Ethyl glucuronide can also be detected in postmortem body fluids and tissues such as gluteal and abdominal fat, liver, brain, cerebrospinal fluid and bone marrow and muscle tissue.

Experiments with 1 g ethanol (taken as champagne, whisky) as well as mouthwash and hand sanitizer gels found EtG concentrations of <1 mg/L in urine. Measurable concentrations in urine were found for up to 11 hours. This aspect is of relevance regarding unintentional exposure of alcohol: sweets (such as pralines), nonalcoholic beer, pharmaceutical products, fruit juice, sauerkraut, mouthwash products, and hand sanitizer gels may contain small amounts of alcohol. Even the intake of 21–42 g yeast with approximately 50 g sugar leads to measureable EtG and EtS concentrations in urine.

A patient's claim of not having consumed alcohol may therefore be true even when EtG is detectable in urine. As patients in withdrawal treatment should avoid even the smallest amount of alcohol, they have to be informed of such hidden sources of ethanol to avoid unintentional alcohol intake. A differential cutoff of 0.1 mg/L in cases where total abstinence is the goal, and 1.0 mg/L if small amounts of alcohol intake are tolerated, have been recommended for practical reasons. The use of EtG in different settings and with different patients has been proven to be practical and beneficial by various studies. EtG determination can be applied in for example high-risk groups as patients in opioid maintenance therapy, monitoring programs as the Physician Health Programs in the United States or pharmacotherapeutic studies. The use of ethanol metabolites allows more possibilities for therapeutic interventions, consequently leading to an improvement in quality of life.

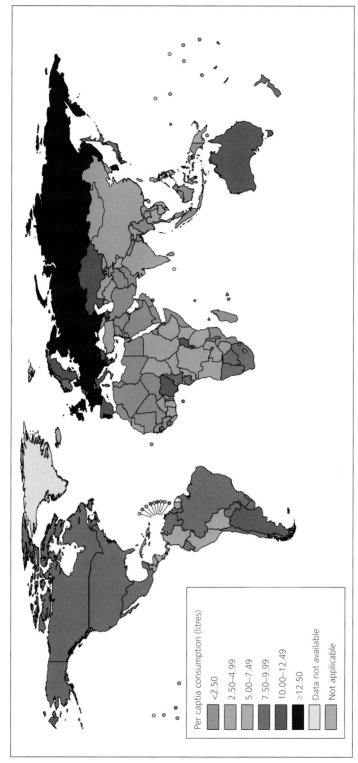

Figure 1.1 Liters of pure alcohol consumed per person aged 15+, from both regulated and unregulated production, 2005. (Source: World Health Organization, 2011 [3])

Per capita consumption (litres)
- <2.50
- 2.50–4.99
- 5.00–7.49
- 7.50–9.99
- 10.00–12.49
- ≥12.50
- Data not available
- Not applicable

Alcohol Abuse and Liver Disease, First Edition. Edited by James Neuberger and Andrea DiMartini.
© 2015 John Wiley & Sons, Ltd. Published 2015 by John Wiley & Sons, Ltd.

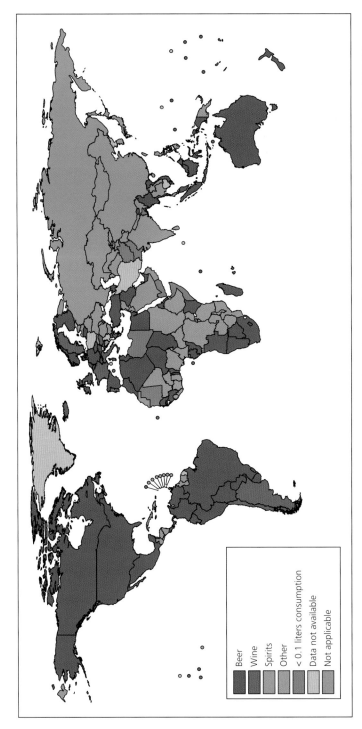

Figure 1.2 Most consumed alcoholic beverages from regulated production in liters of pure alcohol, 2005. (Source: World Health Organization, 2011 [3])

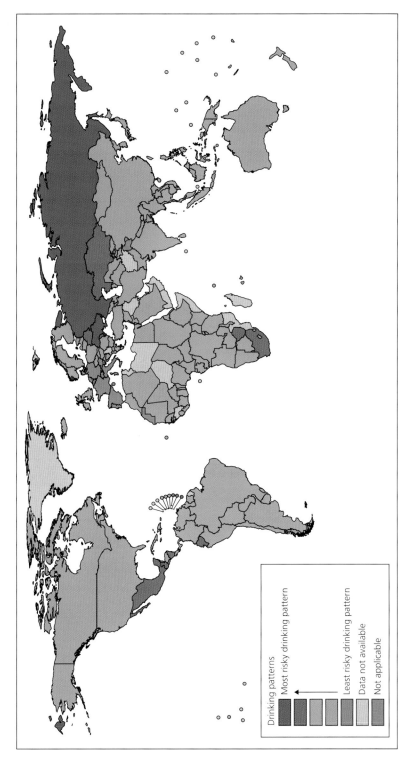

Figure 1.7 Patterns of drinking score, 2005. (Source: World Health Organization, 2011 [3])

Drinking patterns

Most risky drinking pattern

Least risky drinking pattern

Data not available

Not applicable

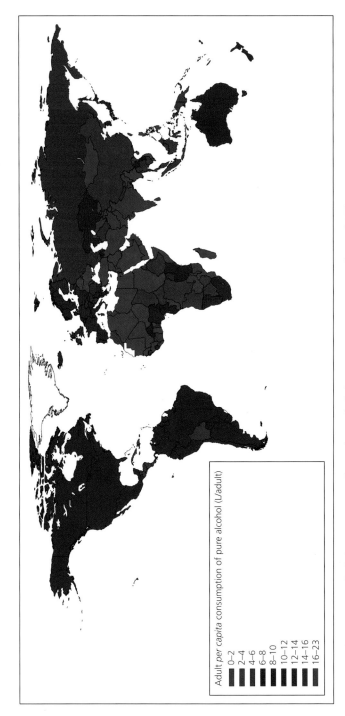

Adult *per capita* consumption of pure alcohol (L/adult)

0–2
2–4
4–6
6–8
8–10
10–12
12–14
14–16
16–23

Figure 2.2 Adult *per capita* alcohol consumption in liters of pure alcohol per year, 2010. (Source: Rehm et al. [8])

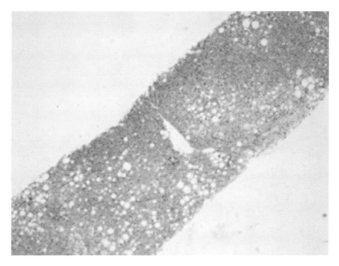

Figure 8.2 Steatosis. Hepatocytes show typical large vacuoles seen in macrovesicular steatosis.

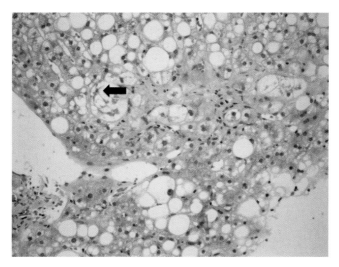

Figure 8.3 Alcoholic hepatitis. The arrow shows a hepatocyte undergoing ballooning degeneration with evidence of Mallory's hyaline accumulation.

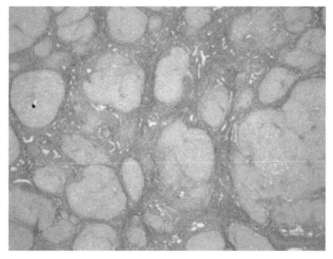

Figure 8.4 Cirrhosis. The liver architecture is disrupted with nodules separated by thick fibrous septa.

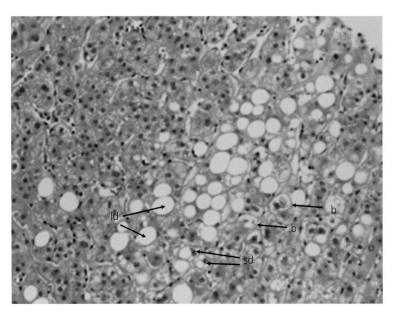

Figure 14.1 Hematoxylin and eosin (H&E) stained section of liver with steatohepatitis. Hepatocyte cytoplasm stains pink, nuclei purple, and fat droplets are clear holes (arrows) as the fat has leached out during processing. A mixture of large (ld) and small (sd) macrovesicular fat is present. The hepatocyte nuclei are pushed to the edge of the cell in large droplets, while they remain central surrounded by variable numbers of smaller vacuoles in small droplet macrovesicular steatosis. Several probably ballooned hepatocytes (b) are present, containing wispy pink Mallory–Denk bodies. Inflammation is minimal, seen as dark blue dots, with morphology of lymphocytes.

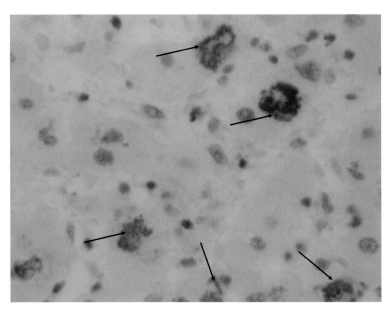

Figure 14.2 Ubiquitin immunostain highlighting Mallory–Denk bodies (MDBs) which are seen as brown wispy material in the hepatocyte cytoplasm (arrows).

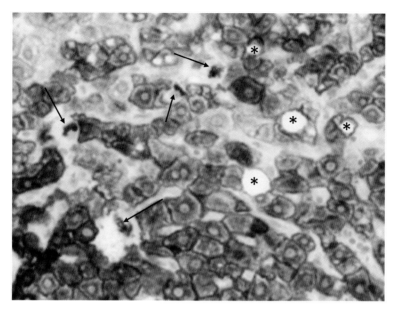

Figure 14.3 Pancytokeratin immunostain which contains cytokeratin 8 and 18. The normal hepatocytes show diffuse brown staining of the cytoplasm with a distinct cell membrane. The ballooned hepatocytes have lost both the diffuse cytoplasmic and membranous staining and contain a clumped brown Mallory–Denk body (arrows). Fat droplets are seen as clear holes (*) within the cytoplasm of some hepatocytes.

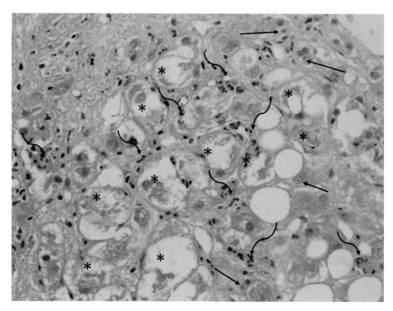

Figure 14.4 Hematoxylin and eosin (H&E) stained section of liver with acute alcoholic hepatitis. There are numerous ballooned hepatocytes (*) containing Mallory–Denk bodies associated with a conspicuous neutrophilic infiltrate (squiggly arrows). Occassional bile plugs (arrows) are present.

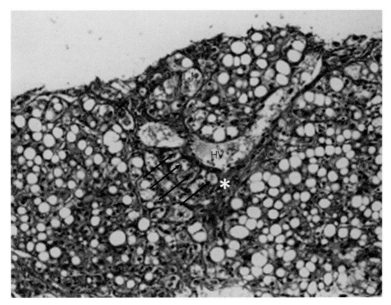

Figure 14.5 Elastic hematoxylin van Gieson (EHVG) stain showing pericellular fibrosis in zone 3. The collagen stains dark pink. Hepatocyte cytoplasm yellow–brown. Fat are clear vacuoles. Arrows point to several hepatocytes surrounded by delicate fibrous tissue. A degree of central hyaline sclerosis (*) is seen adjacent to a hepatic vein (HV).

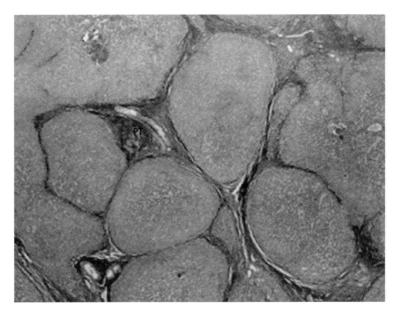

Figure 14.6 Elastic hematoxylin van Gieson (EHVG) stain demonstrating severe fibrosis amounting to established cirrhosis. Islands of hepatocytes are surrounded by fibrous septa (dark pink) and the normal vascular relationships between hepatic veins and portal tracts are lost. Several portal tracts (PT) are identifiable within the fibrous septa.

Methods of determination

A EtG enzyme immunoassay (DRI-EtG EIA) is commercially available. However, in cases with medicolegal relevance, confirmation with forensic toxicologically accepted methods such as liquid chromatography–tandem mass spectrometry (LC/MS-MS) is needed. The use of penta-deuterium labeled EtG as internal standard and LC/MS-MS must be considered to be a gold standard. A simple mass spectrometry would provide less reliable evidence. EtG can also be detected in specimen of dried blood which is of relevance for forensic investigations.

Limitations

Aspects of a potential for *in vitro* formation and degradation of EtG and EtS have been investigated in recent years. Hydrolysis of EtG may occur in the context of urinary tract infections, especially by *Escherichia coli*. Complete degradation of EtG within 3–4 days by *E. coli* and *Clostridium sordellii* was confirmed, although in other contexts EtS may be stable for up to 11 days. Further studies with standardized test procedures for biodegradation showed that EtS in closed bottle test (OECD 301 D) remained stable for even longer periods whereas in the context of a higher bacterial density such as in the in the manometric respiratory test a reduction after 6 days was detected. This problem could be countered by cooling and the addition of stabilizers. A recent study also reported that the bacterial degradation of EtG by *E. coli* can be prevented by the use of dried urine spots on filter paper.

Influences on EtG levels

In the "WHO/ISBRA Study on biological state and trait markers of alcohol use and dependence," nicotine consumption, BMI, cirrhosis, and body water content had no significant influence on EtG concentrations. In contrast, EtG urine concentrations were influenced by age, gender, cannabis consumption, and renal function.

The results concerning renal and liver functions have recently been confirmed:

- In patients with reduced renal function, prolonged elimination may occur.
- In patients with liver diseases, the severity of disease had no influence on the validity of ethyl glucuronide [11].

Ethyl sulfate

EtS is a secondary elimination pathway for alcohol and is detectable in varying inter-individual concentrations. The use of rapid LC/MS-MS procedures as routinely applied allows the combined detection of EtS and EtG.

The formation of EtS is by sulfotransferase and the breakdown by sulfatases. The molecular weight is 126 g/mol and the molecular formula $C_2H_5SO_4H$.

Schneider and Glatt used 2-propylsulphate as an internal standard for a LC/MS-MS method. Helander and Beck used liquid chromatography-electro sprayionization-mass spectrometry (LC-ESI-MS) in a single-quadruple modus and D_5-ethylsulfate as internal standard for the quantification of EtS in urine samples. The disadvantage of this method is a longer period of chromatographic separation. Furthermore, the exclusive monitoring of deprotonated molecules in a single-MS does not meet forensic standards [12]. At any rate, an additional fragment ion would be required for the verification analyses according to forensic guidelines [12]. Even when this requirement from forensic guidelines must not be met in clinical diagnostics, the test remains in demand in workplace drug testing in the United States. In this context, an LC/MS-MS method with penta-deuterium EtS as internal standard and two ion transitions can be used in forensic and medicolegal cases as well as for routine clinical use.

For repeated alcohol consumption, a cutoff of 0.05 mg/L is suggested. As with EtG, there is prolonged elimination in reduced renal function.

Fatty acid ethyl esters

The existence of FAEEs, nonoxidative metabolic products of ethanol in blood and various organs with a reduced or deficient capacity to oxidize ethanol after consumption has been demonstrated. Since these esters can cause damage to subcellular structures, they were postulated to be mediators of organ damage.

Two enzymes – acyl-coenzyme a:ethanol O-acyltransferase (AEAT) and FAEE synthase – catalyze the formation of FAEE and can be isolated from rabbit myocardium, human brain, and rat fat tissue. Furthermore, pancreatic lipase, lipoprotein lipase, and glutathione transferase possess FAEE synthase activity.

In the presence of ethanol, FAEEs are formed from free fatty acids, triglycerides, lipoproteins or phospholipids affected by specific cytosolic or microsomal FAEE synthases or through AEAT. Detectable levels are found in blood shortly after alcohol consumption and remain detectable for more than a day.

There are at least 15 different FAEEs in hair but the sum of four of these (ethyl stearate, ethyl oleate, ethyl myristate, and ethyl palmitate) may act as a reliable marker of alcohol use. Using a cutoff of 0.5 ng/mL, they have a sensitivity and a specificity of 90% and will allow differentiation between abstinent, social, and excessive drinkers. However, the complex gas chromatography (GC)/MS method makes such an approach impractical for routine use.

Phosphatidylethanol

PEth is a phospholipid formed in the presence of alcohol via the action of phospholipase D. The precursor is naturally existing lipid-phosphadidyl choline. The lipid PEth consists of glycerol which is substituted at positions sn1 and sn2 by fatty acids and is esterified at position sn3 with phospho-ethanol. Because of the variations of the fatty acids, various homologs of PEth can be detected. In 2010, 48 PEth homologs were described in the blood of a deceased alcohol-dependent individual for the first time. The PEth homologs 16:0/18:1 und 16:0/18:2 are most prevalent and their combined sum correlates better with PEth than PEth 16:0/18:1 or PEth 16:0/18:2 alone.

Using high-performance liquid chromatography (HPLC) methods, repeated consumption of more than 40–50 g alcohol over 2–3 weeks yielded positive results.

A recent study of healthy volunteers with an alcohol consumption of 1 g/kg body weight on five consecutive days showed PEth levels up to 237 ng/mL [13]. Measurements were made using LC/MS-MS. In contrast, in alcohol-dependent patients, the values were reported to be up to 4200 ng/mL. Thus, even after one episode of alcohol ingestion, PEth is detectable using LC/MS-MS with lower detection limits for several days.

There is a linear relationship between the amount of alcohol consumed and PEth values with no false positives. The sensitivity of PEth is 99%, compared with 40–77% with CDT, MCV, and GGT. PEth also shows a correlation with the amount consumed. In a receiver-operated characteristic (ROC) curve analysis with consumption status (active drinkers versus abstinent drinkers) as a state variable and with PEth, MCV, and GGT as test variables, the area under the curve (AUC) was 0.973 for PEth, the sensitivity was 94.5% and the specificity 100%.

PEth values are not influenced by liver diseases or hypertension. PEth also has proven to be a useful tool in detection of prenatal ethanol intake.

Methods of determination

Initially, a HPLC method in combination with evaporative light scattering detection was used. This method detects a sum of all PEth homologs. In contrast, the new approach is the use of LC/MS and LC/MS-MS methods [13]. These methods facilitate detection and quantification of single homologs, if a reference is available. Furthermore, recent publications suggested liquid chromatography high resolution mass spectrometry (LC-HRMS) method and a metabolic approach using liquid chromatography with quadruple ion trap – time-of-flight-mass spectrometry (LC-MS-IT-TOF).

For routine use, the use of dried blood spots may be of helpful as this method shows results similar to whole blood measures. Furthermore, obtaining samples is easier since untrained staff can obtain capillary blood, the risks for transmitting infections such as HIV or hepatitis C are decreased, and storage and transport are simplified.

Limitations

The formation of PEth in blood and tissues containing ethanol may occur under certain conditions. Blood samples can be stored in the refrigerator for up to 72 hours or frozen at –80°C without affecting the assay.

In vitro formation of PEth in erythrocytes has been reported after addition of ethanol. Further experimental studies in rats showed that ceramide is able to block the activity of phospholipase D and inhibits the synthesis of PEth.

Hair analyses
Ethyl glucuronide and fatty acid ethyl esters

Hair analysis has been established to assess ethanol intake. FAEE and EtG, two metabolic by-products of ethanol, have become valuable alcohol markers in hair. The time frame for detection of alcohol consumption is longer in hair than in blood or urine. Because head hair growth is about 1 cm/month, depending on the length of the hair, evidence of alcohol consumption can be found a long time period. The deposit of lipophilic FAEE in hair occurs in sebum, whereas hydrophilic EtG is incorporated through perspiration and/or from blood.

Measurement of FAEE and EtG allows differentiation between chronic excessive and moderate alcohol consumption or very low levels of alcohol consumption as well as abstinence.

In a consensus of the Society of Hair Testing (SOHT), a FAEE concentration of over 0.5 ng/mg hair and/or EtG concentration of >30 pg/mg hair is interpreted as definite evidence for excessive and regular alcohol consumption (>60 g/day EtOH) [12]. A concentration >7 pg/mg EtG in the 0–3 up to 0–6 cm proximal scalp hair segment strongly suggests repeated alcohol consumption [12]. A lower concentration is not in contradiction to the self-reported abstinence of a person during the corresponding time period before sampling. A negative pubic hair result strongly confirms abstinence.

However, total abstinence cannot be proven by hair analysis, because regular consumption of low amounts (e.g. one drink per day) or single consumption of higher amounts once a week may not give a positive hair result. Pragst and Yegles reported in their study that 32 women who consumed 16 g/day alcohol had EtG values of less than 7 pg/mg in their scalp hair. These divergent results may be explained by the fact that EtG values lower than 7 pg/mg do not exclude alcohol ingestion. Furthermore, scalp hair was preanalytically cut in this study while previous studies pulverized the specimens. The preparation preanalytically cut may have a significant effect on the results.

Other influencing factors

- *Cosmetic treatment:* FAEEs and EtG in hair are sensitive to cosmetic treatment. Both the use of EtG-containing shampoo and regular use of alcohol-containing hair tonic can lead to false positive FAEE results. No such false positive results are reported for EtG. False negative results for both alcohol markers can also be caused by use of hair cosmetics, such as alkaline hair cosmetics for FAEE and bleaching, coloring, and perming agents for EtG.
- *Impaired kidney function:* may lead to higher EtG levels.
- *Hair color:* hair color and melanin content in hair have no role, in contrast to drugs and medications.

Therefore, the type of cosmetic hair treatment must be recorded during sampling, visually controlled during sample preparation, and dealt with in the interpretation of results.

In doubtful cases, for confirmation and for exclusion of false positive and false negative results, the determination of both parameters can be useful. A negative FAEE result cannot overrule an EtG result ≥7 pg/mg. FAEEs may be considered in cases of perm, bleached, or dyed hair.

A FAEE concentration >200 pg/mg in the 0–3 cm proximal hair segment or >400 pg/mg in the 0–6 cm proximal hair segment strongly suggests repeated alcohol consumption [12]. A lower concentration does not contradict self-reported abstinence of a person during the corresponding period before sampling.

In segmental investigations of hair samples, a chronologic correlation to a drinking or abstinent phase with FAEE is not possible but is for EtG. For EtG, there is a correlation between alcohol intake and EtG concentrations in hair. Furthermore, a recent meta-analysis reported a sensitivity of 96% and a specificity of 99% of EtG in hair (HEtG) for assessing chronic excessive drinking.

Overall, hair analysis for FAEE or EtG is currently a sensible tool to clarify retrospective alcohol consumption, as shown in many studies.

Applications

Hair analysis for FAEE or EtG is applicable in several contexts including judging driving ability, liver disease or transplantation [14,15], and forensic psychiatry. Another clinical use of alcohol metabolites measures is the screening for alcohol use in medication assisted treatment of opioid-dependent subjects.

Ethanol metabolites and liver transplantation

Alcohol-related liver disease accounts for up to 30% of liver transplants. Postoperatively, 20–25% of patients lapse or relapse to alcohol intake. As patients' self-reports are often unreliable, objective and accurate indicators of abstinence are required. Measurement of ethanol metabolites offers a reliable and practical approach to detect alcohol consumption.

Ethyl glucuronide in urine

In a study of 18 patients with alcohol-associated liver disease who denied alcohol intake, Erim et al. [16]found one of 127 tests for breath alcohol was positive, whereas 24 of 49 urine samples were positive for EtG (UEtG). Others have reported similar findings.

Ethyl glucuronide in hair

HEtG is a promising ethanol metabolite for the detection of alcohol consumption because it detects alcohol consumption over a longer time period. It allows retrospective determination of alcohol consumption for up to 6 months which is the abstention period often required by transplant programs prior to listing patients. Several studies have evaluated HEtG concentrations in liver transplant patients, proposing it to be a highly specific and useful tool for the monitoring of alcohol use before and after transplant [14] and superior to traditional markers. Further substantial advantages compared with routine methods of alcohol detection in urine or blood are that obtaining samples is noninvasive and storage of the samples is easy. Despite their excellent profile, it is not advisable to use the results of hair testing for alcohol markers in isolation and conclusions should always be corroborated by a clinical assessment and interpretation.

The applications mentioned show that UEtG and HEtG tests are complementary to self-reports and questionnaires, yielding valuable information on alcohol consumption that is relevant to diagnosis and therapy.

Conclusions

Direct ethanol metabolites are highly sensitive and specific, covering the spectrum of short-term intake of small amounts and long-term use of large amounts of alcohol, and are routinely used. Thus, they open new perspectives in the prevention, interdisciplinary cooperation, diagnosis, and therapy of alcohol-related disorders.

Appropriate methods of analysis and preanalytics are crucial for valid and reliable detection of markers. For EtG, the most frequently used marker, the best methods for detection are chromatographic approaches which are considered a standard method especially in forensic cases. A commercial test kit is available and has contributed to widespread distribution of the test. Of course, laboratory values always require clinical interpretation. EtG is detectable in urine using LC/MS-Ms even after an ingestion of low amounts of alcohol (1 g), which also occurs in some food, drugs, and disinfectants. Therefore individuals with the motivation or obligation for abstinence have to be informed about these "hidden sources" to avoid involuntary intake of alcohol. For forensic purposes, the current cutoff value of 0.1 mg/L should be adapted to exclude cases of involuntary alcohol use. With respect to differences in formation and degradation, EtG and EtS should be analyzed together, if

possible. As for HEtG values there are only rare factors generating false positive results, HEtG should be recommended as a marker for alcohol intake for the last 3–6 months. FAEEs may be considered in case of permed, bleached, or dyed hair. Detailed guidelines for interpretations of values are available from the International Society of Hair Testing [12].

While positive urine values of EtG and EtS can be in accordance with innocent or unintentional alcohol intake, positive values of PEth are related to previous intoxications of 0.5‰ and more. The use of "dried blood spots" is promising and may facilitate sample taking, storage, distribution, and decrease of infection risk.

When using traditional biomarkers, marker combinations such as the Antilla Index can be recommended. Among ethanol metabolites, UEtG is suggested for assessing recent ethanol intake and PEth and HEtG for longer lasting or chronic ethanol consumption.

References

[1] Thon N, Weinmann W, Yegles M, Preuss U, Wurst FM. Direct metabolites of ethanol as biological markers of alcohol use: basic aspects and applications. *Fortschr Neurol Psychiatr* 2013; **81**(9): 493–502.

[2] Conigrave KM, Davies P, Haber P, Whitfield JB. Traditional markers of excessive alcohol use. *Addiction* 2003; **98**(Suppl 2): 31–43.

[3] Wurst FM, Yegles M, Weinmann W, Thon N, Piro J, Preuss UW. Biologische Zustandsmarker für Alkoholkonsum. In: Singer VM, Batra A, Mann K, eds. *Alkohol und Tabak, Grundlagen und Folgeerkrankungen*. Georg Thieme Verlag, Stuttgart, New York; 2011.

[4] Schmidt LG. Biologische Marker des Alkoholismus und alcoholassoziierter Organschäden In: Singer VM, Teyssen S, eds. *Alkohol und Alkoholfolgekrankheiten: Gundlagen, Diagnostik, Therapie*, 2nd edn. Springer, Heidelberg; 2005.

[5] Sillanaukee P, Strid N, Jousilahti P, et al. Association of self-reported diseases and health care use with commonly used laboratory markers for alcohol consumption. *Alcohol Alcohol* 2001; **36**: 339–345.

[6] Brinkmann B, Köhler H, Banaschak S, et al. ROC analysis of alcoholism markers: 100% specificity. *Int J Legal Med* 2000; **113**(5): 293–299.

[7] Helander A. Biological markers in alcoholism. *J Neural Transm* 2003; **66**: 15–32.

[8] Hannuksela ML, Liisanantti MK, Nissinen AE, et al. Biochemical markers of alcoholism. *Clin Chem Lab Med* 2007; **45**: 953–961.

[9] Niemelä O. Biomarkers in alcoholism. *Clin Chim Acta* 2007; **377**: 39–49.

[10] Walsham NE, Sherwood RA. Ethyl glucuronide. *Ann Clin Biochem* 2012; **49**(2): 110–117.

[11] Stewart SH, Koch DG, Burgess DM, et al. Sensitivity and specificity of urinary ethyl glucuronide and ethyl sulfate in liver disease patients. *Alcohol Clin Exp Res* 2013; **37**(1): 150–155.

[12] Society of Forensic Toxicologists and American Academy of Forensic Sciences, SOFT/AAFS. Forensic Toxicology Laboratory Guidelines; 2006. http://www.soft-tox.org/index.php?option=com_content&view=article&id=55&Itemid=62 (accessed 8 December 2014).

[13] Gnann H, Weinmann W, Thierauf A. Formation of phosphatidylethanol and its subsequent elimination during an extensive drinking experiment over 5 days. *Alcohol Clin Exp Res* 2012; **36**(9): 1507–1511.

[14] Sterneck M, Yegles M, von Rothkirch G, et al. Determination of ethyl glucuronide in hair improves evaluation of long-term alcohol abstention in liver transplant candidates. *Liver Int* 2014; **34**(3): 469–476.

[15] Stewart SH, Koch DG, Willner IR, Randall PK, Reuben A. Hair ethyl glucuronide is highly sensitive and specific for detecting moderate-to-heavy drinking in patients with liver disease. *Alcohol Alcohol* 2013; **48**(1): 83–87.

[16] Erim Y, Bottcher M, Dohmen U, et al. Urinary ethyl glucuronide testing detects alcohol consumption in alcoholic liver disease patients awaiting liver transplantation. *Liver Transpl* 2007; **13**: 757–761.

CHAPTER 14
The role of histology

Desley A.H. Neil

Queen Elizabeth Hospital Birmingham, Birmingham, UK

KEY POINTS

- The indication for liver biopsy is ill defined and is at the discretion of the treating clinician.

- Biopsy is undertaken to confirm the role of alcohol, assess additional pathologic processes (which occur in up to 20% of patients), and identify the predominant cause of damage.

- In acute deterioration with jaundice, biopsy is used to confirm or refute a clinical suspicion of acute alcoholic hepatitis and rule out other possible causes of liver damage.

- The majority of heavy drinkers develop fatty liver disease – steatosis.

- A subset of these will develop a steatohepatitis in which hepatocyte injury occurs with progressive fibrosis and potential to develop cirrhosis.

- Steatosis and steatohepatitis due to alcohol cannot be distinguished from that due to nonalcoholic fatty liver disease (NAFLD)/nonalcoholic steatohepatitis (NASH).

- The injury to hepatocytes in steatohepatitis results in damage to the cytoskeleton with ballooning of the cell and the aggregation of cytokeratin in the cytoplasm, termed Mallory–Denk bodies.

- Immunohistochemistry can highlight Mallory–Denk bodies.

- No noninvasive markers of fibrosis are validated in alcoholic liver disease (ALD), so a biopsy is the definitive test to diagnose cirrhosis which is the trigger for hepatocellular carcinoma (HCC) surveillance.

- HCC is currently the only major carcinoma to not require a tissue diagnosis prior to treatment.

- Biopsy of focal lesions in cirrhotic patients with equivocal radiologic findings is used to differentiate a dysplastic nodule from HCC.

- Recent improvements in immunohistochemistry have increased the sensitivity and specificity for diagnosis of HCC in needle biopsies.

- Up to 30% of radiologically diagnosed HCCs turn out not to be malignant.

- Alcohol in combination with HCV, iron accumulation, or homozygous or heterozygous states of alfa-1 antitrypsin deficiency results in an accelerated course of damage.

- Recurrent ALD can occur post-transplant and is indistinguishable histologically from *de novo* NAFLD/NASH.

Alcohol Abuse and Liver Disease, First Edition. Edited by James Neuberger and Andrea DiMartini.
© 2015 John Wiley & Sons, Ltd. Published 2015 by John Wiley & Sons, Ltd.

Background

A liver biopsy is undertaken when the cause of abnormalities in liver tests, liver imaging, or liver appearance is uncertain and is used to make a diagnosis as to the cause or possible causes. It also helps in the acute situation to determine if this is a recent onset process or is an acute exacerbation of a chronic problem. Liver biopsy also has a role in the assessment of focal lesions detected by imaging, often surveillance imaging in the long-term follow-up of cirrhotic patients.

In the United Kingdom, the guidelines from the National Clinical Guideline Centre, Royal College of Physicians, about when to perform a liver biopsy in the assessment of alcoholic liver disease (ALD) are vague and are left open to the treating hepatologist, recognizing that the indications for a biopsy are varied and complex [1]. The guidelines in the United States provided jointly by American Association for the Study of Liver Diseases (AASLD) and American College of Gastroenterology [2] also leave the decision to the treating physician, noting that if treatment is not being considered for ALD or acute alcoholic hepatitis (AAH), a biopsy is usually not necessary. Mortality related to the biopsy procedure is thought to be at the lower end of reported rates at less than 0.4% with transjugular biopsy having a lower risk than percutaneous biopsy which approaches 0% risk [1], although the histologic information obtained may be less.

A history of drinking may suggest ALD but only a subset of patients with excessive alcohol intake progress to liver injury with progressive fibrosis [1,2]. In general, a biopsy is undertaken to confirm the clinical suspicion of ALD, particularly when other possible causes cannot be excluded from the history and serologic findings, or there is the potential for dual pathology when a biopsy will help to identify the cause or the predominant factor if several etiologies are identified. Up to 20% of patients with excessive alcohol intake have an additional etiologic agent in the pathogenesis of their liver disease [2]. It may also be of relevance in the acute setting to identify a nonalcoholic cause for which super-urgent listing for transplantation would be appropriate; an acute alcohol-related cause would usually exclude listing.

In patients who are drinking, an understanding of the amount of tissue injury and degree of scarring will help with management and allow an informed discussion with the patient on the merits of stopping or limiting alcohol intake. The earlier in the disease process injury can be detected, the more likely that progression can be stopped and potentially changes reversed towards normal; however, not all will normalize histologic findings and some will continue to progress to cirrhosis [2].

Clinical and biochemical parameters do not accurately correlate with the severity of liver injury [1,2] and liver biopsy remains the gold standard for the assessment of fibrosis and separation of steatosis (fat within hepatocytes) from steatohepatitis (steatosis with hepatocyte injury and inflammation or fibrosis). Separation of steatosis from steatohepatitis cannot be reliably done without a liver biopsy. A liver biopsy is often undertaken to determine or confirm the stage of the fibrosis. ALD can reach the stage of severe fibrosis with cirrhosis while still clinically compensated and as a result it is difficult to separate out patients with cirrhosis from lesser degrees of scaring on clinical and biochemical grounds. A knowledge of the degree of fibrosis is used to help with management, in particular identifying individuals with cirrhosis who are at risk of developing hepatocellular carcinomas (HCCs) requiring HCC surveillance. Noninvasive methods of detecting fibrosis are not validated for any stage of ALD [3]. Measures of liver stiffness such as transient elastography are influenced by inflammation as well as fibrosis. Serologic markers, such as hyaluronic acid, appear to be reliable for detecting advanced fibrosis but are less so for less severe or early fibrosis.

Acute alcoholic hepatitis

This is a severe form of alcoholic liver disease with a high mortality rate, usually presenting with jaundice but with nonspecific symptoms which can occur for other reasons in heavy drinkers including sepsis and decompensation of cirrhosis, making the clinical diagnosis difficult [1,2,4] and each scenario has a different management strategy. In this setting a liver biopsy is the most accurate way to make or confirm the diagnosis, but usually requires a transjugular approach resulting in generally small fragmented pieces of liver which can be difficult to interpret, particular for nonspecialist pathologists [4]. Consideration should be given to getting these biopsies referred for evaluation by a specialist liver pathologist.

Clinical grounds based on systemic inflammatory response are unreliable at predicting histologically proven AAH [1,2], with only 50% of patients clinically thought to have AAH having the diagnosis confirmed by biopsy and 41% of patients thought not to be AAH having features of AAH on biopsy.

Pathology of alcoholic liver disease

The changes seen in the liver from alcohol vary from the accumulation of large fat droplets within hepatocytes, called steatosis, to the development of hepatocyte injury, inflammation, and scarring when the histologic pattern is termed steatohepatitis. The scarring can progress to the development of cirrhosis at which stage the internal architecture of the liver is lost and there are nodules of surviving hepatocytes in a sea of fibrous tissue with loss of vascular relationships due to obliteration of many of the veins by the fibrosis.

Steatosis occurs in the majority of heavy drinkers, but with simple steatosis there is no hepatocyte injury and therefore no fibrosis or scarring. Up to 5% of hepatocytes containing fat droplets is generally regarded as being within normal limits. Steatosis is graded into mild (up to one-third), moderate (one-third to two-thirds), and severe (more than two-thirds) based on the number of hepatocytes containing large fat droplets (macrovesicular steatosis) see Table 14.1 and Figure 14.1. Steatosis occurring within the setting of ALD can take two forms both designated macrovesicular steatosis but subdivided into large droplet and small droplet macrovesicular steatosis (Figure 14.1), the latter also termed mediovesicular steatosis to avoid confusion with the term microvesicular steatosis.

- Large droplet macrovesicular steatosis is defined as a single or several fat vacuoles occupying the majority of the hepatocyte cytoplasm and producing displacement of the nucleus to the edge of the cell.
- Small droplet steatosis is the presence of several to moderate numbers of readily identified vacuoles that do not cause displacement of the nucleus.

True microvesicular steatosis is associated with mitochondrial dysfunction, hepatic encephalopathy and the hepatocyte cytoplasm has a foamy appearance and discrete fat vacuoles are not readily discerned. This is not generally a feature of ALD.

Table 14.1 Grading: nonalcoholic steatohepatitis (NASH) activity score.

Feature graded	Description	Score
Steatosis	Parenchymal involvement	
	<5%	0
	5–33%	1
	>33–66%	2
	>66%	3
Lobular inflammation	Overall assessment at high power	
	No foci of inflammation	0
	<2 foci per average high power field	1
	2–4 foci per high power field	2
	>4 foci per high power field	3
Ballooning/ Mallory–Denk bodies	No cells ballooned/contain MDBs	0
	Very occasional ballooned cells	1
	Prominent/many ballooned cells	2

Source: adapted from Kleiner et al. 2005 [9].
This is the grading of activity used for research and now often management decisions in NASH. A formal grading is not generally given or required for management of alcoholic steatohepatitis.

It is thought that the natural history of fat accumulation in the liver starts as mediovesicular or small droplet macrovesicular and that as the amount of fat increases within a cell the vacuoles fuse to form large droplet macrovesicular steatosis. It is this latter type of steatosis, present in donors, which causes short-term problems in transplanted organs and may lead to primary nonfunction.

In steatohepatitis, the hepatocytes become injured, with damage to the cytoskeleton resulting in:
- Ballooning (swelling) of the cell; and
- The aggregation of cytokeratin within the cytoplasm [5,6] – termed Mallory's hyaline, Mallory bodies, or Mallory–Denk bodies (MDBs) (Figure 14.1).

The injured hepatocytes evoke an inflammatory response in the form of lobular inflammation, generally relatively mild. The MDBs may be difficult to see on routinely stained sections but can be highlighted by immunohistochemistry using antibodies again ubiquitin (Figure 14.2) and cytokeratin 8/18 (Figure 14.3) or P62. On the cytokeratin 8/18 immunostain, the ballooned hepatocytes lose their normal membranous staining (Figure 14.3).

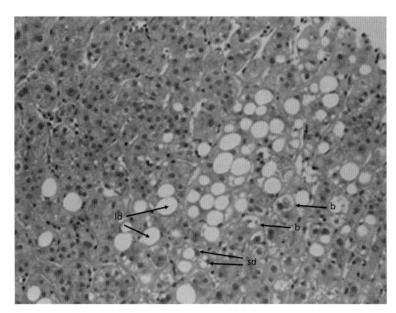

Figure 14.1 Hematoxylin and eosin (H&E) stained section of liver with steatohepatitis. Hepatocyte cytoplasm stains pink, nuclei purple, and fat droplets are clear holes (arrows) as the fat has leached out during processing. A mixture of large (ld) and small (sd) macrovesicular fat is present. The hepatocyte nuclei are pushed to the edge of the cell in large droplets, while they remain central surrounded by variable numbers of smaller vacuoles in small droplet macrovesicular steatosis. Several probably ballooned hepatocytes (b) are present, containing wispy pink Mallory–Denk bodies. Inflammation is minimal, seen as dark blue dots, with morphology of lymphocytes. *(See insert for color representation of the figure)*

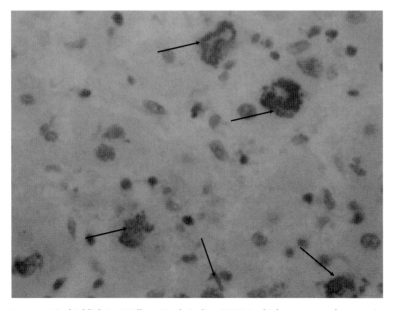

Figure 14.2 Ubiquitin immunostain highlighting Mallory–Denk Bodies (MDBs) which are seen as brown wispy material in the hepatocyte cytoplasm (arrows). *(See insert for color representation of the figure)*

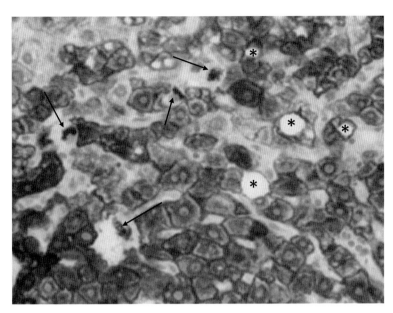

Figure 14.3 Pancytokeratin immunostain which contains cytokeratin 8 and 18. The normal hepatocytes show diffuse brown staining of the cytoplasm with a distinct cell membrane. The ballooned hepatocytes have lost both the diffuse cytoplasmic and membranous staining and contain a clumped brown Mallory–Denk body (arrows). Fat droplets are seen as clear holes (*) within the cytoplasm of some hepatocytes. *(See insert for color representation of the figure)*

During AAH, a severe form of steatohepatitis occurs in which there are large numbers of ballooned hepatocytes containing Mallory's hyaline; many of these injured hepatocytes are surrounded by infiltrating neutrophils (Figure 14.4). The fat is often lost during AAH and bilirubinostasis is generally apparent as canalicular bile plugs (Figure 14.4).

The hepatocyte injury occurs in perivenular regions (zone 3) and may lead to progressive fibrosis if the injurious process (drinking) continues. Initially, fibrosis is perisinusoidal in zone 3, then develops a pericellular pattern with delicate strands of collagen surrounding individual zone 3 hepatocytes (Figure 14.5). Fibrosis can also develop in a periportal distribution driven by the development of a ductular reaction. With time, fibrous bridges between central veins, central veins and portal tract, and between portal tracts develop, at this stage the degree of fibrosis is termed moderate. Progression of the fibrosis results in nodules of hepatocyte becoming surrounded by fibrous bridges or septa at which stage the fibrosis is severe and is termed cirrhosis (Figure 14.6).

Many of the histologic clues to the etiology can be absent or very focal and subtle in cirrhosis. This is because the interpretation of zonation of changes is difficult or impossible when vascular relationships are lost, with the incorporation of the affected areas into the fibrous septa. This is made more difficult when alcohol intake is minimized or stopped, as in the case of examination of an explanted liver at the time of transplantation, abstinence being a prerequisite for transplant listing. The fat disappears first, followed by the MDBs which may persist for many months, probably at least 1 year. The only clue remaining may be the pattern of fibrosis, but this may be lost in advanced fibrosis when it just becomes part of the fibrous septa.

Summary of typical features of steatosis, steatohepatitis, and AAH

In practice, typical features seen to indicate a steatohepatitis are:
- Fat and MDB;
- Fat and pericellular fibrosis; or
- Fat with both MDBs and pericellular fibrosis.

If neither MDBs nor pericellular fibrosis are present then it is a simple steatosis. The amount of inflammation

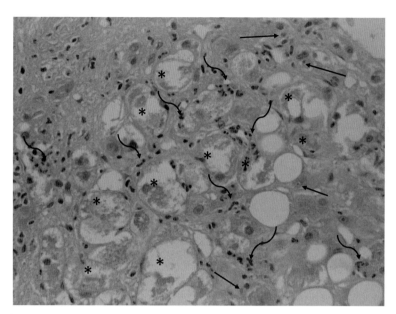

Figure 14.4 Hematoxylin and eosin (H&E) stained section of liver with acute alcoholic hepatitis. There are numerous ballooned hepatocytes (*) containing Mallory–Denk bodies associated with a conspicuous neutrophilic infiltrate (squiggly arrows). Occassional bile plugs (arrows) are present. *(See insert for color representation of the figure)*

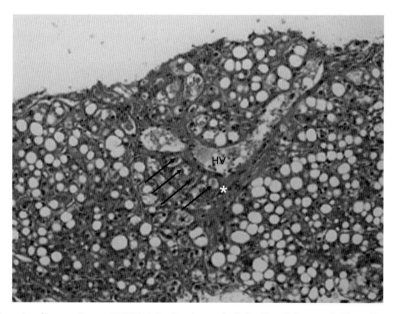

Figure 14.5 Elastic hematoxylin van Gieson (EHVG) stain showing pericellular fibrosis in zone 3. The collagen stains dark pink. Hepatocyte cytoplasm yellow–brown. Fat are clear vacuoles. Arrows point to several hepatocytes surrounded by delicate fibrous tissue. A degree of central hyaline sclerosis (*) is seen adjacent to a hepatic vein (HV). *(See insert for color representation of the figure)*

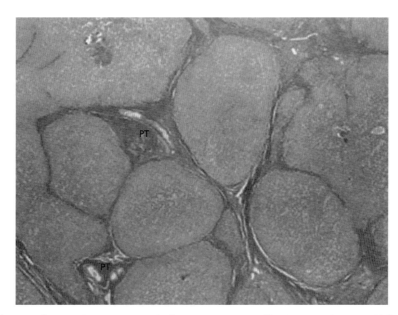

Figure 14.6 Elastic hematoxylin van Gieson (EHVG) stain demonstrating severe fibrosis amounting to established cirrhosis. Islands of hepatocytes are surrounded by fibrous septa (dark pink) and the normal vascular relationships between hepatic veins and portal tracts are lost. Several portal tracts (PT) are identifiable within the fibrous septa. *(See insert for color representation of the figure)*

Table 14.2 Steatosis, steatohepatitis, and alcoholic hepatitis.

	Steatosis	Steatohepatitis	Acute alcoholic hepatitis
Fat	+ − +++	+ − +++	+/−
Fibrosis (PCF)	0	0 − +++	0 − +++
MDB	0	0 − +++	+++
Neutrophils	0	+/−	+++
Non-neutrophilic lobular inflammation	+/−	+ − ++	+/−

Source: adapted from Kleiner et al. 2005 [9].
Steatosis without Mallory–Denk bodies (MDBs) and pericellular fibrosis (PCF) indicates simple steatosis and the report is usually worded as "steatosis without typical features of a steatohepatitis." The presence of MDBs and/or PCF in conjunction with steatosis indicates the presence of a steatohepatis. Both MDBs and PCF may be difficult to identify and fibrous stains and immunohistochemistry for MDBs (ubiquitin, cytokeratin 8/18, and/or p62) can be helpful in their identification. In both steatosis and steatohepatitis, inflammation is relatively mild and neutrophils are not a conspicuous component on any inflammatory infiltrate. In acute alcoholic hepatitis, the most striking feature is ballooned cells with prominent MDBs, usually readily identifiable on H&E stain, associated with a conspicuous neutrophilic infiltrate around these damaged cells. Fat is often not present or minimal.

in a typical alcohol-related steatohepatitis is minimal, can be described as spotty lobular inflammation, and neutrophils are sparse if at all present. Neutrophils around ballooned hepatocytes containing MDBs, irrespective of the amount of fat, are the features that suggest the diagnosis of AAH, although this should be a clinicopathologic diagnosis. The differences between steatosis, steatohepatitis, and AAH are shown in Table 14.2.

Differentiation of ALD from NASH and other diseases with overlaping features

The histologic features of steatohepatitis from alcohol and nonalcoholic causes (nonalcoholic steatohepatitis, NASH) are the same and it is not possible confidently to distinguish between them as to the cause of the steatohepatitis. However, there are some features that favors one over the other: prominent fibrosis with obliteration of the hepatic vein termed sclerosing hyaline necrosis or central hyaline sclerosis is more typical of alcohol-related steatohepatitis, while glycogenation of hepatocyte nuclei is more prominent in NASH.

MDB may also occur in chronic biliary processes; however, they are in a different location to those that occur in steatohepatitis being periportal/periseptal rather than zone 3/perivenular. In cirrhosis when vascular relationships are lost other features of a chronic biliary process such as significant quantities of copper-associated protein, a periseptal halo zone, and a paucity of bile ducts are required to make the distinction.

Steatosis is also a feature of hepatitis C virus (HCV) infection, particularly genotype 3. MDBs are not typically seen in HCV, so if present this is an indication that a steatohepatitis is also present for which both alcohol and nonalcoholic factors must be considered as etiologic agents contributing to the pathologic process.

Cofactors

Iron

Heavy alcohol intake is associated with the accumulation of iron in hepatocytes [7], termed siderosis, most likely related to alcohol downregulating hepcidin expression. Hepcidin is the central regulator for iron homeostasis. A decrease in hepcidin results in an increase in iron accumulation and as hepcidin is synthesized in the liver this occurs in chronic liver injury. Alcoholics have a twofold increase in gut iron absorption. The iron accumulation is generally mild but may be so marked that genetic hemochromatosis enters the differential diagnosis of possible etiologic agents, particular as the degree of fibrosis increases, although can be readily diagnosed using genetic analysis for *HFE* genes.

Both iron and alcohol act synergistically to exacerbate iron burden and liver injury and the accumulation of iron can produce a vicious circle of hepatocyte injury. Alcohol induces hepatocyte injury and death and fibrosis by several pathways: oxidative stress, lipopolysaccharide toxicity, and endoplasmic reticulum stress. Iron generates free radical production which leads to oxidative cell death via damage to membranes, proteins, and DNA. Additionally, iron accumulates in Kupffer cells leading to the production of a proinflammatory environment with the release of tumor necrosis factor alfa (TNF-α) and activation of the transcription factor nuclear factor kappa beta (NF-$\kappa\beta$).

Hepatitis C virus

Steatosis and inflammation are features of hepatitis C; the fat is generally mild and is most pronounced with genotype 3. HCV produces an environment in which there are reactive oxygen species (ROS) and reactive nitrogen species (RNS) with inhibition of hepcidin leading to an accumulation of iron. ROS and RNS produce oxidative and nitrosative stress, respectively. Alcohol also leads to ROS and RNS production and the alcohol and HCV act synergistically in their production. Alcohol, even in small amounts, exacerbates the HCV-induced liver injury and HCV exacerbates alcohol-induced liver injury. Patients who are drinking have increased viral load, respond less well to HCV treatment, and are more likely to develop cirrhosis at an accelerated rate, so the finding of steatohepatitis (MDBs and/or pericellular fibrosis) on a biopsy, particularly when there are no or minimal risk factors for NASH, will aid in management discussions with the patient.

A-1-antitrypsin globules

The accumulation of periodic acid–Schiff positive diastase resistant (PASD) globules within the hepatocyte cytoplasm are characteristic of alpha-1 antitrypsin deficiency (a-1-AT), but can occur in both homozygous and heterozygous individuals, and also PASD positive globules are seen in unrelated conditions so are not pathognomonic for a-1-AT deficiency. Immunohistochemistry with an antibody against a-1-AT can rule out accumulation of different proteins; however, genetic testing or isoelectric focusing is required for the diagnosis and differentiation between the different mutations and whether individuals are homozygous or heterozygous for the pathogenic alleles. The presence of PASD globules does not exclude a diagnosis of ALD and indeed even the heterozygous carriers are at increased risk of injury from alcohol with acceleration of the process, so identification early on is important.

Information in the pathology report

The biopsy is able to assess the severity of the inflammatory process at the time of the biopsy, termed the grade, and the severity of the fibrosis, termed the stage. There are numerous systems for scoring fibrosis

[8], with 0 indicating no fibrosis and the upper end of each scoring system indicating severe fibrosis with established cirrhosis. There are no specific scoring systems designed for the evaluation of alcoholic liver disease, the nearest system that was developed for research trials in NASH is the Kleiner system [9]. From a management perspective, unless specific research projects are being undertaken, a more general indication of fibrosis – nil, mild, moderate, and severe (Table 14.3) – will allow appropriate management to be determined.

Table 14.3 Stage of fibrosis.

General fibrosis stage for clinical management		Kleiner fibrosis stage for NASH trials	
Stage	Meaning	Stage	Meaning
Nil	No fibrosis present	0	No fibrosis present
Mild	Periportal and/or pericellular without bridging fibrosis	1A	Delicate zone 3 (perisinusoidal/pericellular)
		1B	Dense zone 3 (perisinusoidal/pericellular)
		1C	Periportal
		2	Periportal and zone 3
Moderate	Bridging fibrosis (P-C, C-C, or P-P)	3	Bridging fibrosis (P-P, P-C, or C-C)
Severe	Nodule formation = cirrhosis	4	Cirrhosis (nodule formation)

The amount of fibrosis is usually given as nil, mild, moderate, or severe in reports where the diagnosis is alcoholic liver disease. This is shown in the left of the table with the type/extent of fibrosis corresponding to these grades in the second column. In NASH, a more formal staging of fibrosis is given, shown in the two right-hand columns. The corresponding more generic stage can be seen by looking which corresponding row it falls into. Mild comprises Kleiner stage 1a, 1b, 1c and 2; moderate equates to Kleiner stage 3; and severe is Kleiner stage 4. P-C, portal–central; C-C, central–central; P-P, portal–portal.

Table 14.4 Ishak system for staging fibrosis.

Ishak stage	Description	General stage
0	No fibrosis	No fibrosis
1	Periportal septa in occasional portal tracts	Mild
2	Periportal septa in majority of portal tracts	Mild
3	occasional foci of P-P bridging fibrosis	Mild to moderate
4	Marked bridging P-P and/or P-C	Moderate
5	Marked bridging with occasional nodules (incomplete cirrhosis)	Moderate to severe
6	Cirrhosis	Severe

The Ishak fibrosis staging system provides a more detailed breakdown of the amount of fibrosis and the corresponding general fibrosis stages are indicated on the right. P-P, portal–portal; P-C, portal–central.

The Ishak staging of fibrosis provides more information, being a seven-point scale (Table 14.4), but reproducibility decreases [8].

In the pathology report an indication of the amount of fat present and extent of ballooning with MDBs is provided; however, a detailed grade of the inflammatory process is not usually given or required for management of ALD. If required, the grading system used for NASH trials would be the most appropriate (Table 14.1), due to the overlapping pathologic pathways present.

HCC diagnosis

HCC is the only clinically significant tumor that does not require a tissue diagnosis, based on historical issues related to the inability to offer effective treatments and the worry of seeding along the biopsy tract. Seeding occurs in less than 0.5% of HCCs biopsied and tumor seeds are amenable to surgical resection. Current international guidelines do not require histologic confirmation for the diagnosis of a focal lesion within a cirrhotic liver detected by surveillance unless imaging findings are equivocal. However, there is a significant false positive rate on radiologic criteria with up to 30% of radiologically diagnosed HCCs not being confirmed as malignant by examination of livers removed at the time of transplantation [10]. A biopsy of radiologically equivocal lesions is undertaken to differentiate a high grade dysplastic nodule from a HCC, this can be very difficult in needle biopsies, particularly if small and the lesion is well differentiated. The identification of portal stromal invasion can be very focal in early HCCs and can be missed by sampling. The diagnostic accuracy of needle biopsies is increased with the use of a panel of immunohistochemical markers: glypican 3, glutamine synthetase, and heat shock protein 70 (HSP70), with at least two of three being positive giving a sensitivity of 72% and a specificity of 100% for the diagnosis of HCC [10]. A biopsy of the lesion and assessment of any adjacent liver is also able to provide increased prognostic information, improving management.

It is likely that liver biopsy will have an increasing role in the diagnosis and assessment of focal lesions in cirrhotic livers to allow appropriate listing for organ transplantation only when a lesion is definitely a HCC and to obtain increased prognostic information to aid management as newer treatments become available.

Post-transplant liver histology

Recurrent disease and *de novo* NAFLD or NASH

Relapse to drinking occurs in a subset of patients transplanted for ALD, although only some of these relapse to harmful drinking patterns. Graft loss due to recurrent ALD, however, appears to be rare (3–6%). *De novo* NAFLD occurs in up to one-third of liver transplant recipients, risk factors being obesity, new onset diabetes after transplant, hyperlipidemia, and hypertension. NASH develops in 3–4%. As in the pretransplant setting, it is not possible to distinguish recurrent ALD from *de novo* NAFLD or NASH histologically.

Conclusions

The role of a biopsy in patients with an excessive alcohol intake is to confirm that alcohol has a role in the pathologic process occurring within the liver or to identify another cause. If alcohol does have a role and there any additional etiologic factors these must also be taken into account in managing the patient. The coexistence of a-1-AT globules, siderosis, or HCV infection will accelerate the development of fibrosis. The biopsy is used to identify where in the spectrum of pathologic processes of ALD an individual patient is – to differentiated simple fatty change (steatosis) from fatty change with injury (steatohepatitis). Within the spectrum of steatohepatitis it is used to determine the degree of fibrosis (scarring). In patients who present acutely with decompensation and jaundice, a liver biopsy is able to differentiate AAH from other potential causes of a similar presentation – decompensation of alcoholic cirrhosis and sepsis. There are no reliable features to differentiate steatosis caused by alcohol from NAFLD or steatosis caused by alcohol from NASH, thus differentiation of recurrent ALD from *de novo* NASH is also problematic post-transplant. In a subset of focal lesions identified in cirrhotic patients, liver biopsy has a role in differentiating high grade dysplastic nodules from HCCs.

References

[1] National Clinical Guideline Centre for Acute and Chronic Conditions. *Alcohol-use disorders: physical complications: full guidance*. London: National Clinical Guideline Centre; 2010. Report No.: CG100.

[2] O'Shea RS, Dasarathy S, McCullough AJ. Alcoholic liver disease. *Hepatology* 2010; **51**(1): 307–328.

[3] Stevenson M, Lloyd-Jones M, Morgan MY, Wong R. Non-invasive diagnostic assessment tools for the detection of liver fibrosis in patients with suspected alcohol-related liver disease: a systematic review and economic evaluation. *Health Technol Assess* 2012; **16**(4): 1–174.

[4] Dhanda AD, Collins PL, McCune CA. Is liver biopsy necessary in the management of alcoholic hepatitis? *World J Gastroenterol* 2013; **19**(44): 7825–7829.

[5] Goodman ZD. The impact of obesity on liver histology. *Clin Liver Dis* 2014; **18**(1): 33–40.

[6] Lackner C, Gogg-Kamerer M, Zatloukal K, Stumptner C, Brunt EM, Denk H. Ballooned hepatocytes in steatohepatitis: the value of keratin immunohistochemistry for diagnosis. *J Hepatol* 2008; **48**(5): 821–828.

[7] Corradini E, Pietrangelo A. Iron and steatohepatitis. *J Gastroenterol Hepatol* 2012; **27**(Suppl 2): 42–46.

[8] Goodman ZD. Grading and staging systems for inflammation and fibrosis in chronic liver diseases. *J Hepatol* 2007; **47**(4): 598–607.

[9] Kleiner DE, Brunt EM, Van NM, et al. Design and validation of a histological scoring system for nonalcoholic fatty liver disease. *Hepatology* 2005; **41**(6): 1313–1321.

[10] Roskams T. Anatomic pathology of hepatocellular carcinoma: impact on prognosis and response to therapy. *Clin Liver Dis* 2011; **15**(2): 245–259.

CHAPTER 15

General assessment and management

Patrizia Burra and Giacomo Germani

Multivisceral Transplant Unit, Department of Surgery, Oncology and Gastroenterology, Padova University Hospital, Padova, Italy

---

KEY POINTS

- A thorough medical history is crucial when evaluating a patient with liver disease, independently of its etiology. The history should determine if the patient has had exposure to any potential risk for liver disease and if he or she has other disorders associated with liver disease.

- Most physical findings and serologic tests in patients with chronic liver disease are not specific for the etiology of liver disease. However, some signs – such as spider angiomas, gynecomastia, and parotid gland enlargement – may be more frequently seen in those with alcohol-related liver disease. Moreover, the interpretation of abnormal biochemical patterns together with the presence of clinical alterations can lead to the suspicion of specific liver diseases.

- Ultrasonography should always be considered as the initial mode of imaging as it is the least expensive. CT scan and MRI are second line studies, which should be performed when focal lesions or other complications such as portal vein thrombosis are detected at ultrasonography and further evaluation is warranted.

- Alcoholic liver disease should not be considered a disease confined to the liver. All the potential extrahepatic manifestations of alcoholic liver disease should be properly assessed and treated when necessary. A multidisciplinary approach with close collaboration between the hepatologist and other specialists is crucial.

Introduction

Chronic alcohol consumption is a major cause of liver disease worldwide and the strongest risk factor for liver cirrhosis [1,2]. Alcoholic liver disease is a complex disease, and its diagnosis is usually based on a combination of features, including a history of significant alcohol intake, clinical evidence of liver disease, and supporting laboratory abnormalities [3]. However, it is common for patients with alcoholic liver disease to have other risk factors for liver disease (such as chronic viral hepatitis) so a thorough medical history and specific laboratory tests should always be performed [4].

Determining the severity of liver disease and the presence of extrahepatic manifestations is a crucial step in the assessment and management of patients with alcohol abuse and alcohol-related liver disease because it may influence treatment choices, and help predict the patient's prognosis.

Therefore, the successful assessment and management of patients with alcoholic liver disease requires not only the integration of all the competences in public health, epidemiology, and addiction behavior, but also an active collaboration between the hepatologist and the specialists involved in this process.

The aim of this chapter is to describe the different aspects of assessment of patients with alcoholic liver disease and to explore how to assess and manage the most important extrahepatic complications of alcohol abuse and alcoholic liver disease.

Alcohol Abuse and Liver Disease, First Edition. Edited by James Neuberger and Andrea DiMartini.
© 2015 John Wiley & Sons, Ltd. Published 2015 by John Wiley & Sons, Ltd.

Medical history

A thorough medical history is crucial when evaluating a patient with liver disease, independently of its etiology. The history should determine if the patient has had exposure to any potential risk for liver disease or if he or she presents with other disorders associated with liver disease.

The quantity of alcohol intake, duration of drinking, and modality of alcohol consumption should always be investigated. The diagnosis of alcoholic liver disease is frequently suspected upon documentation of excess alcohol consumption >30g/day alcohol [5]. Drinking habits should be screened with reliable tools [6], such as Alcohol Use Disorders Identification Test (AUDIT) and CAGE questionnaires.

Alcohol intake can be calculated counting standard drink units [7]: although the content of a standard drink may differ from country to country, this method is reliable and easy to use [5]. Risk factors associated with virus-related chronic liver disease – such as multiple sexual partners, drug use, tattooing, and past blood transfusions – should always be investigated as multiple causes of liver disease can coexist in the same patient. Questioning about drug use should seek to identify all drugs used as well as the durations of use. Drug use is not limited to prescription medications, but includes over-the-counter medications, herbal and dietary supplements, and illicit drug use.

Other important factors to be considered include diabetes mellitus, hypertension, hyperlipidemia, and body weight, as these are linked to the development of nonalcoholic fatty liver disease (NAFLD). The diagnosis of NAFLD also requires the exclusion of other causes of liver disease (viral, autoimmune, genetic, etc.) and an alcohol intake ≤20–30g/day [8].

Lastly, patient and family history of autoimmune or hepatic diseases should always be investigated, as well as all those conditions that are potentially associated with hepatobiliary disease such as right-sided heart failure, diabetes mellitus and obesity, inflammatory bowel disease, and early onset emphysema.

Physical examination

Most patients with chronic liver disease remain asymptomatic until decompensation occurs. Weight loss, weakness, and anorexia are typical clinical manifestation of patients with compensated liver disease; however, when decompensation occurs patients can present with jaundice, ascites, hepatic encephalopathy, and variceal bleeding [9].

Most physical findings in patients with chronic liver disease are not specific of the etiology. However, some signs such as spider angiomas (vascular spiders), gynecomastia, and parotid gland enlargement may be more frequently seen in those with alcohol-related liver disease [5].

Vascular spiders are vascular lesions usually found on the trunk, face, and upper extremities. Overall, 33% of patients with cirrhosis present with spider angiomas [10], being more frequent amongst patients with alcohol-related liver disease than nonalcoholic cirrhotic patients (50% vs. 27%) [11]. However, vascular spiders are not specific for chronic liver disease as they can also occur during pregnancy, in patients with severe malnutrition, and in healthy persons.

The prevalence of gynecomastia in patients with chronic liver disease has been reported to be about 45% [12]. It is caused by reduced catabolism of androstenedione, with consequent shunting of estrogen precursor and increasing plasma levels of estradiol [13]. Gynaecomastia may also be caused by drugs such as spironolactone.

Parotid gland enlargement is typically seen in patients with alcoholic liver disease and is probably a direct effect of alcohol, rather than cirrhosis. Liver enlargement is usually secondary to fatty infiltration, fibrosis, and edema rather than a hyperfunctioning organ [14].

Abdominal examination should focus on the size and consistency of the liver, the size of the spleen, and assessment for ascites. Patients with chronic liver disease and portal hypertension may develop the so-called caput medusa, which appears as tortuous vessels that radiate from the umbilicus. Several other common physical findings such as asterixis, jaundice, clubbing, testicular atrophy, and Dupuytren's contracture can be detected in patients with chronic liver disease.

Laboratory evaluation

Although no serologic test is specific for diagnosing chronic liver disease, the interpretation of abnormal biochemical patterns together with the presence of clinical alterations can lead to the suspicion of alcohol-related liver disease.

Liver function tests include aspartate transaminase (AST), alanine transaminase (ALT), alkaline phosphatase, gamma-glutamyl transferase (GGT), and serum bilirubin. Serum albumin, a complete blood count with platelets, and prothrombin time test should also be measured [15]. The ALT is thought to be the most cost-effective screening test for identifying metabolic or drug-induced hepatic injury but, like other liver function tests, it is of limited use in predicting the degree of inflammation and of no use in estimating severity of fibrosis [16]. A prospective study showed a strong correlation between elevated liver function tests for at least 6 months and histologically proven underlying liver disease [17]. If the clinical suspicion for liver disease is high, then additional serologic studies should be performed to evaluate for various etiologies of cirrhosis [15,16].

In nearly 70% of patients with alcoholic liver disease the AST:ALT ratio is greater than 2, but this may be more useful in detecting patients before the development of cirrhosis [18]. In patients with alcoholic liver disease, the mitochondria are damaged, releasing AST, which is added to that released from the cytoplasm. Therefore, in cases of mild alcoholic liver disease, the AST level may be 1.5–2 times the normal level, whereas the ALT level is normal. In patients with severe alcoholic hepatitis, AST is typically elevated to a level of 2–6 times the upper limit.

Noninvasive tests

Several blood tests, combining different markers of fibrosis, are available for patients with hepatitis C, but they can be also applied to patients with alcoholic liver disease but cutoff values to distinguish varying levels of fibrosis will vary according to etiology [5].

FibroTest is a serum biomarker of fibrosis combining α-2-macroglobulin, haptoglobin, GGT, ApoA1, and bilirubin, corrected for age and sex [19]. In one study of 221 patients with histology-proven alcoholic liver disease, the FibroTest area under the curve (AUROC) for the diagnosis of cirrhosis was at 0.95 [20]. Therefore this test seems to have high diagnostic potential for the detection of significant fibrosis in this group of patients. In contrast, the aspartate aminotransferase to platelet ratio index (APRI) score is of limited use in patients with alcoholic liver disease because of its very low sensitivity (13.2%).

Other markers, such as Fibrometer [21] and Hepascore, were compared with Fibrotest, and their diagnostic accuracy did not differ from that of FibroTest both for advanced fibrosis and for cirrhosis [22].

Noninvasive tests may be also useful in predicting liver-related mortality. Several studies have shown that liver stiffness measurement is a reliable tool for assessing hepatic fibrosis in patients with alcoholic liver disease [23–25]. However, the estimates of liver stiffness in patients with alcoholic liver disease were significantly higher than patients with viral cirrhosis. Despite these data showing a correlation between the etiology and the amount of fibrosis, recent studies have showed that the presence of alcoholic steatohepatitis increases liver stiffness measurement independently of the fibrosis stage [26,27]. Therefore the interpretation of liver stiffness measurement in patients with alcoholic liver disease should always consider not only the degree of inflammation, but also of cholestasis and liver congestion [26,27].

Lastly, alcohol consumption itself may also modify liver stiffness measurement as shown by the decrease in liver stiffness among abstainers and the increase in relapsers [28].

Imaging techniques

The main roles of imaging techniques such as ultrasonography, magnetic resonance imaging (MRI), and computed tomography (CT) are to contribute to the assessment of complications of advanced liver disease, such as ascites, portal vein thrombosis, and hepatocellular carcinoma (HCC) and to exclude other causes of abnormal liver tests such as obstructive biliary pathology. Imaging studies usually do not have a role in diagnosis of the specific etiology of liver disease, although magnetic resonance cholangiography will allow diagnosis of primary sclerosing cholangitis [29].

When evaluating patients with liver disease, ultrasonography should always be considered the first imaging study to perform as it is the least expensive, does not expose the patient to radiation nor to intravenous contrast. Recent guidelines from the European Association for the Study of the Liver suggest that cirrhotic patients, independently from the severity of liver disease, as well as noncirrhotic hepatitis B virus carriers with active hepatitis or family history of HCC and noncirrhotic patients with chronic hepatitis C and advanced liver fibrosis F3 should participate in a surveillance program [30].

CT scan and MRI are second line studies, when focal lesions or other complications such as portal vein thrombosis are detected at ultrasonography, and further evaluation is warranted.

Assessing the severity of liver disease

The clinical tools most widely used to determine prognosis in patients with liver diseases are the Child–Turcotte–Pugh classification and the Model for end-stage liver disease (MELD) score. The prognostic MELD score was adopted in 2002 to prioritize patients on the waiting list for liver transplantation [31]. Other disease-specific scores have been developed for primary biliary cirrhosis and primary sclerosing cholangitis [32].

The Child–Pugh classification was originally developed to stratify the risk of portacaval shunt in patients with variceal bleeding [33,34]. It is based on five empirically selected variables: ascites, encephalopathy, serum bilirubin, albumin, and prothrombin time. It is simple and easy to use for determining the prognosis of patients with chronic liver disease. More than one-third of patients with Child–Pugh score ≥10 can be expected to die within 1 year [35], whereas patients with scores of 7–9 and 5–6 have a 90% and 80% chance of surviving at 5 years, respectively [36,37]. Although the Child–Pugh score has been widely adopted for risk-stratifying patients with cirrhosis because of its simplicity, it presents several limitations, such as the subjective measurement of ascites and encephalopathy. Moreover, there is no variable in the Child–Pugh score that reflects renal function, which is a well-established prognostic marker in end-stage cirrhosis [38,39].

The MELD was initially developed to predict survival in patients undergoing elective transjugular intrahepatic portosystemic shunt [40]. This score was later modified to predict survival in patients with cirrhosis according to the severity of liver disease [31]. The main advantage of MELD score is that it uses objective and widely available laboratory tests such as serum bilirubin, serum creatinine, and the international normalized ratio (INR) of prothrombin time. In a study by Wiesner et al. [41], MELD score was stated to be better than Child–Pugh classification for predicting 3-month survival. However,

a further study including patients from the same UNOS database but evaluating patients with Child–Pugh class 2A, 2B and 3, showed that the ROC curves for 90-day mortality for Child–Pugh score and MELD were the same [42].

Lastly, considerable variations of MELD score occur due to different laboratory methodologies for INR [43,44] and creatinine measurement [45]. These variations can have a negative impact on the correct evaluation of patients' prognosis, but most importantly on the correct prioritization of patients for liver transplantation. Moreover, some conditions such as HCC or other complications of cirrhosis, are not well described by the MELD system. For these "MELD exceptions, " extra-MELD points are needed in other to guarantee patients the correct prioritization on the waiting list [46].

Assessment and management of extrahepatic manifestations

Digestive tract

Nearly 50% of patients with advanced liver disease, independently from its etiology, have gastroesophageal varices as a result of portal hypertension. This represents a serious complication as variceal bleeding is associated with a 6-week mortality of 10–20% [47]. Moreover, alcohol consumption can interfere with the function of all parts of the gastrointestinal tract. Chronic alcohol abuse can damage the salivary glands interfering with saliva secretion, it can increase the incidence of esophageal mucosal inflammation with the potential development of Barret's esophagus, and it can alter gastric acid secretion and motility, inducing gastric mucosal injury.

Considering all these alcohol-related gastrointestinal complications, it is reasonable to consider performing esophagogastroduodenoscopy in patients with alcohol abuse when they present with specific gastroesophageal symptoms. This becomes mandatory when evaluating patients with cirrhosis, independently of etiology. In patients with compensated cirrhosis, the main objective for screening is to prevent variceal hemorrhage. If no varices are seen on the initial endoscopy, the esophagogastroduodenoscopy should be repeated in 2–3 years, whereas if small varices are seen, then it should be repeated in 1–2 years [47].

Chronic pancreatitis with periodic episodes of acute pancreatitis is the most frequent pancreatic disorder in patients with alcoholic abuse with or without alcohol-related liver disease. The mortality rate of patients with alcoholic pancreatitis is about one-third higher than the general population. A study showed that repeated episodes of acute pancreatitis in rats produced chronic changes in the pancreas, including fat deposits, atrophy, and fibrosis [48]. In humans, changes in the pancreas related to chronic pancreatitis are more likely to occur in alcoholics who had recurrent acute inflammation of the pancreas [49]. Therefore all patients with alcohol abuse should have an assessment of pancreatic function with regular evaluation of pancreatic enzymes and abdominal ultrasound to assess pancreas morphology.

Heart and vascular system

The most common cardiovascular complications in patients with liver disease are ischemic coronary artery disease and cardiomyopathy [50]. Cardiomyopathy is frequent amongst patients with alcohol abuse and with alcohol-related liver disease. Recent studies suggest that not only the quantity of alcohol intake, but also the drinking patterns and genetic factors may influence the relation between alcohol consumption and cardiovascular disease [51].

Although the prevalence of angiographically proven critical coronary artery stenosis in patients with end-stage liver disease is unknown, some studies have reported that at least one critical coronary artery lesion occurs in 5–26% of asymptomatic cirrhotic patients undergoing evaluation for liver transplantation [52–54]. The diagnosis of ischemic artery disease in patients with advanced liver disease is difficult as they usually have poor exercise capacity, and they may not experience common symptoms provoked by exercise such as chest pain or shortness of breath [55]. Some investigators argue that the prevalence of coronary artery disease in patients with end-stage liver disease undergoing evaluation for liver transplantation is insufficient to warrant testing all asymptomatic patients over 50 years of age [56]. Therefore the decision to proceed with a specific test must be based not only on the number of risk factors present, but also, and most importantly, on the relative predicting strength of each risk factor [50].

In patients with alcohol abuse, but not necessarily alcoholic liver disease, the most common cardiac complication is alcoholic cardiomyopathy. The reported prevalence of alcoholic cardiomyopathy is variable, with men representing the largest proportion of alcoholic cardiomyopathy cases [57]. Alcoholics can present with either asymptomatic or a symptomatic alcoholic cardiomyopathy and the symptoms of congestive heart failure do not differ from those in patients with congestive heart failure from other etiologies. Alcoholic patients consuming >90 g/day alcohol for >5 years are at risk for developing asymptomatic alcoholic cardiomyopathy [58], whereas those who continue to drink may develop signs and symptoms of heart failure.

The early recognition of alcoholic cardiomyopathy is essential, as abstinence may improve, at least partially, the cardiac situation relatively quickly. The diagnosis can be made on the combined presence of alcoholism and a dilated hypocontractile heart in the absence of any other cause of dilated cardiomyopathy. Patients with acute alcohol intoxication often present with pathologic ECG changes, therefore ECG can also be useful in the diagnosis [59].

The first therapeutic step is abstinence from alcohol intake. Abstinence after development of mild heart failure can stop progression or even reverse symptoms in some cases. Without complete abstinence, the 4-year mortality for acute cardiomyopathy is nearly 50% [60]. In addition to abstinence, treatment of alcoholic cardiomyopathy is based on the standard regimen of therapy for heart failure.

Nutritional status

Alcoholic liver disease has a profound effect on nutrient intake, nutrition status, and metabolism with the results of the development of malnutrition [61]. The pathogenesis of malnutrition in patients with chronic liver disease is multifactorial, including decreased caloric intake, malabsorption, and maldigestion. Patients with alcohol abuse often replace nutrient food with empty calories from alcohol. Moreover, because of the underlying liver disease, these patients often have a reduced nutrient intake because of anorexia, dietary restrictions, and fatigue [61].

The severity of malnutrition correlates with the severity of liver disease, as advanced liver disease is associated with an increased catabolic state. In the study by Carvalho and Parise [62], considering patients with alcohol-related liver disease, the percentage of malnourishment was 46%, 84%, and 95% in Child–Pugh stages A, B, and C, respectively. Moreover, the presence of malnutrition is associated with a higher rate of complications such as variceal bleeding, ascites, encephalopathy, infections, hepatorenal syndrome, and mortality [63–65]. Therefore a proper nutritional assessment should be always performed in patients with chronic liver disease in order to identify potential nutritional risk, which may be modifiable with specific interventions.

The nutritional assessment should start with a detailed medical history with particular attention to patient weight history, dietary intake, gastrointestinal symptoms, severity of liver disease, and features suggestive of micronutrient deficiency (such as dermatitis, paresthesia, or burning of the mouth or tongue). A general physical examination focusing on findings suggestive of macro- and micronutrient deficiency should then be performed. Body mass index can be easily calculated for each patient; however, it may be misleading in patients with end-stage liver disease and those with edema and/or ascites.

Subjective global assessment tool has been proposed as a simple bedside tool to evaluate nutritional status in patients with liver disease. It comprises information on weight, dietary intake, physical appearance, and existing medical conditions. However, its sensitivity in patients with cirrhosis is controversial as it seems to not perform as well as assessment of handgrip strength. Its ability to estimate the prevalence of malnutrition amongst cirrhotic patients is inferior to body composition analysis [66].

Considering evaluation of laboratory tests, those that are routinely used in patients with liver disease (serum albumin, creatinine, prothrombin time) are affected by hepatic function, therefore their role in the nutritional assessment of nutritional status could be helpful in the early phases of liver disease. Two studies found poor correlation between plasma proteins and anthropometric measures such as triceps skinfold thickness and muscle circumference in patients with advanced liver disease [67]. Moreover, albumin is frequently used as therapeutic agent in clinical practice masking the true albumin levels. Other additional and more specific laboratory tests can be obtained in special population such as patients with alcohol-related liver disease (water-soluble vitamins), patients with cholestatic liver disease (fat-soluble vitamins), and patients with evident malnutrition.

Multiple nutritional assessment tools have been assessed in patients with liver disease; however, they should be used on an individual basis in those with evidence of malnutrition. Moreover, other specialized investigations such as dual energy X-ray absorptiometry scan, deuterium oxide dilution, and bioelectrical impedance analysis have been studied but they have high costs and limited availability.

The goal of nutritional management of patients with liver disease it to provide adequate nutrition to reduce complications, reduce hospital stay, and improve outcome of hospitalization, surgery, and possibly of liver transplantation. Patients not meeting their daily needs through diet should receive proper nutritional supplementation according to the European Society for Clinical Nutrition and Metabolism [68]. Referral to a dietitian with experience in patients with chronic liver disease can be helpful.

Bone disorders

Osteoporosis is a common complication amongst patients with liver disease [69], with a prevalence ranging between 12% and 55% [70]. The risk of osteoporosis is increased in postmenopausal women, patients with cholestatic disorders, and patients who have received prolonged corticosteroid therapy [71], but it is also common in patients with chronic hepatitis C and alcoholic cirrhosis [72,73], being associated with a 2.8-fold increase in the risk of hip fractures [74]. In patients with cirrhosis the prevalence of osteoporosis is related to the severity of liver disease [74].

The prevalence of fracture in the same population ranges between 7% and 35% [75]. In a study on patients with alcohol abuse, the prevalence of radiologically proven vertebral fractures was 22%. However, it was not known if there was an underlying liver disease and authors suggested that traumatic fractures accounted for a large proportion of the observed fractures [76].

Patients with cirrhosis or severe cholestasis should always undergo bone mineral density measurement, whereas patients with noncirrhotic liver disease, in the absence of other determined risk factors, should not undergo bone mineral density measurement as there is no evidence that osteoporosis is more prevalent in these groups [74].

Considering the management of patients with chronic liver disease, general measures includes lifestyle measures such as reduction in alcohol intake if excessive, regular weight-bearing exercise, and stopping smoking.

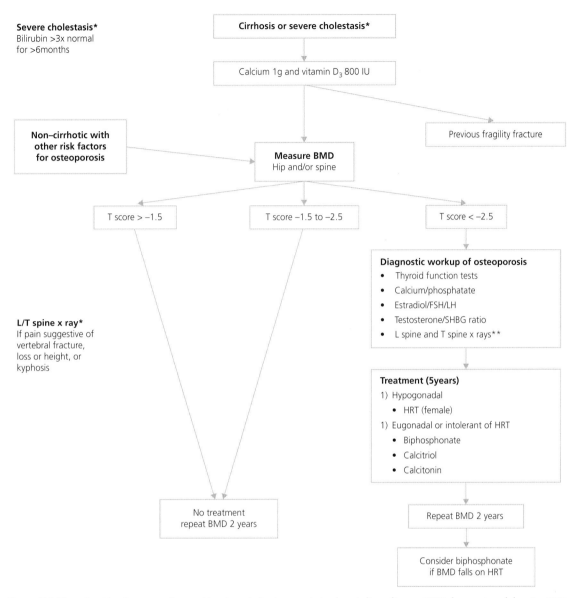

Figure 15.1 Flow chart for the prevention and treatment of osteoporosis in chronic liver disease. BMD, bone mineral density; FSH, follicle stimulating hormone; HRT, hormone replacement therapy; LH, luteinizing hormone; L, lateral; SHBG, sex hormone-binding hormone; T, transverse. (Source: Collier et al. 2002 [74]. Reproduced with permission of BMJ)

Dietary measures, such as ensuring an adequate nutrition and supplementation with calcium and vitamin D, are also recommended [74]. According to the results of the bone density measurement, different therapeutic measures and potential additional assessment are required (Figure 15.1).

Nervous system

Patients with liver disease often have neurologic signs and symptoms. The most common is hepatic encephalopathy, but other conditions such as acquired hepatocerebral degeneration and hepatic myelopathy have also been described.

Hepatic encephalopathy is a reversible neuropsychiatric and functional syndrome, occurring in 50–70% of patients with advanced liver disease. It manifests with progressive deterioration of neurologic functions ranging from mental status to deep coma. The overall prognosis for patients who develop overt hepatic encephalopathy is poor. Following the first episode of overt hepatic encephalopathy, 1-year survival is approximately 40%. In the diagnosis of encephalopathy, other etiologies of altered mental status must be ruled out. The first step in the treatment strategy of patients with hepatic encephalopathy is the identification and removal of underlying precipitating factors such as infections, gastrointestinal bleeding, and constipation. Protein restriction and treating constipation may be effective; however, there is lack of evidence to support aggressive dietary protein restriction. Oral antibiotics such as rifaximin are also used and have been proved to be effective in maintaining remission from hepatic encephalopathy, and in reducing the risk of hospitalization for hepatic encephalopathy [77].

In patients with alcohol abuse and alcohol-related liver disease, neurologic damage is related to the direct effects of ethanol on neural tissue, combined with thiamine deficiency and malnutrition. Alcohol can have a negative effect on certain neurologic processes, such as temperature regulation, sleep, and coordination. Moreover, alcohol-related brain changes can cause abnormalities in mental functioning that are detectable using specialized neuropsychologic tests. These include a wide range of diseases such as Wernicke–Korsakoff syndrome (Wernicke's encephalopathy and Korsakoff psychosis), alcoholic neuropathy, alcoholic cerebellar degeneration, alcoholic myopathy, fetal alcohol syndrome, alcohol withdrawal syndrome, dementia, and other cognitive deficits. These complications are characterized by changes in emotions and personality as well as impaired perception, learning, and memory (i.e. cognitive abilities).

Early diagnosis and intervention is important to prevent permanent neurologic damage. Brain damage may be clinically suspected by cognitive impairment, and confirmed by CT, nuclear magnetic resonance, and cognitive tests. In a study on 50 patients with end-stage liver disease, single-positron-emission tomography (SPECT) was used to assess changes in regional blood flow according to etiology of liver disease. SPECT showed significantly lower changes in regional blood flow in the frontal superior, medial, and temporal inferior regions amongst patients with previous alcohol abuse [78].

Considering the management of neurologic complications in alcoholic patients, a slow recovery of cognitive functioning can occur in patients who remain abstinent for at least 4 weeks. Moreover, CT and MRI images and brain glucose metabolism have been shown to improve with prolonged abstinence. Prolonged supplementation with thiamine, cobalamine, pyridoxine, and folate in addition to physiotherapy can also improve recovery.

Psychiatric disorders

Patients with alcohol abuse, and particularly patients with alcohol dependence, have a high prevalence of psychiatric comorbidities such as anxiety, depression, and affective disorders [79]. Moreover, alcoholics have a higher risk of developing other addictions such as nicotine [80].

Therefore the coordination between hepatologist and addiction specialists such as psychiatrists, psychologists, and social workers is crucial to reduce the time interval between the first manifestations of alcohol dependence and referral [5]. Because cigarette smoking and alcohol abuse are synergistic in causing cardiovascular diseases and cancer, including HCC, hepatologists are encouraged to promote and assist smoking cessation among patients with alcoholic liver disease [81].

Endocrine system

The liver and its pleotropic functions have a fundamental role in regulating metabolism, and are also an inevitable target of multiple metabolic disorders. The numerous and constant relationships and feedback mechanisms between the liver and all endocrine organs are reflected by the fact that an alteration of one often results in the malfunction of the other [82].

Alcoholic liver disease is commonly associated with abnormalities in circulating levels of thyroid hormones. In a study on 31 patients with alcoholic liver disease, a reduction in circulating free T3, in association with normal or reduced levels of thyroid-stimulating hormone (TSH), was noted in subjects with alcoholic hepatitis and cirrhosis. The absence of abnormalities in subjects with fatty changes despite similar alcohol intake suggested that changes in free T3 reflect the severity of the underlying liver disease [83]. Patients with autoimmune hepatitis or primary biliary cirrhosis have a higher than expected incidence of thyroid dysfunction. From a series of patients with different etiologies of liver disease, the prevalence of thyroid dysfunction was reported to be 13% in primary biliary cirrhosis, 11% in primary sclerosing cholangitis, and 25% in NAFLD [84]. In patients with cirrhosis, adrenal insufficiency is reported during sepsis and septic shock, and is associated with increased mortality.

Pseudo-Cushing's syndrome has been described in patients with alcohol-induced liver disease. This condition may develop as a result of continuing oral cortisol secretion in the presence of impaired cortisol metabolism. The latter is mediated by defective hepatic 11β-hydroxysteroid dehydrogenase activity, while the former might be due to either an abnormal glucocorticoid feedback or to stimulation of cortisol secretion at the level of the hypothalamus or pituitary [85].

The normal function of the hypothalamic–pituitary–gonadal axis is affected in liver disease. Alcoholic liver disease is associated with abnormalities in circulating levels of gonadal steroid hormones. Increasing circulating estradiol and reduction in testosterone have been found in male patients with alcohol-related hepatic fatty changes, hepatitis, and cirrhosis. Testicular atrophy, decreased libido, infertility, and gynecomastia are common findings in men with cirrhosis.

Among women, alcohol abuse causes disturbances in the hormonal status and reproductive performance. Chronic alcohol consumption is associated with hypogonadism, loss of secondary sexual characteristics, amenorrhea, and early menopause, as a result of a reduction in estrogen and gonadotropin secretion [86]. Female patients with cirrhosis show significantly lower levels of total testosterone and higher levels of prolactin and δ4-androstenedione than patients who have undergone liver transplantation [87].

Conclusions

Alcohol remains the main cause of liver disease worldwide; however, it is common for patients with alcoholic liver disease to share risk factors for coexisting liver diseases such as NADLD or chronic viral hepatitis. Moreover, extrahepatic complications are often present in patients with alcoholic liver disease. In addition to a complete medical history and physical examination, emphasis during clinical assessment should be placed on all the potential extrahepatic manifestations which should be treated when necessary.

Therefore, the successful assessment and management of patients with alcoholic liver disease requires not only the integration of all the competences in public health, epidemiology, and addiction behavior, but also an active collaboration between the hepatologist and all the specialists involved in this process.

References

[1] Mann RE, Smart RG, Govoni R. The epidemiology of alcoholic liver disease. *Alcohol Res Health* 2003; **27**: 209–219.

[2] Rehm J, Taylor B, Mohapatra S, et al. Alcohol as a risk factor for liver cirrhosis: a systematic review and meta-analysis. *Drug Alcohol Rev* 2010; **29**: 437–445.

[3] Levitsky J, Mailliard ME. Diagnosis and therapy of alcoholic liver disease. *Semin Liver Dis* 2004; **24**: 233–247.

[4] O'Shea RS, Dasarathy S, McCullough AJ. Alcoholic liver disease. *Hepatology* 2010; **51**: 307–328.

[5] EASL clinical practical guidelines: management of alcoholic liver disease. *J Hepatol* 2012; **57**: 399–420.

[6] Zakhari S, Li TK. Determinants of alcohol use and abuse: impact of quantity and frequency patterns on liver disease. *Hepatology* 2007; **46**: 2032–2039.

[7] Miller WR, Heather N, Hall W. Calculating standard drink units: international comparisons. *Br J Addict* 1991; **86**: 43–47.

[8] Scaglioni F, Ciccia S, Marino M, Bedogni G, Bellentani S. ASH and NASH. *Dig Dis* 2011; **29**: 202–210.

[9] Heidelbaugh JJ, Bruderly M. Cirrhosis and chronic liver failure: part I. Diagnosis and evaluation. *Am Fam Physician* 2006; **74**: 756–762.

[10] Li CP, Lee FY, Hwang SJ, et al. Spider angiomas in patients with liver cirrhosis: role of alcoholism and impaired liver function. *Scand J Gastroenterol* 1999; **34**: 520–523.

[11] Diehl AM. Alcoholic liver disease. *Med Clin North Am* 1989; **73**: 815–830.

[12] Cavanaugh J, Niewoehner CB, Nuttall FQ. Gynecomastia and cirrhosis of the liver. *Arch Intern Med* 1990; **150**: 563–565.

[13] Braunstein GD. Gynecomastia. *N Engl J Med* 1993; **328**: 490–495.

[14] Dutta SK, Dukehart M, Narang A, Latham PS. Functional and structural changes in parotid glands of alcoholic cirrhotic patients. *Gastroenterology* 1989; **96**: 510–518.

[15] Dufour DR, Lott JA, Nolte FS, Gretch DR, Koff RS, Seeff LB. Diagnosis and monitoring of hepatic injury. I. Performance characteristics of laboratory tests. *Clin Chem* 2000; **46**: 2027–2049.

[16] Dufour DR, Lott JA, Nolte FS, Gretch DR, Koff RS, Seeff LB. Diagnosis and monitoring of hepatic injury. II.

Recommendations for use of laboratory tests in screening, diagnosis, and monitoring. *Clin Chem* 2000; **46**: 2050–2068.

[17] Skelly MM, James PD, Ryder SD. Findings on liver biopsy to investigate abnormal liver function tests in the absence of diagnostic serology. *J Hepatol* 2001; **35**: 195–199.

[18] Cohen JA, Kaplan MM. The SGOT/SGPT ratio: an indicator of alcoholic liver disease. *Dig Dis Sci* 1979; **24**: 835–838.

[19] Imbert-Bismut F, Ratziu V, Pieroni L, Charlotte F, Benhamou Y, Poynard T. Biochemical markers of liver fibrosis in patients with hepatitis C virus infection: a prospective study. *Lancet* 2001; **357**: 1069–1075.

[20] Naveau S, Raynard B, Ratziu V, et al. Biomarkers for the prediction of liver fibrosis in patients with chronic alcoholic liver disease. *Clin Gastroenterol Hepatol* 2005; **3**: 167–174.

[21] Cales P, Oberti F, Michalak S, et al. A novel panel of blood markers to assess the degree of liver fibrosis. *Hepatology* 2005; **42**: 1373–1381.

[22] Naveau S, Gaude G, Asnacios A, et al. Diagnostic and prognostic values of noninvasive biomarkers of fibrosis in patients with alcoholic liver disease. *Hepatology* 2009; **49**: 97–105.

[23] Foucher J, Chanteloup E, Vergniol J, et al. Diagnosis of cirrhosis by transient elastography (FibroScan): a prospective study. *Gut* 2006; **55**: 403–408.

[24] Nahon P, Kettaneh A, Tengher-Barna I, et al. Assessment of liver fibrosis using transient elastography in patients with alcoholic liver disease. *J Hepatol* 2008; **49**: 1062–1068.

[25] Nguyen-Khac E, Saint-Leger P, Tramier B, Coevoet H, Capron D, Dupas JL. Noninvasive diagnosis of large esophageal varices by Fibroscan: strong influence of the cirrhosis etiology. *Alcohol Clin Exp Res* 2010; **34**: 1146–1153.

[26] Mueller S, Millonig G, Sarovska L, et al. Increased liver stiffness in alcoholic liver disease: differentiating fibrosis from steatohepatitis. *World J Gastroenterol* 2010; **16**: 966–972.

[27] Mueller S, Sandrin L. Liver stiffness: a novel parameter for the diagnosis of liver disease. *Hepat Med* 2010; **2**: 49–67.

[28] Gelsi E, Dainese R, Truchi R, et al. Effect of detoxification on liver stiffness assessed by Fibroscan® in alcoholic patients. *Alcohol Clin Exp Res* 2011; **35**: 566–570.

[29] Chapman R, Fevery J, Kalloo A, et al. Diagnosis and management of primary sclerosing cholangitis. *Hepatology* 2010; **51**: 660–678.

[30] EASL–EORTC clinical practice guidelines: management of hepatocellular carcinoma. *J Hepatol* 2012; **56**: 908–943.

[31] Kamath PS, Wiesner RH, Malinchoc M, et al. A model to predict survival in patients with end-stage liver disease. *Hepatology* 2001; **33**: 464–470.

[32] Murray KF, Carithers RL Jr. AASLD practice guidelines: evaluation of the patient for liver transplantation. *Hepatology* 2005; **41**: 1407–1432.

[33] Pugh RN, Murray-Lyon IM, Dawson JL, Pietroni MC, Williams R. Transection of the oesophagus for bleeding oesophageal varices. *Br J Surg* 1973; **60**: 646–649.

[34] Trey C, Burns DG, Saunders SJ. Treatment of hepatic coma by exchange blood transfusion. *N Engl J Med* 1966; **274**: 473–481.

[35] Shetty K, Rybicki L, Carey WD. The Child–Pugh classification as a prognostic indicator for survival in primary sclerosing cholangitis. *Hepatology* 1997; **25**: 1049–1053.

[36] Lucey MR, Brown KA, Everson GT, et al. Minimal criteria for placement of adults on the liver transplant waiting list: a report of a national conference organized by the American Society of Transplant Physicians and the American Association for the Study of Liver Diseases. *Liver Transpl Surg* 1997; **3**: 628–637.

[37] Propst A, Propst T, Zangerl G, Ofner D, Judmaier G, Vogel W. Prognosis and life expectancy in chronic liver disease. *Dig Dis Sci* 1995; **40**: 1805–1815.

[38] Durand F, Valla D. Assessment of the prognosis of cirrhosis: Child–Pugh versus MELD. *J Hepatol* 2005; **42**(Suppl): S100–107.

[39] D'Amico G, Garcia-Tsao G, Pagliaro L. Natural history and prognostic indicators of survival in cirrhosis: a systematic review of 118 studies. *J Hepatol* 2006; **44**: 217–231.

[40] Malinchoc M, Kamath PS, Gordon FD, Peine CJ, Rank J, ter Borg PC. A model to predict poor survival in patients undergoing transjugular intrahepatic portosystemic shunts. *Hepatology* 2000; **31**: 864–871.

[41] Wiesner R, Edwards E, Freeman R, et al. Model for end-stage liver disease (MELD) and allocation of donor livers. *Gastroenterology* 2003; **124**: 91–96.

[42] Heuman DM, Mihas A. Utility of the MELD score for assessing 3-month survival in patients with liver cirrhosis: one more positive answer. *Gastroenterology* 2003; **125**: 992–993; author reply 994–995.

[43] Porte RJ, Lisman T, Tripodi A, Caldwell SH, Trotter JF. The International Normalized Ratio (INR) in the MELD score: problems and solutions. *Am J Transplant* 2010; **10**: 1349–1353.

44] Trotter JF, Brimhall B, Arjal R, Phillips C. Specific laboratory methodologies achieve higher model for endstage liver disease (MELD) scores for patients listed for liver transplantation. *Liver Transpl* 2004; **10**: 995–1000.

[45] Cholongitas E, Marelli L, Kerry A, et al. Different methods of creatinine measurement significantly affect MELD scores. *Liver Transpl* 2007; **13**: 523–529.

[46] Freeman RB Jr, Gish RG, Harper A, et al. Model for end-stage liver disease (MELD) exception guidelines: results and recommendations from the MELD Exception Study Group and Conference (MESSAGE) for the approval of patients who need liver transplantation with diseases not considered by the standard MELD formula. *Liver Transpl* 2006; **12**: S128–136.

[47] de Franchis R. Revising consensus in portal hypertension: report of the Baveno V consensus workshop on methodology of diagnosis and therapy in portal hypertension. *J Hepatol* 2010; **53**: 762–768.

[48] Elsasser HP, Haake T, Grimmig M, Adler G, Kern HF. Repetitive cerulein-induced pancreatitis and pancreatic fibrosis in the rat. *Pancreas* 1992; **7**: 385–390.

[49] Ammann RW, Muellhaupt B. Progression of alcoholic acute to chronic pancreatitis. *Gut* 1994; **35**: 552–556.

[50] Mandell MS, Lindenfeld J, Tsou MY, Zimmerman M. Cardiac evaluation of liver transplant candidates. *World J Gastroenterol* 2008; **14**: 3445–3451.

[51] Maron BJ, Towbin JA, Thiene G, et al. Contemporary definitions and classification of the cardiomyopathies: an American Heart Association Scientific Statement from the Council on Clinical Cardiology, Heart Failure and Transplantation Committee; Quality of Care and Outcomes Research and Functional Genomics and Translational Biology Interdisciplinary Working Groups; and Council on Epidemiology and Prevention. *Circulation* 2006; **113**: 1807–1816.

[52] Carey WD, Dumot JA, Pimentel RR, et al. The prevalence of coronary artery disease in liver transplant candidates over age 50. *Transplantation* 1995; **59**: 859–864.

[53] Tiukinhoy-Laing SD, Rossi JS, et al. Cardiac hemodynamic and coronary angiographic characteristics of patients being evaluated for liver transplantation. *Am J Cardiol* 2006; **98**: 178–181.

[54] Senzolo M, Bassanello M, Graziotto A, et al. Microvascular autonomic dysfunction may justify false-positive stress myocardial perfusion imaging in patients with liver cirrhosis undergoing liver transplantation. *Transplant Proc* 2008; **40**: 1916–1917.

[55] Mandell MS, Tsou MY. Cardiovascular dysfunction in patients with end-stage liver disease. *J Chin Med Assoc* 2008; **71**: 331–335.

[56] Kryzhanovski VA, Beller GA. Usefulness of preoperative noninvasive radionuclide testing for detecting coronary artery disease in candidates for liver transplantation. *Am J Cardiol* 1997; **79**: 986–988.

[57] Fernandez-Sola J, Estruch R, Nicolas JM, et al. Comparison of alcoholic cardiomyopathy in women versus men. *Am J Cardiol* 1997; **80**: 481–485.

[58] Fauchier L, Babuty D, Poret P, et al. Comparison of long-term outcome of alcoholic and idiopathic dilated cardiomyopathy. *Eur Heart J* 2000; **21**: 306–314.

[59] Laonigro I, Correale M, Di Biase M, Altomare E. Alcohol abuse and heart failure. *Eur J Heart Fail* 2009; **11**: 453–462.

[60] Skotzko CE, Vrinceanu A, Krueger L, Freudenberger R. Alcohol use and congestive heart failure: incidence, importance, and approaches to improved history taking. *Heart Fail Rev* 2009; **14**: 51–55.

[61] DiCecco SR, Francisco-Ziller N. Nutrition in alcoholic liver disease. *Nutr Clin Pract* 2006; **21**: 245–254.

[62] Carvalho L, Parise ER. Evaluation of nutritional status of nonhospitalized patients with liver cirrhosis. *Arq Gastroenterol* 2006; **43**: 269–274.

[63] Alvares-da-Silva MR, Reverbel da Silveira T. Comparison between handgrip strength, subjective global assessment, and prognostic nutritional index in assessing malnutrition and predicting clinical outcome in cirrhotic outpatients. *Nutrition* 2005; **21**: 113–117.

[64] Campillo B, Richardet JP, Scherman E, Bories PN. Evaluation of nutritional practice in hospitalized cirrhotic patients: results of a prospective study. *Nutrition* 2003; **19**: 515–521.

[65] Sam J, Nguyen GC. Protein-calorie malnutrition as a prognostic indicator of mortality among patients hospitalized with cirrhosis and portal hypertension. *Liver Int* 2009; **29**: 1396–1402.

[66] Figueiredo FA, Perez RM, Freitas MM, Kondo M. Comparison of three methods of nutritional assessment in liver cirrhosis: subjective global assessment, traditional nutritional parameters, and body composition analysis. *J Gastroenterol* 2006; **41**: 476–482.

[67] Piquet MA, Ollivier I, Gloro R, Castel H, Tiengou LE, Dao T. Nutritional indices in cirrhotic patients. *Nutrition* 2006; **22**: 216–217; author reply 218–219.

[68] Plauth M, Cabre E, Riggio O, et al. ESPEN Guidelines on enteral nutrition: liver disease. *Clin Nutr* 2006; **25**: 285–294.

[69] Sokhi RP, Anantharaju A, Kondaveeti R, Creech SD, Islam KK, Van Thiel DH. Bone mineral density among cirrhotic patients awaiting liver transplantation. *Liver Transpl* 2004; **10**: 648–653.

[70] Collier J. Bone disorders in chronic liver disease. *Hepatology* 2007; **46**: 1271–1278.

[71] Menon KV, Angulo P, Weston S, Dickson ER, Lindor KD. Bone disease in primary biliary cirrhosis: independent indicators and rate of progression. *J Hepatol* 2001; **35**: 316–323.

[72] Carey EJ, Balan V, Kremers WK, Hay JE. Osteopenia and osteoporosis in patients with end-stage liver disease caused by hepatitis C and alcoholic liver disease: not just a cholestatic problem. *Liver Transpl* 2003; **9**: 1166–1173.

[73] Floreani A, Mega A, Tizian L, et al. Bone metabolism and gonad function in male patients undergoing liver transplantation: a two-year longitudinal study. *Osteoporos Int* 2001; **12**: 749–754.

[74] Collier JD, Ninkovic M, Compston JE. Guidelines on the management of osteoporosis associated with chronic liver disease. *Gut* 2002; **50**(Suppl 1): i1–9.

[75] Guanabens N, Pares A, Ros I, et al. Severity of cholestasis and advanced histological stage but not menopausal status are the major risk factors for osteoporosis in primary biliary cirrhosis. *J Hepatol* 2005; **42**: 573–577.

[76] Peris P, Guanabens N, Pares A, et al. Vertebral fractures and osteopenia in chronic alcoholic patients. *Calcif Tissue Int* 1995; **57**: 111–114.

[77] Bass NM, Mullen KD, Sanyal A, et al. Rifaximin treatment in hepatic encephalopathy. *N Engl J Med* 2010; **362**: 1071–1081.

[78] Burra P, Senzolo M, Pizzolato G, et al. Does liver-disease aetiology have a role in cerebral blood-flow alterations in liver cirrhosis? *Eur J Gastroenterol Hepatol* 2004; **16**: 885–890.

[79] Bourdon KH, Rae DS, Locke BZ, Narrow WE, Regier DA. Estimating the prevalence of mental disorders in US adults from the Epidemiologic Catchment Area Survey. *Public Health Rep* 1992; **107**: 663–668.

[80] Grant BF, Hasin DS, Chou SP, Stinson FS, Dawson DA. Nicotine dependence and psychiatric disorders in the United States: results from the national epidemiologic survey on alcohol and related conditions. *Arch Gen Psychiatry* 2004; **61**: 1107–1115.

[81] Altamirano J, Bataller R. Cigarette smoking and chronic liver diseases. *Gut* 2010; **59**: 1159–1162.

[82] Burra P. Liver abnormalities and endocrine diseases. *Best Pract Res Clin Gastroenterol* 2013; **27**: 553–563.

[83] Burra P, Franklyn JA, Ramsden DB, Elias E, Sheppard MC. Severity of alcoholic liver disease and markers of thyroid and steroid status. *Postgrad Med J* 1992; **68**: 804–810.

[84] Silveira MG, Mendes FD, Diehl NN, Enders FT, Lindor KD. Thyroid dysfunction in primary biliary cirrhosis, primary sclerosing cholangitis and non-alcoholic fatty liver disease. *Liver Int* 2009; **29**: 1094–1100.

[85] Stewart PM, Burra P, Shackleton CH, Sheppard MC, Elias E. 11 beta-hydroxysteroid dehydrogenase deficiency and glucocorticoid status in patients with alcoholic and non-alcoholic chronic liver disease. *J Clin Endocrinol Metab* 1993; **76**: 748–751.

[86] Karagiannis A, Harsoulis F. Gonadal dysfunction in systemic diseases. *Eur J Endocrinol* 2005; **152**: 501–513.

[87] Burra P, Germani G, Masier A, et al. Sexual dysfunction in chronic liver disease: is liver transplantation an effective cure? *Transplantation* 2010; **89**: 1425–1429.

CHAPTER 16

Brief alcohol interventions

Stephanie Scott[1] and Eileen Kaner[2]

[1]*Human Nutrition Research Centre and Institute of Health and Society, Newcastle University, Newcastle upon Tyne, UK*
[2]*Institute of Health and Society, Newcastle University, Newcastle upon Tyne, UK*

KEY POINTS

- Rapidly increasing incidence of liver problems in the United Kingdom, including an increase in both younger patients and women, mean it is important to develop upstream preventive approaches to help tackle liver damage before it becomes too established.

- A large body of research supports the effectiveness and cost-effectiveness of brief intervention at reducing alcohol-related problems across a range of population groups and settings, particularly in primary health care.

- Current evidence does not generally indicate an additional benefit of longer or more intensive brief intervention as opposed to shorter, less intensive input. Therefore, practitioners should emphasize risk identification and short, simple interventions that focus on promoting patients' awareness and self-regulation of alcohol intake.

Background

Alcohol consumption contributes to over 60 diseases and is responsible for almost 4% of deaths worldwide [1]. Risky drinking is also one of the five leading risk factors for global disease burden [2] and the second in high income countries after tobacco use [1]. Alcohol consumption is estimated to cause 20–50% of liver cirrhosis cases worldwide [1] and death certification data show that more than 80% of UK liver deaths are due to alcohol-related cirrhosis [3]. Furthermore, liver disease causes a greater loss of working years of life than chest disease, lung cancer, cerebrovascular disease, or diabetes [4]. The United Kingdom has seen distinct changes in patterns of alcoholic liver disease over the past 30 years, with doctors and the wider hepatology community reporting an increase in both younger patients and women presenting with alcoholic liver disease [5]. In contrast to many parts of continental Europe, which have seen a decrease in liver mortality over the same period of time, UK liver disease death rates increased by more than 400% between 1970 and 2010 [6]. Between 2001 and 2012 alone, UK deaths from liver disease rose by 40% from 7841 to 10 948, with a fivefold increase in cirrhosis among young people aged 35–55 [7]. Thus, while there remains a clear link between worldwide alcohol consumption and liver death rates, this relationship differs between countries [8]. For example, while Finland, the United Kingdom, and France have higher liver mortality rates for a given alcohol consumption, Spain and Italy remain at a more intermediate level. Reasons for between-country differences are yet to be fully determined with a number of cofactors thought to influence the relationship between alcohol consumption and liver mortality, including diet, genetics, and drinking patterns [8]. In addition to these acute health problems, wider societal

---

Alcohol Abuse and Liver Disease, First Edition. Edited by James Neuberger and Andrea DiMartini.
© 2015 John Wiley & Sons, Ltd. Published 2015 by John Wiley & Sons, Ltd.

consequences of alcohol consumption include the exacerbation of mental health problems, self-harm and/or suicidal behavior, crime and disorder, domestic violence, accidents and trauma, and unintended or unprotected sexual experiences. Thus, burden relating to alcohol consumption is costly. For example, recent estimates calculate the total cost to the UK economy to be £25.1 ($40.2) billion each year [9]. Given this extensive array of damage caused by excessive alcohol use, intervening to reduce its risk and harm is a global public health priority.

Epidemiologic data have long suggested that it is those who drink at hazardous and harmful levels (rather than dependent drinkers) who contribute the majority of alcohol-related problems at a population level. Hazardous drinking is a repeated pattern of drinking that increases the risk of physical or psychologic problems [10], whereas harmful drinking is defined by the presence of these problems [11]. As hazardous and harmful drinkers outnumber dependent drinkers by a ratio of 7 : 1 in the United Kingdom, achieving the greatest impact in reducing alcohol problems at a population level is widely regarded to be made by focusing on this larger group rather than the smaller group of dependent drinkers. This is known as the *preventative paradox* [12], although recent work has challenged such a strong emphasis on hazardous as well as harmful drinking, by suggesting that small changes amongst very heavy drinkers can also bring substantive health gain, an effect largely explained by increased levels of comorbidity amongst very heavy drinkers [13]. Nevertheless, it is still the case that only focusing on dependent drinkers would miss a high burden of morbidity and social harm. The paradox is the fact that, while dependent drinkers each experience higher individual levels of alcohol-related damage, society incurs a greater burden from a larger group of hazardous and harmful drinkers often due to an accumulate of a wide range of public sector services costs. Nondependent drinkers are likely to experience less severe problems, at least for much of their drinking life, but the aggregate impact of social, chronic, and acute health problems in this group affects both the drinkers themselves and often a wide range of other people (this is often called collateral damage). Thus, there is a clear need for an effective preventative measure to help reduce excessive drinking in this larger sector of society which covers a wide range of drinking patterns and intensities.

Preventative medicine is typically described on three basic levels – primary, secondary, and tertiary. Primary prevention involves attempts to stop the disease or behavior from occurring in the first place (e.g. educational initiatives) while tertiary prevention is treatment focused. Although there is a large volume of evidence on primary prevention, only a relatively small number of programs are reportedly effective, while specialist treatment is suitable for dependent drinkers only. Thus, of interest in this chapter are *secondary* preventative measures which consist of interventions to improve health behavior at an early stage of risk or harm, when it is likely to be most amenable to change. Such measures tend to include screening to identify relevant individuals, followed by the delivery of individual feedback, advice, and/or counseling. Such interventions have been demonstrated to be effective and cost-effective at reducing harm at a population level. The rest of this chapter focuses on brief interventions as a secondary preventative approach to reduce alcohol-related risk or harm amongst hazardous and harmful drinkers. In essence, this approach aims to prevent individuals progressing to liver damage later in life by trying to promote lower risk drinking at an earlier point. Thus, we consider the theory and practice behind brief alcohol interventions, the available evidence base for brief intervention across a variety of settings, and conclude with an overview of the key debates, new directions, and knowledge gaps in the field of brief intervention research.

What is brief intervention?

Brief alcohol intervention refers to the use of structured, talk-based counseling or advice aimed at reducing alcohol consumption or risky drinking behavior. In most circumstances, the goal of brief intervention is generally to reduce drinking to lower risk levels rather than promote abstinence. Brief interventions can also focus on reducing alcohol-related problems with or without reduced consumption such as by promoting drinking in lower risk settings. Sessions can be accompanied by additional components such as information leaflets, web-based resources, drinking diaries, and booster sessions to reinforce messages from the original brief intervention activity. Given the size of the group potentially requiring attention, it is necessary to have an intervention that is feasible to deliver in community-based settings by generalist practitioners. To this end, brief alcohol intervention is designed to be delivered to opportunistic, nontreatment-seeking populations by nonaddictions specialists, in a wide variety of settings but often in primary care. Moreover, potential recipients may not be aware of their alcohol-related risk or harm, are yet to develop chronic or dependent patterns of drinking, and are unlikely to have come into contact with specialist treatment services. Thus, interventions need to be effective and feasible to deliver to a large population, but also acceptable and practically relevant to those in receipt of the intervention.

Brief intervention theory

Importantly, brief intervention does not simply consist of traditional (psychologic or psychiatric) treatment squeezed into a shorter duration of time [14]. Rather, it has a specific theoretical underpinning and practical structure of its own. Brief intervention is based on social cognitive theory, drawn from the wider discipline of psychology, which is concerned with understanding, predicting, and changing human behavior. Social cognitive theory itself is broadly founded on the concept of social learning [15] which regards behavior as a dynamic and reciprocal interaction between the individual, their actions, and the physical and social environment around them. In this approach, the individual's cognitive (thinking) and affective (feeling) attributes affect how they respond to the external world and are reinforced by it. Hence, all individuals are seen as having the capacity to observe and learn from the behavior of other people around them and the situations they encounter. Thus, drinking behavior is influenced not only by an individual's attitudes towards alcohol and their awareness of risk, but also by social norms or patterns of use in relevant social groups, and the attitudes of friends and family members. All of these factors influence an individual's motivation or ability to change their drinking behavior; brief intervention focuses on both personal and contextual facets of drinking behavior. Of importance is that the individual is recognized to be the expert in their own lives and so brief intervention encourages them to examine their beliefs and attitudes towards drinking, their self-efficacy (or sense of personal confidence) about being able to

change, and draws attention to how their drinking sits in relation to other people's (normative comparisons). As such, empathy and rapport are key principles of brief intervention and practitioners must honor an individual's sense of autonomy. Thus, if an individual is not ready or does not wish to change, this must be respected – in fact, acknowledging the individual's right to make this decision can enhance motivation as this reinforces personal responsibility for health behavior change. Hence, the final step in brief alcohol intervention (making a plan for change) may not always be reached. If this is the case, practitioners will instead assist individuals to consider their own personal barriers and facilitators of change.

Brief intervention structure and practice

Brief interventions generally consist of two broad modalities [16]: *simple structured advice*, in the form of personalized feedback following screening and practical steps on how to reduce drinking and/or avoid its adverse consequences; and *extended brief intervention*, which generally takes the form of counseling such as behavior change counseling or Motivational Interviewing (MI). The former is a distilled and often manualized version of MI while the latter is more person-centered and it aims to highlight conflicts regarding the pros and cons of behavior change and use empathy and an avoidance of direct confrontation to encourage change. Both forms of brief intervention share the aim of motivating people to change drinking behavior to promote health gain but differ in the precise means by which this is achieved. Brief intervention for nontreatment-seeking populations tends to be delivered in a single appointment or a series of related sessions (typically exceeding no more than five sessions) lasting between 5 and 60 minutes [17]. Despite this variability, its content should be based on the FRAMES structure [18], characterized by the acronym:

F – personalized *feedback* on the individual's risk from their drinking;

R – promoting personal *responsibility* for change;

A – providing *advice* on risk reduction or give explicit direction to change;

M – provide a *menu* of options or strategies for behavior change;

E – delivering advice or counseling using *empathy* and avoiding judgment;

S – promoting *self-efficacy* or encouraging optimism about the scope for behavior change.

While traditionally delivered face-to-face, practitioner to patient, increasingly brief alcohol intervention has been delivered electronically via the internet or computer-based apps, and there are seven reviews that have examined computer or web-based brief alcohol intervention. Although better than no intervention controls, electronic forms of brief intervention rarely produce superior outcomes in comparison to other, active, face-to-face interventions. The duration of effect is also unclear. Nevertheless, augmenting more traditional brief intervention approaches with technology may achieve moderate health benefits and represent a low cost method of reaching individuals who tend not to present to services, such as the working population, young people, or those involved in the criminal justice sector. Lastly, while some have used the term brief intervention to describe shorter forms of therapy within a specialist care context in drinkers who are aware that they have an alcohol problem, this is best referred to as *brief treatment* to avoid confusion.

Evidence for brief interventions

There is a large evidence base supporting the effectiveness of brief alcohol intervention at reducing alcohol-related problems across a range of population groups and settings. Indeed, it represents one of the most robust areas of alcohol interventions compared with other psychologic and pharmacologic approaches. Thus, in 2010, the US Preventative Services Task Force gave brief alcohol intervention a "B" recommendation meaning "there is strong evidence supporting the need for primary care providers to do it." The most comprehensive systematic review of brief interventions was conducted by Moyer et al. [19], comprising 56 controlled trials conducted in a range of settings, with treatment-seeking and nontreatment-seeking patients. This review identified 34 trials comparing brief intervention (defined as no more than four sessions) to control conditions in nontreatment-seeking populations; 20 trials comparing brief interventions to more extended interventions within treatment-seeking populations; one comparing brief intervention to more extended treatment in a nontreatment-seeking sample; and one

final report examining both brief intervention versus control and brief intervention versus extended treatment comparisons. Meta-analyses demonstrated that brief intervention led to a significant reduction in both alcohol consumption and other alcohol-related outcomes in comparison to control conditions at <3 months, 3–6 months, and 6–12 months follow-up.

This review does not stand alone. A recent review of systematic reviews highlighted that there have been 24 published systematic reviews (covering a total of 56 randomized controlled trials reported across 80 papers) of brief alcohol interventions in primary health care settings, all coming to similar conclusions, with evidence for beneficial effects (e.g. reductions in drinking quantity, frequency, and intensity) particularly strong amongst middle-aged male drinkers [20]. Brief intervention appears most impactful in nontreatment-seeking populations, with directly delivered, individually focused brief intervention (i.e. structured and face-to-face) generally producing greater positive effects than indirect delivery. A recent review and meta-analysis also suggests that success can be achieved via practitioners other than doctors [21]. Further, while the effects from a single session brief intervention have been found still to be present at 2 and 4 years post intervention, another study found no evidence at 10 years follow-up. Moreover, Chisholm et al. [22] have estimated that, if brief interventions were successfully delivered to 25% of the at-risk population within primary care throughout Europe, 408 000 years of disability and premature death would be avoided, representing an estimated saving of £639 million each year.

Nevertheless, while the effects from brief intervention have been found still to be present at 2 and 4 years post intervention (this was an initial 15-minute session followed up by a booster telephone call), another study found no evidence at 10 years follow-up. Further, in certain population groups (such as younger adolescents) and contexts (such as emergency care, the workplace, and the criminal justice sector), evidence is weaker (because of small numbers of individual trials) or more equivocal, with both positive and null findings reported. Thus, while one systematic review based in emergency care found that brief intervention had a significant effect upon alcohol intake, risky drinking practices, alcohol-related negative outcomes, and injury frequency [23], another found insufficient evidence of superior impact [24]. A further systematic review in general hospital settings found that brief intervention reduced alcohol consumption by up to 69 g/week compared with controls at 6 months, with a significant effect also demonstrated at 12-month follow-up [25]. However, the small number of studies with comparable outcomes (n = 3) resulted in only weak evidence. Thus, evidence for brief alcohol intervention is plentiful, and generally positive, but stronger in some settings than others.

Targeting key groups

Targeting interventions at young people who are already drinking excessively is more effective than primary prevention, because the interventions will have more salience for the individuals receiving them. Further, in light of the overlapping effect of drinking and high body mass inex (BMI), brief intervention has the added potential to focus on comorbidity of both alcohol and weight management. However, most research has focused on older adolescents attending educational establishments where there have now been approximately 16 controlled trials [26], while work with younger adolescents remains limited. The most effective forms of brief intervention with older adolescents appear to be those involving MI approaches and elements of personalized feedback about a young person's alcohol consumption and level of alcohol-related risk, with a normative component. Nevertheless, few brief intervention effects in this age group seem to persist beyond 6 months post intervention, and booster or repeated sessions might be needed amongst this population to sustain change.

A key consideration when comparing preventative and treatment options for younger people is that they often have a number of other difficulties including social, emotional, family, and criminologic needs, which generally compound their alcohol needs and the inefficacy of treatment interventions. There are also a number of general challenges inherent in the delivery of brief interventions to young people who drink, related to both the setting in which the intervention can occur and its traditional face-to-face format. For example, brief interventions with adults have primarily been delivered in health settings, with this approach often missing individuals who do not frequently engage with health services, such as young people. To this end, it has been suggested that young people may prefer self-directed or minimal-contact methods of alcohol intervention,

and there is a burgeoning field using information technology, mobile phone technology, and the internet, where initial results are conflicting yet promising.

Evidence gaps have also been identified in other key population groups including older drinkers, female drinkers (especially pregnant women), minority ethnic groups, dependent or comorbid drinkers, and those living in transitional, low income, and developing countries, with the evidence base dominated by English and Nordic speaking countries [20]. Further, despite an association between alcohol use and offending behavior, there has been relatively little research in the criminal justice sector. The SIPS probation trial (a large cluster randomized trial) included over 500 offenders and found reduced drinking in all three conditions (leaflet-based control, 5 minutes structured advice, and 20 minutes of behavior change counseling) at 6 and 12-month follow-up [27]. Despite the lack of between-group differences at follow-up, those in the brief advice (36%) or counseling (38%) groups were less likely to reoffend than controls (50%) in the year following brief intervention.

Finally, evidence for the efficacy of brief interventions among dependent drinkers is inconsistent, with one review concluding that benefits cannot be extended to very heavy and dependent drinkers [28], and another demonstrating that brief interventions had a greater effect when applied to heavy drinkers than moderate drinkers [29]. Nevertheless, there are scenarios in which brief intervention would no longer be sufficient. When patients have already developed a chronic alcohol-related health problem (such as alcoholic cirrhosis or hepatitis), abstinence rather than harm reduction is usually recommended. Thus, it is important for clinicians to consider the needs of this specific group of patients if brief intervention proves ineffective. In such circumstances, referral to formal treatment within a specialist hepatology unit may be required (see Chapter 18) [30]. To this end, interventions have the best track record with adult heavy drinkers in health settings and additional support may need to be provided to some vulnerable groups.

Implementing brief interventions

Compelling and robust evidence for the effectiveness and cost-effectiveness of brief intervention for hazardous and harmful drinkers in primary health care has led to recommendations that it should be implemented into practice and this has been supported by three sets of NICE guidelines focusing on prevention, physical and mental health management [31–33]. To date, primary care is the setting where the majority of brief intervention work occurred; thus, it is here where the richest detail on the implementation of brief alcohol intervention has accumulated. Primary health care is the ideal context for the early detection and secondary prevention of alcohol-use disorders because of high contact-exposure to the population, the fact that patients tend to return regularly for follow-up appointments, and the ability to build long-term relationships with staff. Ballesteros et al. [29] found that the number of hazardous and harmful drinkers within this setting needing to be treated before one person showed a benefit was 8–12.

Delivery of brief intervention within primary care capitalizes on a "teachable moment," whereby patients can consider alcohol use within the context of an alcohol-related illness with a credible health care professional. In this setting, individuals present for a wide range of reasons, not always (at least consciously) for alcohol-related care. Thus, there are many opportunities for brief intervention delivery in primary care because patients are routinely asked about alcohol during new patient registrations, general health checks, and specific disease clinics (e.g. hypertension, diabetes). Nevertheless, brief alcohol intervention can only be effective as a public health strategy if widespread implementation is achieved [34]. Despite efforts to persuade practitioners to adopt brief interventions in practice many have yet to do so, although recent evidence suggests that practitioners are starting to do more in this area [35]. There is an established international literature on barriers to the implementation of brief alcohol intervention:

- A lack of time within busy, time-limited consultations;
- Role insecurity (lack of appropriate skills, knowledge, or training);
- A lack of suitable screening and intervention materials;
- A lack of support from government health policies;
- A lack of incentivization or reimbursement from government health schemes;
- Scepticism of the effect of brief intervention;
- A belief that patients will not take advice to change drinking behavior; and

- A fear amongst practitioners of offending patients by discussing alcohol.

Some of these obstacles are relatively straightforward to overcome. Research suggests that practitioner anxiety about discussing alcohol use with patients is not supported by evidence. Rather, patients are more likely to believe that questions about their alcohol use are justified and expected within a health care setting. High patient acceptance of alcohol screening and brief intervention was also found in a large, pragmatic trial (the SIPS trial) in the United Kingdom [36]. Further, other barriers can be overcome by translating and disseminating the evidence base supporting brief intervention effectiveness to public health practitioners; national guidance such as that produced in England has supported this process. However, the most difficult obstacles to brief intervention delivery are related to a lack of time and lack of reimbursement for this work. Thus, in order to find ways of embedding this work in busy practice, there is a need to encourage national and local policymakers to prioritize alcohol issues and to identify relevant means to incentivize brief intervention delivery.

Key messages for practitioners

First, evidence does not generally indicate an additional benefit of longer or more intensive brief intervention as opposed to shorter, less intensive input. Findings from SIPS demonstrated no additional benefit of delivering 5 minutes' brief advice or 20 minutes' brief lifestyle counseling compared with providing personalized feedback and an alcohol information leaflet, regardless of readiness to change [36]. In other words, it does not appear that length, complexity, and intensity are essential to brief intervention effects. Second, positive effects in terms of consumption reduction have consistently been reported for control groups (screening or assessment only) in brief intervention trials. There are a number of explanations for this effect including regression to the mean (wherein extreme measures of behavior tend to shift to less extreme positions from one time point to another) and assessment reactivity or a response to merely being asked about alcohol consumption. In the latter, the process of helping an individual to become aware of their alcohol-related risk or harm may be beneficial in itself, suggesting that screening per se may be an important element of positive behavior change. Nevertheless, good screening practice is that identification of risk or harm should be followed through with an evidence-supported intervention. Indirect or generalized feedback is rarely enough to achieve robust behavior change. Thus, directly delivered, personalized feedback and relevant written patient information about alcohol should be delivered as a minimum if there is not time for simple structured advice or brief counseling approaches. However, referral to formal treatment may be required in circumstances where patients have already developed a chronic alcohol-related health problem and brief intervention has proven ineffective. Finally, a strength of primary care is that patients are likely to return in the future and so other opportunities for intervention are likely to present themselves. Evidence in this field suggests even delivering the basics could have an effect. In other words, for maximum impact with minimal input, time-pressed clinicians should focus on short, simple interventions that focus on prompting individuals to record their alcohol intake, and that these are likely to be most effective in middle-aged male drinkers in a primary health care setting [20].

Conclusions

Given the rapidly increasing incidence of liver problems in the United Kingdom, it is important to develop upstream preventive approaches to help tackle liver damage before it becomes too established. Recent research has shown that young people may be influenced by alcohol marketing by mid-adolescence, thus there is a need to focus earlier in the life course than practitioners generally expect and as drinking patterns are becoming established [37]. Once cirrhosis occurs damage cannot simply be reversed. However, the majority of liver disease cases have preventable origins such as heavy drinking and excess weight gain. Thus, there is considerable scope for benefit from lifestyle interventions. Evidence is sufficiently robust to indicate that we should be doing more brief interventions for heavy drinking, and we should consider extending this focus into other areas of lifestyle. Brief alcohol interventions of between 5 and 20 minutes, typically delivered to nontreatment-seeking individuals attending generalist health settings offer an effective approach for practitioners and are endorsed in UK public health policy.

Evidence of impact is particularly clear for nontreatment-seeking adult males in a primary care setting. Although brief interventions in other health and social care settings show promise, existing research findings are equivocal being based on a much smaller number of trials; future research should concentrate on these key evidence gaps. Finally, current evidence does not generally indicate an additional benefit of longer or more intensive brief intervention as opposed to shorter, less intensive input. Therefore, and somewhat unusually, in the area of alcohol risk reduction less can often be more and practitioners should emphasize risk identification and short, simple interventions that focus on promoting patients' awareness and self-regulation of alcohol intake.

References

[1] World Health Organization. *Global Status Report on Alcohol and Health*. World Health Organization, Geneva; 2011.

[2] Lim SS, Vos T, Flaxman AD, et al. A comparative risk assessment of burden of disease and injury attributable to 67 risk factors and risk factor clusters in 21 regions, 1990–2010: a systematic analysis for the Global Burden of Disease Study 2010. *Lancet* 2012; **380**(9859): 2224–2260.

[3] Flint C. Response by Caroline Flint to a parliamentary question by Alex Salmond. Hansard. 2006; Oct 9 (col 629W).

[4] Office for National Statistics. *Mortality Statistics: Deaths Registered in England and Wales* (Series DR), 2010. Office for National Statistics, Newport, South Wales; 2011.

[5] Sheron N, Olsen N, Gilmore I. An evidence-based alcohol policy. *BMJ* 2008; **57**(10): 1341–1344.

[6] World Health Organization Regional Office for Europe. European Health for All database (HFA-DB). http://www.euro.who.int/en/data-and-evidence/databases/european-health-for-all-database-hfa-db (accessed 10 December 2014).

[7] All-Party Parliamentary Hepatology Group. Liver Disease: Today's Complacency, Tomorrow's Catastrophe. The All-Party Parliamentary Hepatology Group (APPHG) Inquiry into Improving Outcomes in Liver Disease. 2014.

[8] Anderson P, Baumberg B. Alcohol in Europe: A public health perspective. EU Health and Consumer Protection Directorate General, 2007. http://ec.europa.eu/health/index_en.htm (accessed 10 December 2014).

[9] National Audit Office. *Reducing Alcohol Harm: Health Services in England for Alcohol Misuse*. The Stationary Office (TSO), London; 2008.

[10] Saunders JB, Lee NK. Hazardous alcohol use: its delineation as a subthreshold disorder, and approaches to its diagnosis and management. *Compr Psychiatry* 2000; **41**(2): 95–103.

[11] World Health Organization. *International Classification of Diseases*, 10th edn. World Health Organization, Geneva; 1992.

[12] Rose G. Strategy of prevention: lessons from cardiovascular disease. *BMJ* 1981; **282**: 1847–1851.

[13] Rehm J, Roerecke M. Reduction of drinking in problem drinkers and all-cause mortality. *Alcohol Alcohol* 2013; **48**(4): 509–513.

[14] Babor T. Avoiding the horrid and beastly sin of drunkenness: does dissuasion make a difference? *J Consult Clin Psychiatry* 1994; **62**(6): 1127–1140.

[15] Bandura A. *Social Learning Theory*. Prentice-Hall, Englewood Cliffs, NJ; 1997.

[16] National Institute for Clinical and Health Excellence. *Alcohol Use Disorders: Preventing the Development of Hazardous and Harmful Drinking*. NICE public health guidance 24. National Institute for Health and Clinical Excellence, London; 2010.

[17] Kaner E, Beyer F, Dickinson H, et al. Effectiveness of brief alcohol interventions in primary care populations. *Cochrane Database Syst Rev* 2007; **2**: CD004148.

[18] Miller W, Sanchez V. Motivating young adults for treatment and lifestyle change. In Howard GS, Nathan PE, eds. *Alcohol Use and Misuse by Young Adults*. University of Notre Dame Press, Notre Dame, IN; 1993, 55–81.

[19] Moyer A, Finney JW, Swearingen CE, Vergun P. Brief interventions for alcohol problems: a meta-analytic review of controlled investigations in treatment-seeking and non-treatment-seeking populations. *Addiction* 2002; **97**(3): 279–292.

[20] O'Donnell A, Anderson P, Newbury-Birch D, et al. The impact of brief alcohol interventions in primary healthcare: a systematic review of reviews. *Alcohol Alcohol* 2013; **49**(1): 66–78.

[21] Sullivan LE, Tetrault JM, Braithwaite RS, Turner BJ, Fiellin DA. A meta-analysis of the efficacy of nonphysician brief interventions for unhealthy alcohol use: implications for the patient-centered medical home. *Am J Addict* 2011; **20**(4): 343–356.

[22] Chisholm D, Rehm J, Van Ommeren M, Monteiro M. Reducing the global burden of hazardous alcohol use: a comparative cost-effectiveness analysis. *J Stud Alcohol* 2004; **65**: 782–793.

[23] Nilsen P, Baird J, Mello M, et al. A systematic review of emergency care brief alcohol interventions for injury patients. *J Subst Abuse Treat* 2008; **35**: 184–201.

[24] Harvard A, Shakeshaft A, Sanson-Fisher R. Systematic review and meta-analyses of strategies targeting alcohol problems in emergency departments: interventions reduce alcohol-related injuries. *Addiction* 2008; **103**: 368–376.

[25] McQueen J, Howe TE, Allan L, Mains D, Hardy V. Brief interventions for heavy alcohol users admitted to general hospital wards. *Cochrane Database Syst Rev* 2011; **8**: CD005191.

[26] Carney T, Myers B. Effectiveness of early interventions for substance-using adolescents: findings from a systematic review and meta-analysis. *Subst Abuse Treat Prev Policy* 2012; **7**: 25.

[27] Newbury-Birch D, Coulton S, Bland M, et al. Screening and brief interventions for hazardous and harmful alcohol use for offenders: a pragmatic multicentre cluster randomized controlled trial. *Alcohol Alcohol* 2014; **49**: 540–548.

[28] Saitz R. Alcohol screening and brief intervention in primary care: absence of evidence for efficacy in people with dependance or very heavy drinking. *Drug Alcohol Rev* 2010; **29**: 631–640.

[29] Ballesteros JA, Duffy JC, Querejeta I, Arino J, Gonzalez-Pinto A. Efficacy of brief interventions for hazardous drinkers in primary care: systematic review and meta-analysis. *Alcohol Clin Exp Res* 2004; **28**(4): 608–618.

[30] British Association for the Study of the Liver (BASL) BSoGBLS. *A Time to Act: Improving Liver Health and Outcomes in Liver Disease*. National Plan for Liver Services UK, 2009.

[31] National Institute for Health and Care Excellence. *Alcohol-Use Disorders: Preventing Harmful drinking Evidence Update 54 March 2014*. NICE, London; 2014.

[32] National Institute for Health and Care Excellence. *Alcohol-Use Disorders: Diagnosis and Clinical Management of Alcohol-related Physical Complications*. NICE, London; 2010.

[33] National Institute for Clinical and Health Excellence. *Alcohol-Use Disorders: Diagnosis, Assessment and Management of Harmful Drinking and Alcohol Dependence*. NICE, London; 2011.

[34] Nilsen P. Brief alcohol intervention: where to from here? Challenges remain for research and practice. *Addiction* 2010: **105**; 954–959.

[35] O'Donnell A, Haighton K, Chappel D, Shevills C, Kaner E. Can routine data help evaluate the implementation of a brief alcohol intervention in primary health care? 36th Annual Scientific Meeting of the Research Society on Alcoholism. 22–26 June 2013. Orlando, USA. *Alcohol Clin Exp Res* 2013; **35**(S6): 149A.

[36] Kaner E, Bland M, Cassidy P, et al. Effectiveness of screening and brief alcohol intervention in primary care (SIPS trial): pragmatic cluster randomised controlled trial. *BMJ* 2013; **346**: e8501.

[37] Scott S, Baker R, Shucksmith J, Kaner E. Autonomy, special offers and routines: a Q methodological study of industry-driven marketing influences on young people's drinking behaviour. *Addiction* 2014; **109**(11); 1833–1844.

CHAPTER 17

Alcohol withdrawal syndrome: diagnosis and treatment

Julie Taub[1,3] and Thomas P. Beresford[1,2]

[1] University of Colorado School of Medicine, Denver, CO, USA
[2] Laboratory for Clinical and Translational Research in Psychiatry, Department of Veterans Affairs Medical Center, Denver, CO, USA
[3] Department of Medicine, Denver Health Medical Center, Denver, CO, USA

KEY POINTS

- **Alcohol withdrawal syndrome** (AWS) occurs as early as 4–6 hours after drinking slows or stops.

- Symptoms require early, vigorous medication treatment to avoid life-threatening later occurrence of seizures and **delirium tremens** (DTs).

- Ankle clonus and/or hyperreflexia in early AWS often signal oncoming seizures and indicate aggressive medication treatment.

- About one-third of AWS seizure cases will develop DTs.

- About 10–15% of cases of untreated DTs will die from its effects.

- Symptom-driven medication delivery using AWS severity scales is more effective than fixed-dose treatment.

- The long-acting oral benzodiazepines, such as chlordiazepoxide or diazepam, or parenteral lorazepam when indicated, remain the agents of choice in most cases.

- Frequent assessment through repeating scales, such as the Severity of Ethanol Withdrawal Scale, provided here, can deliver needed medication rapidly. Single dose "front-loading" techniques have also been used for this purpose.

- AWS severity over time appears related to the total number of AWS episodes the patient encounters as well as to the neurogenetic makeup of the individual.

- The underlying **alcohol dependence** or **alcohol use disorder** itself must always be addressed as AWS and its potential neurocognitive effects clear.

Epidemiology

Alcohol withdrawal syndrome (AWS) is a major diagnostic criteria of Alcohol Dependence (Addiction). In the United States, the current and lifetime prevalence of alcohol dependence is 4–13% [1]. In 2006, the cost of problematic alcohol consumption reached $223.5 billion in the United States [2].

In the DSM III and IV, alcohol dependence is defined as a clinical syndrome, a concept that remains in use in the internationally applied ICD-10. In the fifth edition of the DSM, the terminology Alcohol Use Disorder has been introduced, with mild, moderate, or severe "specifiers." That is, alcohol dependence is now construed as existing on one end of a clinical spectrum. How useful clinicians will find the spectrum versus the syndrome approach has yet to be established.

Alcohol use disorders account for roughly 2 million hospital admissions in the United States annually, varying in frequency from approximately 15% to 30%

Alcohol Abuse and Liver Disease, First Edition. Edited by James Neuberger and Andrea DiMartini.
© 2015 John Wiley & Sons, Ltd. Published 2015 by John Wiley & Sons, Ltd.

of all admissions [3,4]. In men undergoing treatment for alcoholism, available estimates indicate that up to 86% experience "minor" or early withdrawal, and over 25% experience "major" or more serious late withdrawal, including delirium tremens (DTs), alcoholic hallucinosis, or seizures [5]. Alcohol withdrawal accounts for a significant part of the overall morbidity associated with alcohol consumption, and represents a substantial burden to health care resources.

Alcohol withdrawal syndrome, early experience and syndrome definition

As long ago as Ancient Greece, Hippocrates noted "if from drinking he has trembling hands, it may well be to announce beforehand either delirium or convulsion." But the systematic observation, and clinical definition, of the AWS are very recent occurrences in the history of medicine. It was not until the mid-twentieth century that several prospective studies closely followed subjects who had recently stopped consumption of excessive amounts of alcohol. In 1953, Victor and Adams [6] described symptoms in 266 patients with alcoholism admitted to Boston City Hospital. They found tremulousness alone in 34.6%, hallucinations in 13.6%, seizures in 12%, and DTs in 5.3%. One of the most definitive, if little known, studies occurred in Sweden in the mid-1950s among 1026 male alcoholics who were admitted over the course of 5 years to an inpatient ward specializing in alcohol disorders [7]. Although some patients received phenobarbitone, and often a sedative such as clomethiazole, this study remains one of the most robust sources of data regarding AWS. The investigators divided 1907 encounters into three major subgroups:

1 Those with minor symptoms (termed "syndrome B");
2 Those with hallucinations without delirium; and
3 Those with DTs.

We list their subgroups as follows:

1 A total of 48% (921 of the total encounters) developed syndrome B, described as tremor with no hallucinations. Except for a small percentage of patients who had seizures, this subset experienced only minor symptoms. In 78% of encounters, the patients with syndrome B improved within 3 days (Table 17.1).

2 Charting further AWS severity in a second group of patients, another 22% (419 of the total encounters)

Table 17.1 Syndrome B subset (921 encouners).

Signs/symptoms	Percentage
Tremor	100
Sweating	59
Vomiting or diarrhea	27
Anxiety	77
Depression	65
Irritability	15
Fever >38.0°C	7
Pulse >90	73
Systolic BP ≥160 mmHg	52
Diastolic BP ≥100 mmHg	58
Delirium tremens	0
Hallucinations	0
Seizures	6

Table 17.2 Hallucinations subset (419 encounters).

Signs/symptoms	Percentage
Visual hallucinations	82
Auditory hallucinations	54
Tactile hallucinations	3
Seizures	6

developed hallucinations without delirium. In most cases, the hallucinations occurred within the first 3 days (especially the first 12 hours) of abstinence, and often lasted less than 24 hours. This group also experienced roughly the same frequency of the minor symptoms described in syndrome B, although the intensity of tremor was more severe (Table 17.2).

3 Last, 30% (567 of the total encounters) developed DTs. In 80% of cases, disorientation started 24 hours after abstinence. A more acute onset (<12 hours after abstinence) was associated with symptoms of shorter duration and less severity. In 75% of cases, the delirium resolved within the first 3 days, and often lasted less than 24 hours. Delirium lasting beyond 1 week was rare. The minor symptoms described for syndrome B were the most frequent in this group, especially fever, tachycardia, and hypertension. This finding suggests alterations in vital signs may be a warning sign of impending DTs. Similarly, this subset of encounters accounted for the greatest frequency of hallucinations and seizures. Seizures often preceded the onset of delirium by 1–2 days (Table 17.3).

Table 17.3 Delirium tremens subset (567 encounters).

Signs/symptoms	Percentage
Visual hallucinations	97
Auditory hallucinations	79
Tactile hallucinations	39
Olfactory and gustatory hallucinations	6
Seizures	25

Table 17.4 Symptoms and signs of early and late alcohol withdrawal syndrome (AWS).

Early AWS: 6–12 hours after a rapid decrease in the blood alcohol concentration (BAC)

Symptoms	*Physical signs*
Anxiety	Hyperactive reflexes
Tremor	Ankle clonus

Nausea with vomiting
Sweating

Vital signs
Tachycardia, pulse >110
Tachypnea
Fever >99.6°F, 37.5°C
Hypertension, diastolic >90 mmHg

AWS: from 24–72 hours, and up to 2 weeks after a rapid decrease in the BAC

Seizures, usually grand mal and often in groups of three or more
DTs:
1. Confusion usually with disorientation
2. Malignant increase in vital signs
3. Hallucinations, usually visual or tactile, but in any of the five senses

The early studies found DTs to be the most grave complication of AWS. Patients exhibited profound autonomic hyperactivity and psychomotor agitation, disorientation, frank confusion, and often hallucinations. Victor and Adams [6] found most cases occurred 3–4 days after alcohol cessation, and the majority lasted less than 3 days.

Mortality in the Swedish study was 0.8% of all admissions during the first 2 weeks. In the DTs group, mortality was 2.6% of all admissions, usually with a finding of brain and pulmonary edema on autopsy [7]. Early reported mortality rates for AWS vary. Victor and Adams [6] found a mortality of 15% among patients with DTs, and these cases were usually complicated by other medical illnesses. As pharmacologic treatment has improved, mortality has decreased.

In 1967 another early study reported on the frequency of seizures ("rum fits") in 241 untreated alcoholic patients. Multiple seizures occurred in 55% of patients, usually 2–4 in number, while 42% experienced only one seizure. Only 3% developed status epilepticus. Usually, the seizures were grand mal. In the 5% of patients with focal seizures, there was often evidence of a cerebral lesion. In nearly all the cases the seizures occurred within the first 48 hours [8]. Victor and Adams [6] found similar data, with 57% of seizures occurring within 48 hours of cessation of alcohol. Their reported seizure frequency was 32% single, 44% multiple, and 2% continuous. Similar to the findings by others, about one-third of patients with seizures go on to develop DTs [6–8]. As with more mild AWS symptoms, seizures can occur when patients still have a significant blood alcohol level, especially in the setting of a rapidly decreasing level [8]. Etiologies other than alcohol withdrawal must be considered when patients with alcohol use present with a seizure, including trauma, infection, stroke, long-term neurotoxic effects of alcohol, and rarely acute alcohol intoxication.

The diagnostic criteria for AWS in the DSM-4-TR and the DSM-5 mirror the above studies, as does the ICD-10. Two or more of the following symptoms are required: autonomic hyperactivity (e.g. sweating or tachycardia), hand tremor, insomnia, nausea or vomiting, transient hallucinations or illusions (visual, tactile, or auditory), psychomotor agitation, anxiety, and grand mal seizures. We have grouped them for current clinical use in Table 17.4 and included current definitions, such as nausea with vomiting as preferable to nausea alone, often a nonspecific symptom. Similarly, we list current definitions of vital sign elevation in early or mild AWS and reserve malignant changes, along with confusion and hallucinations, for late or severe AWS. Of special note, the two physical signs listed appear especially useful in indicating an incipient seizure and possible DTs. We will revisit the symptoms and vital signs in the discussion of AWS severity scales for symptom triggered AWS treatment in clinical practice.

Acute AWS is generally thought to subside completely within 14 days of abstinence [7]. Clinically, many providers are concerned about a protracted withdrawal state in which neurocognitive deficits persist beyond the first

2 weeks. However, this is likely better conceptualized as brain healing rather than a remnant of the acute AWS.

Patients should be cared for in an intensive care unit (ICU) when they require close supervision because of uncontrolled signs and symptoms, as in DTs, or if sedation is needed to control symptoms. Patients in ICU can be treated with symptom-guided protocols if they are alert and able to comprehend questions.

Pathophysiology of AWS

During chronic alcohol exposure, the brain appears to undergo a series of neuroadaptations that we conceptualize as an overall attempt at retaining its non-drinking homeostasis. AWS, in this model, occurs when the drinking version of brain homeostatic balance must rapidly readapt to the lack of alcohol. A number of neurochemical changes have been associated with alcohol exposure and withdrawal in animal studies. None have proved definitive as a single pathophysiologic mechanism, or even a consistent group of them, in all cases. For example, ethanol causes sedation by enhancing gamma-aminobutyric acid type A (GABA-A) activity, an inhibitory neurotransmitter. With continued alcohol exposure, GABA-A receptors are downregulated. During withdrawal, GABA levels are increased, but inhibitory effects are mild because of the downregulation of receptors. Alcohol also inhibits N-methyl-D-aspartate (NMDA) receptors, decreasing glutamate excitatory transmission. Due to inhibition during alcohol dependence, NMDA receptors are upregulated. When the inhibitory effects of alcohol are then withdrawn, glutamate neuroexcitation is increased.

Alcohol enhances dopamine activity, and tolerance occurs with these receptors as well. Dopamine is the main neurotransmitter involved with behavioral reward mechanisms during active drinking. During withdrawal, a relative dopamine deficit likely contributes to the high frequency of depression. Adding to the mood changes, serotonin levels are also decreased during alcohol withdrawal.

And in yet other neural systems, norepinephrine and aspartate are also affected by persistent alcohol, and their withdrawal is associated with sympathetic overdrive [9]. In addition, the interaction of individual genetic and environmental differences in AWS are just beginning to be investigated. Genetics likely affords protection to a subset that can sustain heavy drinking while encountering little or no acute AWS on cessation.

However, in most individuals, environmental factors, such as the duration and degree of heavy alcohol use appear to increase the risk of major AWS symptoms. As another example, kindling is an environmental phenomenon defined as repetitive low impact insults to the brain that cause progressively more severe neurologic changes. Applied to alcohol, kindling describes how repeated episodes of withdrawal progressively shorten the time to onset of symptoms, increase the severity of symptoms, and make seizures more likely [10]. Studying rats, Ulrichsen et al. [11] found kindling may be prevented using diazepam. Compared with a control population, rats initially treated with diazepam during several withdrawal episodes experienced less seizure activity when withdrawal episodes continued without treatment.

Methods of treatment of AWS

There are three main pharmacologic approaches to treating alcohol withdrawal: front-loading, fixed-schedule (or gradual taper dosing), and symptom-triggered (see the pharmacology section for specific recommendations in patients with liver disease).

Front-loading
Front-loading involves a schedule such as diazepam 20 mg orally every 1–2 hours until patients experience sedation or symptoms are controlled. A long-acting benzodiazepine is recommended so that the drug can self-taper. This technique rapidly controls withdrawal symptoms, there is less risk of drug-seeking behavior, and it can be used in patients with prior seizures.

Front-loading techniques can be useful in the critically ill. Gold et al. [12] demonstrated that higher doses of front-loaded diazepam resulted in less intubation. In patients critically ill from alcohol withdrawal, front-loading diazepam with an average total dose of 562 mg resulted in a 22% rate of mechanical ventilation, compared with a 47% intubation rate when the average dose was 248 mg diazepam.

A continuous infusion of short-acting benzodiazepines, such as lorazepam or midazolam, is a technique used in many intensive care settings. Continuous infusions have a great risk of oversedation, however, and often patients will require mechanical ventilation. Unlike typical front-loading protocols where there is an assessment of symptoms between dosing intervals, continuous infusion of drugs are often continued for many hours or days, and not stopped once sedation occurs. There is increased risk of drug side effects, such as delirium resulting from massive doses of benzodiazepines, increased cost, increased length of stay [13], increased duration of ventilation and potential for pneumonia [13], and increased risk of significant debility resulting from prolonged sedation and bed rest.

The parenteral form of lorazepam has the added risk of propylene glycol toxicity. Propylene glycol, a diluent, can cause lactic acidosis, an osmolar gap and renal failure when the infusion rate exceeds 6 mg/hour [14].

Fixed-schedule

Fixed-schedule involves a regimen such as chlordiazepoxide 50 mg orally every 6 hours for 2 days, then 25 mg orally every 8 hours for 3 days. A symptom-triggered regimen is often added to the fixed-schedule in the event the patient's withdrawal worsens. Fixed-dosing has the disadvantage of potential under- or overdosing a patient, because the amount of drug given is not tailored to the degree of withdrawal. The technique does not take into account that a significant portion of patients may not require pharmacologic treatment and supportive care may be sufficient. When compared with fixed-schedule, symptom-triggered regimens decrease length of stay and decrease total dose of benzodiazepine required [15–17].

System-triggered

Symptom-triggered regimens utilize a standardized withdrawal severity scale, such as the Clinical Institute Withdrawal Assessment for Alcohol, revised (CIWA-Ar). Medications are given when symptoms exceed a threshold severity. Different doses of medication may be given depending on the degree of withdrawal symptoms. Symptom-triggered regimens are distinct from informal PRN orders for medications such as diazepam 10 mg orally every 4 hours PRN for "alcohol withdrawal." A relaxed approach such as this is not recommended, as it does not standardize treatment.

Symptom-triggered therapy alone is not recommended for patients with seizures [15,18]. Most studies involving symptom-triggered approaches exclude patients with seizures, as patients can develop a seizure as one of the first signs of withdrawal when the blood alcohol level is still significant. It may be appropriate to use a hybrid mixture of techniques, with a baseline amount of fixed-dose benzodiazepine for 48 hours, and symptom-triggered therapy as needed throughout the course. Front-loading has also been recommended in the setting of a prior seizure [18].

There are multiple rating scales that have been developed to guide symptom-triggered therapy, and assess AWS severity. In 1973, Gross et al. [19] developed the Total Severity Assessment (TSA) and Selected Severity Assessment (SSA) scales to quantify the severity of alcohol withdrawal. The TSA was not practical with 30 variables, so the SSA was developed from it with only 11 variables. Almost all rating scales in use today have significant similarities to the SSA. They are usually developed and tested within specialized alcohol detoxification units, and they remain extremely detailed, and often inappropriately burdensome to nursing staff. Furthermore, they are often poorly validated.

The default "gold standard" rating scale is often considered the revised Clinical Institute Withdrawal Scale for alcoho (CIWA-Ar) [20]. The original Clinical Institute Withdrawal Scale for Alcohol (CIWA-A) was developed in 1981 as a research tool to predict severity of AWS, not to dose drugs based on the scale. The CIWA-A was validated by comparing nursing scores with physician scores [21]. Foy et al. [22] showed that a modified version of CIWA could be used to guide pharmacologic treatment.

The CIWA-Ar protocol includes 10 signs and symptoms, including nausea/vomiting, tremor, paroxysmal sweats, anxiety, agitation, tactile disturbances, auditory disturbances, visual disturbances, headache, and orientation/clouding of sensorium. CIWA-Ar has been included in more studies than any other rating scale, but there are only two randomized studies comparing it with another treatment regimen and both were performed in specialized alcohol treatment units. Saitz et al. [15] and Daeppen et al. [16] found symptom-triggered therapy using the CIWA-Ar to be similarly efficacious in reducing AWS symptoms to fixed-schedule benzodiazepines. Both studies found that symptom-triggered therapy decreased duration of detoxification, reduced the dosage of total benzodiazepine required, and resulted in a significant number of patients who required no benzodiazepines. Daeppen et al. [16] reported 60% of patients required no medications when treated with the symptom-triggered approach.

Unfortunately, CIWA-Ar has many limitations. Perplexingly, headache is included as a metric, which is not a sign of AWS. People who become intoxicated with alcohol only once can develop a headache, often in the form of a hangover. Headache was never one of the symptoms described in the original studies of alcohol withdrawal [6,7], nor in the TSA or SSA scales [19].

Conversely, vital signs are not part of the CIWA-Ar, which is an unfortunate absence because fever, tachycardia, and hypertension are often warning signs of impending DTs [7]. Additionally, reported experience is limited in patients with significant medical or trauma comorbidities despite complicated AWS in patients with those issues. Most studies of CIWA-Ar include patients with only mild to moderate withdrawal, and patients are usually excluded if they present in active withdrawal.

Similar to the original SSA protocol, the CIWA-Ar scale is labor intensive for staff, with each item being scored from 0 to 7, except orientation which is scored 0 to 4. CIWA-Ar has never been compared with another symptom-triggered rating scale. There is no standardization of a specific drug or drug dosage to the scale, nor a level at which to dose medication. No drug regimen has ever been compared in a trial. Furthermore, there is no standardized nursing assessment frequency.

In response to the limitations of the CIWA-Ar in hospital practice, we (TPB and colleagues) developed the Severity of Ethanol Withdrawal Scale (SEWS) in order to improve AWS diagnosis and scale-driven treatment (Table 17.5). The SEWS:

1 Requires only a Yes/No observer evaluation;
2 Weights the AWS phenomena with respect to clinical presentation. e.g. emphasizing early, minor AWS signs and symptoms in order to mitigate progression to later, more severe AWS;
3 Deletes headache as a symptom; and
4 Includes vital signs in the scoring system.

In our protocol, patients with a SEWS score <6 receive no medication. Those scoring >6 but <12 receive either chlordiazepoxide 25–50 mg or lorazepam 1–2 mg, while those scoring >12 receive chlordiazepoxide 50–100 mg

Table 17.5 Severity of Ethanol Withdrawal Scale (SEWS).

Severity of Ethanol Withdrawal Scale (SEWS)	Yes	Score
ANXIETY: do you feel that something bad is about to happen to you right now?	3	
NAUSEA or DRY HEAVES and VOMITING?	3	
SWEATING (includes moist palms, sweating now)?	2	
TREMOR: with arms extended, eyes closed	2	
AGITATION: fidgety, restless, pacing	3	
ORIENTATION	1	
Name and place but not date	1	
Name but not place and date	3	
HALLUCINATIONS		
Auditory only (check for major psychotic disorder)	1	
Visual, tactile, olfactory, gustatory (any)	3	
VITAL SIGNS: *any* of the following	3	
Pulse >110		
Diastolic BP >90		
Temp >99.6		
TOTAL SCORE =		
Total Score **<6:** lower risk for withdrawal		
Total Score = or >**6:** higher risk		

or lorazepam 2–4 mg, with the choice of agent dictated by clinical variables including liver status, confusion, and age. Early analysis in a comparison with a CIWA-Ar score driven clinical protocol indicates the SEWS lessens the time on protocol by one hospital day along with significantly greater *de facto* front-loading of the benzodiazepines given, because of the weight given to early AWS recognition.

Pharmacology of treatment

Numerous drug combinations have been used to treat withdrawal in the past 50 years. During the middle of the last century, paraldehyde, barbiturates, and chloral hydrate were the main drugs. Alcohol itself has been considered a treatment but is inappropriate because of a short half-life, narrow therapeutic index, gastric irritation, risk of continued metabolic derangements, and Wernike–Korsakoff syndrome. In mouse models, ethanol is associated with delayed wound closure, decreased collagen content, and impaired angiogenesis [23]. Ethanol is also expensive in parenteral form, and oral alcohol is more expensive than other current options.

Benzodiazepines

Kaim et al. [24] wrote the landmark study that established the efficacy of benzodiazepines for alcohol withdrawal treatment. A double-blind study of 537 alcoholics comparing chlordiazepoxide, chlorpromazine, hydroxyzine, and thiamine found significantly decreased DTs (1%) and seizures (1%) in the chlordiazepoxide group. The incidence of DTs and seizures with the other drugs was 5% and 8.8% [24]. In the past 40 years the GABAergic benzodiazepines have remained the drugs of choice.

Benzodiazepines potentiate the binding of the neurotransmitter GABA to the GABA-A receptor. They produce sedation, sleep, anticonvulsant activity, and decreased anxiety. Paradoxically, they can produce hallucinations and confusion, especially with toxicity.

Long-acting benzodiazepines, such as chlordiazepoxide and diazepam, are preferred as they self-taper and allow a smoother detoxification. Diazepam has an almost immediate onset of action, and is available in multiple routes (PO, IM, IV, rectal). Chlordiazepoxide is only available in oral form in the United States. The intramuscular route is not recommended with these agents because of slow and erratic absorption that increases the risk of dose stacking [25]. Intermediate half-life benzodiazepines, such as alprazolam and oxazepam, are less effective at preventing seizures, and, more importantly, seizures can present after cessation of these shorter-acting benzodiazepines [26,27].

Long-acting benzodiazepines should be avoided in patients for whom oxidation of benzodiazepines is decreased. This occurs most commonly in patients with liver disease and in the elderly, resulting in increased terminal elimination half-life, an increased volume of distribution, and a greater accumulation of metabolites. Chlordiazepoxide and diazepam are metabolized by hepatic oxidation, and then hepatic glucuronidation. Lorazepam and oxazepam only undergo glucuronidation [25].

Chlormethiazole

Chlormethiazole is a sedative, hypnotic, and anticonvulsant that enhances GABA-A activity. It is not available in the United States, but is still used in Europe. It has been found to be equivalent to chlordiazepoxide in two double-blind studies [28,29]. Unfortunately, it has a short half-life and an unpredictable systemic bioavailability. Further, it has been associated with respiratory depression and fatal cardiopulmonary collapse [30]. Because of these concerns, some recommend it be avoided as a first line agent for alcohol withdrawal.

Barbiturates

Barbiturates are not common first line agents. They have no reversal agent. They have a narrower therapeutic window compared with benzodiazepines, and greater risk of respiratory depression. Associated tachycardia, delirium, and coma with barbiturate intoxication can cloud the picture of alcohol withdrawal. Despite the drawbacks with barbiturates, there is evidence for using phenobarbital as an adjunct in individuals refractory to benzodiazepines alone. Rosenson et al. [31] demonstrated the utility of front-loading with phenobarbitol, showing that a single large dose in addition to a benzodiazepine symptom-guided protocol served to decrease ICU admissions and length of stay.

Propofol

Propofol, a GABA-A agonist and glutamate inhibitor, is an intravenous agent used for general anesthesia that is occasionally used to treat alcohol withdrawal. It is not recommended as a first line treatment because of limited evidence in alcohol withdrawal, and almost invariably patients need to be placed on mechanical ventilation [12].

Anticonvulsants

Anticonvulsants have been an area of interest in treating alcohol withdrawal for the past 20 years. Carbamazepine, valproate, and gabapentin have found more recent interest although somewhat equivocal results. The anticonvulsants may have a role as adjunctive agents in complicated cases but their clinical usefulness as first line agents has yet to be established.

Baclofen

Baclofen, a selective GABA-B receptor agonist, has shown promising results in several small studies that suggest it may lessen the benzodiazepine doses needed to manage withdrawal. Larger studies are needed.

Antipsychotics

Antipsychotics, such as haloperidol, may have a role as an adjunct to benzodiazepines to treat severe agitation. However, antipsychotics can lower the seizure threshold and should only be given in low doses as needed to clear hallucinations or to calm agitated patients who may present a danger to themselves or to others.

Beta-blockers

Beta-blockers are not recommended alone. They have been studied in combination with benzodiazepines for mild to moderate withdrawal [32,33], but there is concern they could mask the early symptoms of withdrawal. The tachycardia and hypertension that beta-blockers suppress are important prompts that additional treatment with benzodiazepines are needed. There is also evidence for increased hallucinations, DTs, and seizures in patients treated with beta-blockers [32,34].

α-2 Agonists

α-2 Agonists, most notably clonidine, afford very little evidence supporting the use of this drug class in AWS. Significant complications of clonidine include increased seizures and hallucinations [35]. There is also the concern that it can mask the sympathetic hyperactivity that is a warning sign for DTs, as the drug is associated with suppressed heart rate and blood pressure.

Dexmedetomidine, a selective central α-2 agonist, is a sedative used for procedures in nonintubated patients, and for mechanically ventilated patients who are critically ill. It is an anxiolytic that does not cause respiratory depression. There are case reports of dexmedetomidine being used successfully to treat DTs, but the current evidence is limited.

Supportive care

Vitamins are necessary for all patients going through alcohol withdrawal because of the poor nutrition that often accompanies alcohol use disorders. Patients should be prescribed a multivitamin, thiamine, and folic acid. High doses of IV thiamine should be used if there is concern for Wernicke–Korsakoff syndrome. Potassium, magnesium, and phosphorus should be closely monitored, as patients are at risk for refeeding syndrome when they begin eating.

Conclusions

AWS is a common and serious complication of alcohol consumption. The prospective observational studies from the 1950s through the 1970s, when AWS was less aggressively treated, are a window into its natural course. The early symptoms, such as tremor, sweating, nausea, vomiting, diarrhea, anxiety, hypertension, tachycardia, and fever are common, especially in the first 3 days after abstinence. They may resolve in less severe cases or they may continue into the later, more serious symptoms.

The major withdrawal complications include alcohol hallucinations, seizures, and DTs. Most patients with hallucinations experience visual phenomena, but auditory and tactile hallucinations are also common. Hallucinations tend to occur within the first 3 days of abstinence, especially the first 12 hours [7]. Seizures usually occur within the first 48 hours, and can occur within hours of abstinence when the blood alcohol level is dropping precipitously but is still high [6,8]. One-third of patients with seizures go on to develop DTs, the most life-threatening complication [6–8]. DTs often occur within the first 4 days of abstinence, and usually last less than 3 days [6,7]. DTs present a significant risk of death when untreated and indicate a true medical emergency.

A number of protocols have been proposed and implemented for the treatment of alcohol withdrawal, but further study is necessary to demonstrate the superiority of a specific approach. The current gold standard, the CIWA-Ar, is inadequate. The signs and symptoms included in the CIWA-Ar do not sufficiently mirror the AWS described in many of the landmark studies. The scale is burdensome for staff. There is doubtful benefit to scoring tremor, sweating, and headache on a scale of 0–7. Tactile, auditory, and visual disturbances are significant, but there is doubtful clinical relevance to scoring "moderately severe hallucinations" as 4 and "extremely severe hallucinations" as 6?

Since the article by Kaim et al. [24], benzodiazepines remain the drug of choice for alcohol withdrawal. Further studies on anticonvulsants, especially carbamazepine and baclofen, are warranted.

Given the profound clinical and financial burden of this condition, the development of more effective AWS treatment protocols is both a realistic and worthy goal. Our group has developed the SEWS which appears to convey a useful combination of both symptom-driven and front-loading attributes.

References

[1] Hasin DS, Stinson FS, Ogburn E, Grant BF. Prevalence, correlates, disability, and comorbidity of DSM-IV alcohol abuse and dependence in the United States: results from the National Epidemiologic Survey on Alcohol and Related Conditions. *Arch Gen Psychiatry* 2007; **64**(7): 830–842.

[2] Bouchery EE, Harwood HJ, Sacks JJ, Simon CJ, Brewer RD. Economic costs of excessive alcohol consumption in the US, 2006. *Am J Prev Med* 2011; **41**(5): 516–524.

[3] Smothers BA, Yahr HT, Ruhl CE. Detection of alcohol use disorders in general hospital admissions in the United States. *Arch Intern Med* 2004; **164**(7): 749–756.

[4] Hearne R, Connolly A, Sheehan J. Alcohol abuse: prevalence and detection in a general hospital. *J R Soc Med* 2002; **95**(2): 84–87.

[5] Caetano R, Clark CL, Greenfield TK. Prevalence, trends, and incidence of alcohol withdrawal symptoms: analysis of general population and clinical samples. *Alcohol Health Res World* 1998; **22**(1): 73–79.

[6] Victor M, Adams RD. The effect of alcohol on the nervous system. *Res Publ Assoc Res Nerv Ment Dis* 1953; **32**: 526–573.

[7] Salum I. Delirium tremens and certain other acute sequels of alcohol abuse: a comparative clinical, social and prognostic study. *Acta Psychiatr Scand Suppl* 1972; **235**: 1–145.

[8] Victor M, Brausch C. The role of abstinence in the genesis of alcoholic epilepsy. *Epilepsia* 1967; **8**(1): 1–20.

[9] De Witte P, Pinto E, Ansseau M, Verbanck P. Alcohol and withdrawal: from animal research to clinical issues. *Neurosci Biobehav Rev* 2003; **27**(3): 189–197.

[10] Booth BM, Blow FC. The kindling hypothesis: further evidence from a US national study of alcoholic men. *Alcohol Alcohol* 1993; **28**(5): 593–598.

[11] Ulrichsen J, Bech B, Allerup P, Hemmingsen R. Diazepam prevents progression of kindled alcohol withdrawal behaviour. *Psychopharmacology (Berl)* 1995; **121**(4): 451–460.

[12] Gold JA, Rimal B, Nolan A, Nelson LS. A strategy of escalating doses of benzodiazepines and phenobarbital administration reduces the need for mechanical ventilation in delirium tremens. *Crit Care Med* 2007; **35**(3): 724–730.

[13] Spies CD, Otter HE, Hüske B, et al. Alcohol withdrawal severity is decreased by symptom-orientated adjusted bolus therapy in the ICU. *Intensive Care Med* 2003; **29**(12): 2230–2238.

[14] Nelsen JL, Haas CE, Habtemariam B, et al. A prospective evaluation of propylene glycol clearance and accumulation during continuous-infusion lorazepam in critically ill patients. *J Intensive Care Med* 2008; **23**(3): 184–194.

[15] Saitz R, Mayo-Smith MF, Roberts MS, et al. Individualized treatment for alcohol withdrawal: a randomized double-blind controlled trial. *JAMA* 1994; **272**(7): 519–523.

[16] Daeppen JB, Gache P, Landry U, et al. Symptom-triggered vs fixed-schedule doses of benzodiazepine for alcohol withdrawal: a randomized treatment trial. *Arch Intern Med* 2002; **162**(10): 1117–1121.

[17] Weaver MF, Hoffman HJ, Johnson RE, Mauck K. Alcohol withdrawal pharmacotherapy for inpatients with medical comorbidity. *J Addict Dis* 2006; **25**(2): 17–24.

[18] Lejoyeux M, Solomon J, Adès J. Benzodiazepine treatment for alcohol-dependent patients. *Alcohol Alcohol* 1998; **33**(6): 563–575.

[19] Gross M, Lewis E, Nagarajan M. An improved quantitative system for assessing the acute alcoholic psychoses and related states (TSA and SSA). In Gross MM, ed. Alcohol Intoxication and Withdrawal: Experimental Studies. Plenum Press, New York; 1973: 365–376.

[20] Sullivan JT, Sykora K, Schneiderman J, Naranjo CA, Sellers EM. Assessment of alcohol withdrawal: the revised clinical institute withdrawal assessment for alcohol scale (CIWA-Ar). *Br J Addict* 1989; **84**(11): 1353–1357.

[21] Shaw JM, Kolesar GS, Sellers EM, Kaplan HL, Sandor P. Development of optimal treatment tactics for alcohol withdrawal. I. Assessment and effectiveness of supportive care. *J Clin Psychopharmacol* 1981; **1**(6): 382–389.

[22] Foy A, March S, Drinkwater V. Use of an objective clinical scale in the assessment and management of alcohol withdrawal in a large general hospital. *Alcohol Clin Exp Res* 1988; **12**(3): 360–364.

[23] Radek KA, Ranzer MJ, DiPietro LA. Brewing complications: the effect of acute ethanol exposure on wound healing. *J Leukoc Biol* 2009; **86**(5): 1125–1134.

[24] Kaim SC, Klett CJ, Rothfeld B. Treatment of the acute alcohol withdrawal state: a comparison of four drugs. *Am J Psychiatry* 1969; **125**(12): 1640–1646.

[25] Peppers MP. Benzodiazepines for alcohol withdrawal in the elderly and in patients with liver disease. *Pharmacotherapy* 1996; **16**(1): 49–58.

[26] Hill A, Williams D. Hazards associated with the use of benzodiazepines in alcohol detoxification. *J Subst Abuse Treat* 1993; **10**(5): 449–451.

[27] Mayo-Smith MF, Bernard D. Late-onset seizures in alcohol withdrawal. *Alcohol Clin Exp Res* 1995; **19**(3): 656–659.

[28] Lapierre YD, Bulmer DR, Oyewumi LK, Mauguin ML, Knott VJ. Comparison of chlormethiazole (Heminevrin) and chlordiazepoxide (Librium) in the treatment of acute alcohol withdrawal. *Neuropsychobiology* 1983; **10**(2–3): 127–130.

[29] Burroughs AK, Morgan MY, Sherlock S. Double-blind controlled trial of bromocriptine, chlordiazepoxide and chlormethiazole for alcohol withdrawal symptoms. *Alcohol Alcohol* 1985; **20**(3): 263–271.

[30] Duncan D, Taylor D. Chlormethiazole or chlordiazepoxide in alcohol detoxification. *Psychiatr Bull* 1996; **20**(10): 599.

[31] Rosenson J, Clements C, Simon B, et al. Phenobarbital for acute alcohol withdrawal: a prospective randomized double-blind placebo-controlled study. *J Emerg Med* 2013; **44**(3): 592–598. e2.

[32] Zilm D, Jacob MS, MacLeod SM, Sellers EM, Ti TY. Propranolol and chlordiazepoxide effects on cardiac arrhythmias during alcohol withdrawal. *Alcohol Clin Exp Res* 1980; **4**(4): 400–405.

[33] Kraus ML, Gottlieb LD, Horwitz RI, Anscher M. Randomized clinical trial of atenolol in patients with alcohol withdrawal. *N Engl J Med* 1985; **313**(15): 905–909.

[34] Worner TM. Propranolol versus diazepam in the management of the alcohol withdrawal syndrome: double-blind controlled trial. *Am J Drug Alcohol Abuse* 1994; **20**(1): 115–124.

[35] Robinson B, Robinson GM, Maling TJ, Johnson RH. Is clonidine useful in the treatment of alcohol withdrawal? *Alcohol Clin Exp Res* 1989; **13**(1): 95–98.

CHAPTER 18

Psychosocial treatments of alcohol use disorders

Terry D. Schneekloth

Mayo Clinic, Rochester, MN, USA

> **KEY POINTS**
>
> - Establishing abstinence should be followed by treatment interventions that develop insight into the drinking problem and alcohol relapse prevention skills promoting long-term abstinence.
>
> - Strategies for strengthening the individual's sober support include partner and family therapy, support network development, and self-help community meetings.
>
> - Liver transplant candidates with alcoholic liver disease (ALD) often lack insight into potential benefits from psychosocial treatment interventions, necessitating mandated treatment by the transplant program.
>
> - The medical field of Addictions has well-characterized the chronic, relapsing nature of alcohol use disorders and efficacy of multiple theoretical frameworks of treatment including cognitive behavioral therapy, motivational enhancement therapy, 12-step facilitation, and Alcoholics Anonymous involvement.
>
> - Though limited, the medical literature on psychosocial treatments specific to patients with ALD indicates prolonged abstinence in patients receiving a combination of both pre- and post-transplant treatments and treatment embedded within the transplant program.
>
> - Psychosocial interventions reduce maladaptive defenses of denial, minimization, and rationalization of drinking, maladaptive coping, increasing insight into the addiction, developing relapse prevention skills, and building a sober support system.

The primary concern over transplanting patients with alcohol-induced liver disease (ALD) is return to drinking, particularly in doses directly injuring the graft and contributing to nonadherence with medication and medical care directives.

Early proponents of transplanting patients with ALD sought to determine the most appropriate candidates through examination of positive predictive factors for medical care adherence and long-term abstinence. Length of pretransplant abstinence was the initial focus and remains the primary issue of concern in many transplant centers. Transplantation of patients with ≥6 months of abstinence became the standard practice in the United States after a series of studies suggested that patients reaching this milestone had a lower likelihood of relapse to drinking [1–3]. This "6-month rule" was generally codified in 1997 when the American Society of Transplantation and the American Association for the Study of Liver Diseases determined that "there is a strong consensus for requiring that most alcoholic

Alcohol Abuse and Liver Disease, First Edition. Edited by James Neuberger and Andrea DiMartini.
© 2015 John Wiley & Sons, Ltd. Published 2015 by John Wiley & Sons, Ltd.

patients should be abstinent from alcohol for at least 6 months before they can be listed for liver transplantation" [4].

Within the medical field of Addiction, establishing abstinence is only the starting point. The focus is on treatment interventions that develop insight into the drinking problem and alcohol relapse prevention skills promoting long-term abstinence. Moreover, the field of Addictions offers multiple strategies for strengthening the individual's sober support, including partner and family therapy, support network development, and self-help community meetings. These programs and various interventions fall under the category of psychosocial treatments.

Liver transplant centers have drawn to varying degrees on these traditional treatments and interventions for alcohol use disorders (AUD) without clearly established protocols or standards across programs. The research into psychosocial treatments most effective for patients with ALD remains limited. This chapter considers challenges specific to patients with AUD and ALD. It reviews the medical literature on evidence-based treatment interventions of AUD in the general population and those specific to transplant patients with AUD. In addition, we examine the role of Alcoholics Anonymous (AA) in the maintenance of long-term alcohol abstinence.

Challenges unique to ALD patients with alcohol use disorders

There are several challenges to engaging patients with end-stage ALD in psychosocial treatments or AA for their AUD. The majority of patients with ALD presenting for transplant center assessment have established several weeks to months of abstinence in the context of their acute health decline. In general, they deny cravings to drink in their decompensated state, and few have entered formal treatment programs or engaged in self-help meeting involvement. They have jumped from a "precontemplative" stage of change while drinking into a forced "action" stage of change (abstinence) when acutely ill, without the sobriety skills generally necessary to maintain long-term abstinence.

Understandably, the focus of the patients and their family members is on the management of their acute medical problems and the life-threatening liver decompensation. These factors complicate the collection of the alcohol use history. Patients and their families may fear that full disclosure of the drinking history will decrease the likelihood of transplant listing, leading to their minimization or denial of the use history. This minimization may undermine attempts to match the severity and extent of their addiction with the proper intensity of treatment.

Additional factors complicating engagement in psychosocial treatments are physical debilitation and hepatic encephalopathy. Residential and outpatient treatment programs often require up to several hours of sitting daily, and the patient's level of concentration, attention, and memory must be sufficient to meaningfully engage in psychoeducation and facilitated treatment groups. Patients must be able to retain the information learned and apply these skills to appropriate situations. Moreover, multiple medical appointments and hospitalizations often disrupt the course of treatment programming and continuity of care.

Patients with ALD present with a wide range of drinking patterns, though the majority tend to either drink in isolation or in settings with other high dose drinkers including drinking with a spouse or partner. In both cases, they have a limited sober support system in early abstinence, which may place them at greater risk for return to former drinking patterns and relationships post-transplant. In the United States, health insurance coverage for treatment provides an additional barrier; some plans allow for insurance coverage only when the most recent consumption has occurred within the past 1–3 months. Insurance companies may limit the intensity, number, and duration of treatments. Moreover, clinicians with the proper addiction expertise may not be available locally or may not be immediately available (e.g. wait-lists for treatment).

Patients with limited insight into the extent of their drinking problem and their risk of relapse may resist, either overtly or more covertly, a proscribed treatment program by the liver program, viewing it as unnecessary. Ideally, addiction treatment should be voluntary when individuals have sufficient intrinsic motivation for change to actively engage in the therapeutic process. In patients with alcohol-induced liver disease, mandated treatment is generally necessary. While they may still benefit substantially from the treatment, as they develop insight into the nature of addiction and their own relapse vulnerability, initial resistance may negatively affect their therapeutic alliance with the transplant center psychosocial care providers.

Rationale for treatment

The American Medical Association first defined alcoholism as a disease in 1956, and it has been increasingly well-characterized as a chronic and relapsing medical condition over the past half century. The definition of alcoholism has evolved through extensive epidemiology. The International Classification of Diseases (ICD-10) distinguishes Alcohol Dependence from Harmful Use, a category of drinking that causes physical or psychologic harm, though not meeting criteria for addiction. The current nomenclature of the Diagnostic and Statistical Manual of Mental Disorders (DSM-V) [5] moved away from two diagnoses (Alcohol Dependence and Alcohol Abuse) to a single diagnosis of Alcohol Use Disorder, which captures a spectrum of alcohol problem severity (see page 490 of DSM-V for diagnostic criteria of alcohol use disorder). Moderate to severe AUD are characterized by loss of control, or an inability to consistently stop drinking after the first drink. This symptom is pathognomonic of addiction and the rationale for establishment of complete abstinence.

Vaillant [6] longitudinally studied the natural history of alcoholism in two demographically dissimilar cohorts of white males over 40 years. He also followed a cohort of men and women hospitalized for alcoholism over 8–12 years [7]. The results are striking. With conventional treatment for alcoholism, 2-year relapse rates of 60–80% are common and long-term prognosis for alcoholism is difficult to predict. Vaillant et al. [8] found only two characteristics distinguishing stable abstinence from chronic relapsing; abstinent men were more likely to have a clear diagnosis of alcoholism (as opposed to alcohol abuse) and were somewhat more likely to attend AA.

Post-transplant relapse rates of 20–40% over 2–5 years are not nearly as grim [9,10]. Vaillant et al. [8] have attributed the improved prognosis after liver transplantation to several factors including the compulsory supervision, the treatment team's continued care, and the group support among liver transplant survivors. Another likely factor is the extensive selection process in transplant centers which excludes the candidates at

highest risk for relapse. Nonetheless, harmful drinking is reported in 15–20% of cases [11], and 10-year survival is worse in those who relapse [12]. Determination of negative prognostic factors and treatment interventions to disrupt the natural course of alcoholism hold promise for further improving outcomes in this population. While patients may initially resist treatment recommendations and AA as punitive, unnecessary hurdles to obtaining a liver, these psychosocial interventions aim to foster adaptive relapse prevention skills and strengthen sober support systems.

Relapse predictors

Survival rates of liver recipients who resume abusive drinking are significantly lower than those maintaining abstinence [9]. This finding necessitates a focus on relapse predicators and modifiable factors to target with treatment interventions.

Early studies of predictive factors implicated a varying range of clinical characteristics. Roggla et al. [13] found insight into the necessity of abstinence, motivation for treatment, and compliance with psychiatric counseling as predictive of survival , while Tringali et al. [14] reported female gender and pretransplant unemployment as factors doubling relapse rates. Neither of these studies found abstinence of 6 months as a significant predictor of sobriety. Others found a family history of alcoholism in first degree relatives as a significant predictor [15,16].

As multiple centers reviewed their clinical experience, they found length of pretransplant abstinence was repeatedly associated with decreasing risk of relapse. Clinical characteristics associated with increased relapse risk included diagnosis of alcohol dependence, younger age, history of other substance use, and prior alcohol rehabilitation [9,10,16–18]. In 2006, McCallum and Masterton [19] reviewed published studies of factors associated with post-transplant abstinence: social stability, older age, and good compliance with medical care. They also concluded that current polydrug misuse, coexisting severe mental disorder, and close relatives with an alcohol problem predicted return to drinking [19]. Two years later, Dew et al. [20] completed a meta-analysis of risk to relapse after solid organ transplantation, which included 50 liver studies. Their findings associated poorer social support, family alcohol history, and pretransplantation abstinence of ≤6 months with post-transplantation relapse [20].

Rodrigue et al. [21] hypothesized 25 possible risk factors for post-transplant relapse to drinking. They found nine predictive risk factors for alcohol relapse. These factors included limited social support, continued alcohol use after liver disease diagnosis, low motivation for alcohol treatment, no rehabilitation relationship, and continued engagement in social activities with alcohol present. Rodrique's group developed an Alcohol Relapse Risk Assessment tool for identifying pretransplant candidates at increased risk for post-transplant alcohol use [21].

Addiction treatment interventions specifically target an individual's risk factors for relapse. Several of the factors associated with higher risk for liver transplant patients are addressed in standard substance use counseling or alcohol treatment programs. Future treatment trials for liver transplant candidates would optimally address relapse factors most problematic for this patient group.

Psychosocial treatments and Alcoholics Anonymous for alcohol use disorders in the general population

The medical field of AUD has an extensive evidence-based literature on the efficacy of multiple psychosocial treatments. A separate branch of the National Institutes of Health, the National Institute on Alcohol Abuse and Alcoholism (NIAAA), has guided this research and provides essential funding. In Europe, the European Union, other governmental agencies, and private foundations provide comparable funding for clinical investigations into alcoholism. Research findings over the past two decades include procedures to characterize, measure, and monitor the fidelity to a particular conceptual psychotherapeutic approach, allowing clear comparisons of treatment methodologies [22]. Specific psychotherapies for the treatment of alcoholism have been reviewed by several authors [22,24], and help-seeking through either treatment or AA has been associated with long-term remission [25].

Psychosocial treatments have multiple objectives with the ultimate goal of reducing the risk of return to drinking and fostering rapid re-establishment of

abstinence in the event of relapse. Across conceptual frameworks of treatment, psychosocial interventions reduce maladaptive defenses of denial, minimization, and rationalization of drinking commonly seen in AUD. Through engagement with a treatment provider, and particularly in group treatment settings, patients experience identification with others who share the same problem. These treatment modalities enhance motivation to change long-time behavioral patterns, provide new skills for coping with life stressors, identify triggers to drink, heal and strengthen marital and family relationships, and foster development of sober support networks and activities.

Treatment is available at multiple levels of care including a continuum of structure and intensity. These levels range from individual counseling and outpatient programs to residential treatment centers and inpatient hospitalization. Placement in the appropriate level of care allows for establishment of sobriety skills in a setting most likely to promote long-term abstinence. Patients who present with ongoing alcohol use, especially those at risk for complicated withdrawal, require a residential or inpatient treatment setting. These programs provide monitored withdrawal and sufficient structure to establish abstinence and prevent surreptitious drinking. Patients often present to transplant centers several weeks or months after discontinuing alcohol use. Intensive outpatient programs, which provide psychoeducation on addiction and psychotherapeutic interventions over the course of several weeks, are generally the optimal approach for these patients. Debilitated or cognitively compromised patients may better tolerate outpatient programs with briefer sessions offered over the course of several weeks to months. While individual counseling may be the only option available in some locations, it is not the treatment of choice. Group settings in addiction programs help patients break from the shame and isolation often associated with alcoholism; feedback from peers also helps to diminish patient denial and minimization of the drinking problem.

Intensive outpatient and residential treatment programs often range 4–6 weeks in duration. Upon completion, patients are encouraged to pursue continuing care programming or "aftercare" for several months. These programs continue the development of relapse prevention skills and provide sober support with a decreased frequency of treatment sessions. Many primary treatment and continuing care programs encourage attendance of

AA or other self-help meetings in the community in addition to the professionally monitored sessions. Most patients to not initially perceive a need for these maintenance therapies; however, they have been repeatedly associated with prolongation of abstinence. If a patient is pursuing liver transplantation, it is critical for the treatment team to reassess the patient upon completion of primary addiction treatment and optimally with ongoing visits to the transplant center. Through reassessment, the team learns whether patients have developed insight into their addiction, learned sober skills, strengthened their sober support system, and completed treatment goals.

The following sections review evidence-based psychosocial interventions for relapse prevention including cognitive behavioral therapy (CBT), motivational interviewing or motivational enhancement therapy (MET), 12-step facilitation, and social network behavior therapy [26]. These treatment interventions promote motivation and insight, and strengthen sober skills, from several theoretical frameworks. We also examine the role of AA in the maintenance of long-term alcohol abstinence.

Cognitive behavioral therapy

CBT and relapse prevention therapies have been consistently found to reduce the rates of return to drinking. A program of CBT might include strategies for self-monitoring, goal setting, functional analysis of drinking situations and triggers, practice of alternative, adaptive coping skills and alcohol refusal skills, and social skills training [23]. Magill and Ray [24] performed a meta-analysis of 53 controlled trials of CBT for adults with substance use disorders. They found a statistically significant treatment effect ($p = 0.005$) across a large and diverse sample of studies and rigorous conditions for establishing efficacy [24]. A multisite study examining the efficacy of pharmacologic and behavioral interventions (The COMBINE Study) found the cognitive behavioral intervention independently associated with improved drinking outcomes [27]. New studies continue to identify specific behavioral and cognitive coping strategies significantly related to drinking outcomes including urge-specific and general lifestyle strategies [28]. Examples include positive outcomes associated with drink refusal training [29].

Motivational enhancement therapy

Motivational interviewing and MET are generally brief therapies of one to four sessions aimed at enhancing the patient's intrinsic desire to change or motivation to engage in addiction treatment. This conceptual framework incorporates an understanding of mechanisms of change in behavior and stages of change. Stages of change include precontemplative, contemplative, readiness, and action stages. Many transplant candidates were precontemplative of alcohol discontinuation before becoming acutely ill. They abruptly discontinue drinking, sometimes during hospitalization, without progressing through contemplative, readiness, and action stages of change and relapse prevention skill acquisition. Given their abstinence, they perceive little need for treatment programs or counseling. MET individualizes or matches patient care interventions to the appropriate level of their motivation. For the general population, this therapeutic approach has been found efficacious in most studies, including the multisite Project MATCH [30,31]. Analysis of Project MATCH data supported a motivational matching hypothesis; individuals with lower baseline motivation had better outcomes with MET than CBT [32]. This finding may have implications for transplant patients lacking motivation for treatment interventions at the time of presentation. MET may help them overcome their ambivalence about beginning treatment.

Network support and couples therapy

Development of a sober support system has been a central component of several conceptual frameworks. Socially focused treatment targeting change in network support to favor abstinence has been significantly associated with drinking outcomes [33]. The COMBINE study measured alcohol-specific support and found it prognostic of drinking outcomes [34]. Behavioral couples therapy (BCT) is another evidence-based intervention for alcoholism focusing on relationships. A review of 12 randomized, controlled trials of this treatment intervention, which focuses on behavioral self-control, coping skills, and relationship functioning, showed better outcomes than individual-based treatments [35]. These therapies may be especially important if the patient has an actively drinking spouse or partner or family member in the household who drinks at home.

12-step facilitation and AA

AA is an international organization founded by a stockbroker, Bill Wilson, and a physician, Dr. Bob Smith, in Akron, Ohio in 1935. They established AA's 12-steps of spiritual and character development, which became the core principles for achieving and maintaining abstinence through AA. Prior to that time, the medical community had struggled to provide effective treatments for individuals with chronically relapsing alcoholism. This "self-help" or mutual aid organization has the primary purpose to help individuals "stay sober and help other alcoholics achieve sobriety"; "the only requirement for membership is a desire to stop drinking" [36]. This organization has spread worldwide and now includes daily meetings for men and women in most towns and cities across the United States and many other countries. While AA is not a treatment per se, the 12-steps of AA shaped some of the early models of residential addiction treatment in the United States, which remain in widespread practice. This model of professional treatment is commonly characterized as "12-step facilitation."

Although the effectiveness of AA has not been demonstrated in randomized studies, AA participation has been shown to reduce relapse risk [37–39]. Over the past decade, several studies have investigated the mechanisms of change through AA involvement and individuals most likely to benefit from participation. Analysis of the Project MATCH data (n = 1726) found AA attendance positively associated with prolonged abstinence, explained primarily by adaptive social network changes and increases in abstinence self-efficacy. For more impaired alcoholics, it also improved outcomes through increasing spirituality or religiosity and by reducing negative affect [40].

As a mutual help organization, AA encourages those who participate to help others stay sober. Pagano et al. [41] examined the role of helping others as a mediator of maintaining abstinence and found compelling evidence that those who help other alcoholics maintain long-term sobriety are themselves better able to maintain sobriety. Others have explored the role of gender in benefits from AA. Although founded by men, women benefit even more than men from AA participation [42]. While both men and women benefit from changes in social factors, this mechanism is more important among men. Another mediator of sobriety, negative affect self-efficacy, was shown to have a strong relationship to outcome for women but not men [43]. In addition, 12-step participation may have a protective role through reduction of frequency and intensity of drinking in the event of relapse [44].

AA is a tremendous resource for maintaining alcohol abstinence. It is widely available, not limited by insurance coverage, and at no cost to the participants. AA meetings are often held in medical settings or hospitals, and they can function as long-term maintenance therapy. Other mutual help groups, such as SMART Recovery, Celebrate Recovery, and Native American spirituality-based groups may have similar mechanisms of change and benefit, though they have not been systematically studied and are frequently less available.

Pre-liver transplant alcohol treatment interventions

Few studies have examined the efficacy of psychosocial treatment interventions specifically for liver transplant populations. In 1996, Wagner et al. [45] called for empirical studies into modified relapse prevention therapies for patients with ALD. They contrasted the transplant population, often with only external motivation for treatment, focus on gaining transplant, declining health, and a precontemplative stage of change, to the standard substance use population, which presents with a degree of internal motivation, focus on abstinence, improving health, and a contemplative or readiness stage of change [45].

In 2003, a group of investigators in Birmingham, UK, reported a pilot study of three 1-hour social behavior and network therapy sessions for patients with ALD awaiting transplantation. The key concept of the intervention was development of positive social support for change in people attempting to modify drinking behavior. Twenty individuals pursued this voluntary intervention. Eight of 19 (42%) drank alcohol post-transplantation. Some experienced this intervention as less stigmatizing and judgmental than other local treatment options [46]. More recently in Germany, a cohort of 89 alcoholic patients with liver disease took part in a manualized 6-month group psychotherapy. Only 56% of these patients reported 6 months of abstinence during the pretransplant intervention. Thirty-five (39.3%) of the patients showed positive ethyl glucuronide results while denying alcohol use [47]. Neither of these interventions appeared superior to standard treatments.

Weinreib et al. [48] pursued the first randomized, controlled study of treatment for alcohol use disorders in patients with ALD awaiting transplant. In this trial, they compared MET with "treatment as usual" (TAU) in the community. A total of 69 subjects completed 24 weeks of observation. Twenty-five percent of the sample drank after randomization and before transplant. MET provided no significant benefit over TAU in relapse to drinking, mood, general health outcomes, or survival [48]. The results of this study were striking for the persistence of pretransplant drinking in a substantial percentage of those awaiting transplantation and the failure of an evidence-based psychosocial treatment (MET), with an intervention specifically targeting motivational issues in transplant patients, to improve outcome over standard community interventions.

In contrast, Addolorato et al. [49] in Rome developed a psychosocial treatment program embedded in the liver transplant center with significantly improved rates of abstinence. They randomized 92 patients between community treatment by psychiatrists with addiction expertise and outpatient treatment in the transplant center Alcohol Addiction Unit (AAU), described as a "multimodal approach" to treatment provided by a psychologist with "expertise in alcoholism." Patients who received treatment in the embedded AAU were significantly more likely to remain abstinent ($p = 0.038$) and had lower mortality ($p = 0.01$) [49]. While this study does not specify the theoretical framework of the treatment interventions, it suggests that an alcohol treatment unit directly associated with the transplant center and addiction therapy providers engaged in the transplant process have therapeutic benefits for patients with ALD.

Post-liver transplant alcohol treatment interventions

The first comparison study of a psychosocial intervention with pharmacotherapy for alcoholism was pursued by Weinrieb et al. [50] in post-transplant liver recipients. They compared MET with the opioid antagonist naltrexone and placebo in a three-arm pilot study [50]. Naltrexone has been associated with reduced cravings

for alcohol and drinks per drinking day in patients who relapse [51]. Unfortunately, Weinreib's group closed the study because of recruitment difficulties. Patients with ALD feared potential naltrexone-induced hepatotoxicity and expressed the belief that alcohol was no longer a problem for them.

Beresford et al. [52] developed an instrument, the Brief Active Focused Follow-Up protocol, for monitoring alcohol use post-transplant. They piloted this intervention in a feasibility study examining relapse in ALD transplant recipients and alcohol-dependent nontransplant patients. This manualized, brief monitoring technique was well-received by the patients. Notably, the average length of abstinence from all substances in the pilot post-transplant group was over 6 years, whereas 8% reported drinking within the last 30 days [52].

Rodrigue et al. [53] at Beth Israel Deaconess Medical Center and Harvard Medical School recently published a retrospective review of substance abuse treatment, pre- and post-transplant, in a cohort with ALD, and its association with post-transplant sobriety. AA was included in the definition of "treatment." Of 118 liver recipients, 61 (52%) engaged in some form of substance abuse treatment, and 40 (34%) relapsed to any alcohol use. There was no significant difference in post-transplant relapse rates between those who received pretransplant treatment and those who did not ($p = 0.20$). However, recipients who pursued both pre- and post-transplant treatment had significantly lower rates of alcohol relapse ($p = 0.03$) [53]. These findings suggest the importance of ongoing or post-transplant professional treatment or AA. They also reinforce the principle of ongoing recovery work for management of a chronic, relapsing disorder.

Conclusions

ALD patients pose a unique challenge for the transplant team. They manifest liver disease as a consequence of an AUD, whose natural course is chronic and relapsing. Yet, they present with little insight into their risk for relapse and often are not motivated to engage in treatment, nor do they see the value of alcohol rehabilitation. Moreover, physical debility and the cognitive impairment related to hepatic encephalopathy often compromise their capacity to participate fully in treatment.

While there is no single predictor of long-term absti- nence for patients with ALD, there are several factors associated with relapse to alcohol use. Standard community treatments for AUD address many of these common relapse factors, and help-seeking through addiction treatment and AA has been consistently associated with remission in community populations. Individuals with alcoholism have been successfully treated by a variety of psychosocial therapies including MET, CBT, network support, couples therapy, and 12- step facilitation.

While there are few transplant-specific studies to guide the choice of optimal psychosocial treatments for ALD patients, the extensive data on efficacious inter- ventions from the addiction field, including AA partici- pation, strongly suggests the potential benefit of pre- and post-transplant treatment interventions. Confirming this assumption, Rodrigue et al. [53], in their recent retro- spective review, found that ALD patients participating in pre- and post-transplant treatment, including AA, are significantly less likely to relapse [53].

In care of the patient with ALD, the treatment team has the dual goals of long-term patient survival and graft preservation. These goals can optimally be met through effective psychosocial treatments for AUD, both pre- and post-transplant, which equip the patient with insight, relapse prevention skills, and a strengthened sober support system.

References

[1] Bird G, O'Grady J, Harvey F, Calne R, Williams R. Liver transplantation in patients with alcoholic cirrhosis: selection criteria and rates of survival and relapse. *BMJ* 1990; **301**: 15.

[2] Kumar S, Stauber R, Gavaler J, et al. Orthotopic liver trans- plantation for alcoholic liver disease. *Hepatology* 1990; **11**: 159–164.

[3] Krom R. Liver transplantation and alcohol: who should get transplants? *Hepatology* 1994; **20**: 28S.

[4] Lucey MR, Brown KA, Everson GT, et al. Minimal criteria for placement of adults on the liver transplant waiting list: a report of a national conference organized by the American Society of Transplant Physicians and the American Association for the Study of Liver Diseases. *Liver Transpl Surg* 1997; **3**: 628–637.

[5] American Psychiatric Association. *Diagnostic and Statistical Manual of Mental Disorders*, 5th edn. American Psychiatric Publishing, Arlington, VA; 2013.

[6] Vaillant G. *The Natural History of Alcoholism Revisited*. Harvard University Press, Cambridge, MA; 1995.

[7] Vaillant G, Clark W, Cyrus C, et al. Prospective study of alcoholism treatment: eight-year follow-up. *Am J Med* 1983; **75**: 455–463.

[8] Vaillant G. The natural history of alcoholism and its rela- tionship to liver transplantation. *Liver Transpl Surg* 1997; **3**(3): 304–310.

[9] Pfitzmann R, Schwenzer J, Rayes N, Seehofer D, Neuhaus R, Nussler N. Long-term survival and predictors of relapse after orthotopic liver transplantation for alcoholic liver disease. *Liver Transpl* 2007; **13**: 197–205.

[10] DiMartini A, Day N, Dew MA, et al. Alcohol consumption patterns and predictors of use following liver transplantation for alcoholic liver disease. *Liver Transpl* 2006; **12**: 813–820.

[11] Singal A, Chaha K, Rasheed K, Anand B. Liver transplanta- tion in alcoholic liver disease current status and contro- versies. *World J Gastroenterol* 2013; **19**(36): 5953–5963.

[12] Parker R, Armstrong M, Corbett C, Day E, Neuberger J. Alcohol and substance abuse in solid-organ transplant recipients. *Transplantation* 2013; **96**: 1015–1024.

[13] Roggla H, Roggla G, Muhlbacher F. Psychiatric prognostic factors in patients with alcohol-related end-stage liver dis- ease before liver transplantation. *Wien Klin Wochenschr* 1996; **108**(9): 272–275.

[14] Tringali R, Trzepacz P, DiMartini A, Dew MA. Assessment and follow-up of alcohol-dependent liver transplantation patients. *Gen Hosp Psych* 1996; **18**: 70S–77S.

[15] Jauhar S, Talwalkar J, Schneekloth T, Jowsey S, Wiesner R, Menon K. Analysis of factors that predict alcohol relapse following liver transplantation. *Liver Transpl* 2004; **10**(3): 408–411.

[16] Perney P, Bismuth M, Sigaud H, et al. Are preoperative patterns of alcohol consumption predictive of relapse after liver transplantation for alcoholic liver disease? *Transplant Int* 2005; **18**: 1292–1297.

[17] Miguet M, Monnet E, Vanlemmens C, et al. Predictive factors of alcohol relapse after orthotopic liver transplanta- tion for alcoholic liver disease. *Gastroenterol Clin Biol* 2004; **28**: 845–851.

[18] DiMartini A, Dew MA, Fitzgeral MG, Fontes P. Clusters of alcohol use disorders diagnostic criteria and predictors of alcohol use after liver transplantation for alcoholic liver disease. *Psychosomatics* 2008; **49**: 332–340.

[19] McCallum S, Masterton G. Liver transplantation for alcoholic liver disease: a systematic review of psychosocial selection criteria. *Alcohol Alcohol* 2006; **41**(4): 358–363.

[20] Dew MA, DiMartini A, Steel J, et al. Meta-analysis of risk for relapse to substance use after transplantation of the liver or other solid organs. *Liver Transpl* 2008; **14**: 159–172.

[21] Rodrigue J, Hanto D, Curry M. The alcohol relapse risk assessment: a scoring system to predict the risk of relapse to any alcohol use after liver transplant. *Prog Transplant* 2013; **23**: 310–318.

[22] Willenbring M. The past and future of research on treatment of alcohol dependence. *Alcohol Res Health* 2010; **33**(1): 55–63.

[23] Mill W, Wilbourne P. Mesa grande: a methodological analysis of clinical trials of treatments for alcohol use disorders. *Addiction* 2002; **97**: 265–277.

[24] Magill M, Ray L. Cognitive-behavioral treatment with adult alcohol and illicit drug users: a meta-analysis of randomized controlled trials. *J Stud Alcohol Drugs* 2009; **70**: 516–527.

[25] Moos R, Moos B. Sixteen-year changes and stable remission among treated and untreated individuals with alcohol use disorders. *Drug Alcohol Depend* 2005; **30**: 337–347.

[26] Mann K, Hermann D. Individualised treatment in alcohol-dependent patients. *Eur Arch Psychiatry Clin Neurosci* 2010; **260**(Suppl 2): S116–S120.

[27] Donovan D, Anton R, Miller W, Longabaugh R, Hosking J, Youngblood M. Combined pharmacotherapies and behavioral interventions for alcohol dependence (the COMBINE study): examination of posttreatment drinking outcomes. *J Stud Alcohol Drugs* 2008; **69**: 5–13.

[28] Dolan S, Rohsenow D, Martin R, Monti P. Urge-specific and lifestyle coping strategies of alcoholics: relationships of specific strategies to treatment outcome. *Drug Alcohol Depend* 2013; **128**: 8–14.

[29] Witkiewitz K, Donovan D, Hartzler B. Drink refusal training as part of a combined behavioral intervention: effectiveness and mechanisms of change. *J Consult Clin Psychol* 2012; **80**(3): 440–449.

[30] American Psychiatric Asociation. Practice guideline for the treatment of patients with substance use disorders. *Am J Psych Suppl* 2007: **164**(4): 66.

[31] Project MATCH Research Group. Matching alcoholism treatments to client heterogeneity: Project MATCH posttreatment drinking outcomes. *J Stud Alcohol* 1997; **58**: 7–29.

[32] Witkiewitz K, Hartzler B, Donovan D. Matching motivation enhancement treatment to client motivation: re-examining the Project MATCH motivation matching hypothesis. *Addiction* 2010; **105**: 1403–1413.

[33] Litt M, Kadden R, Kabela-Cormier E, Petry N. Changing network support for drinking: initial findings from the network support project. *J Consult Clin Psychol* 2007; **75**(4): 542–555.

[34] Longabaugh R, Wirtz P, Zywiak W, O'Malley S. Network support as a prognostic indicator of drinking outcomes: The COMBINE study. *J Stud Alcohol Drugs* 2010; **71**: 837–846.

[35] Powers M, Vedel E, Emmelkamp P. Behavioral couples therapy (BCT) for alcohol and drug use disorders: a meta-analysis. *Clin Psychol Rev* 2008; **28**: 952–962.

[36] Alcoholics Anonymous. *AA Preamble*. AA Grapevine, Inc.

[37] Ferri M, Amato L, Davoli M. Alcoholic Anonymous and other 12-step programmes for alcohol dependence. *Cohrane Databse Syst Rev* 2006; **3**: CD005032.

[38] Moos R, Moos B. Participation in treatment and Alcoholics Anonymous: a 16-year follow-up of initially untreated individuals. *J Clin Psychol* 2006; **62**: 735–750.

[39] Humphreys K, Moos R. Encouraging posttreatment self-help group involvement to reduce demand for continuing care services: two-year clinical and utilization outcomes. *Alcohol Clin Exp Res* 2007; **31**: 64–68.

[40] Kelly J, Hoeppner B, Stout R, Pagano M. Determining the relative importance of the mechaisms of behavior change within Alcoholics Anonymous: a multiple mediator analysis. *Addiction* 2011; **107**: 289–299.

[41] Pagano M, Friend K, Tonigan J, Stout R. Helping other alcoholics in Alcoholics Anonymous and drinking outcomes: findings from Project MATCH. *J Stud Alcohol* 2004; **65**: 766–773.

[42] Krentzman A, Brower K, Cranford J, Bradley J, Robinson E. Gender and extroversion as moderators of the association between Alcoholics Anonymous and sobriety. *J Stud Alcohol Drugs* 2012; **73**: 44–52.

[43] Kelly J, Hoeppner B. Does Alcoholics Anonymous work differently for men and women? A moderated multiple-mediation analysis in a large clinical sample. *Drug Alcohol Depend* 2013; **103**: 186–193.

[44] Tonigan J, Beatty G. Twelve-step program attendance and plysubstance use: interplay of alcohol and illicit drug use. *J Stud Alcohol Drugs* 2011; **72**: 864–871.

[45] Wagner C, Haller D, Olbrisch ME. Relapse prevention treatment for liver transplant patients. *J Clin Psychol Med Settings* 1996; **3**(4): 387–398.

[46] Georgiou G, Webb K, Griggs K, Copello A, Neuberger J, Day E. First report of a psychosocial intervention for patients with alcohol-related liver disease undergoing liver transplantation. *Liver Transpl* 2003; **9**(7): 772–775.

[47] Erim, Y, Beckmann M. Bottcher M, Paul A, Senf W. Alcohol abuse in the context of end stage liver disease and transplantation: results of a comprehensive psychotherapeutic care program [Abstract]. *J Psychosom Res* 2012; **72**: 478.

[48] Weinrieb R, Van Horn D, Lynch K, Lucey M. A randomized, controlled study of treatment for alcohol dependence in patients awaiting liver transplantation. *Liver Transpl* 2011; **17**: 539–547.

[49] Addolorato G, Mirijello A, Leggio L, et al., Gemelli OLT Group. Liver transplantation in alcoholic patients: impact of an alcohol addiction unit within a liver transplant center. *Alcohol Clin Exp Res* 2013; **37**(9): 1601–1608.

[50] Weinrieb R, Van Horn D, McLellan A, et al. Alcoholism treatment after liver transplantation: Lessons learned from a clinical trial that failed. *Pschosomatics* 2001; **42**: 111–115.

[51] Volpicelli J, Alterman A, Hayashida M, O'Brien C. Naltrexone in the treatment of alcohol dependence. *Arch Gen Psychiatry* 1992; **49**: 876–880.

[52] Beresford T, Martin B, Alfers J. Developing a brief monitoring procedure for alcohol-dependent liver graft recipients. *Psychosomatics* 2004; **45**(3): 220–223.

[53] Rodrique J, Hanto D, Curry M. Substance abuse treatment and its association with relapse to alcohol use after liver transplantation. *Liver Transpl* 2013; **19**(12): 1387–1395.

CHAPTER 19
Pharmacologic interventions

Renata Yang and Marian Fireman

Oregon Health and Science University, Portland, OR, USA

KEY POINTS

- Benzodiazepines remain the pharmacologic treatment of choice for alcohol withdrawal. Short-acting benzodiazepines without active metabolites are recommended for patients with liver disease.

- No agent has been shown to be highly effective for the treatment of alcohol use disorders. Baclofen is the only agent studied in patients with advanced liver disease.

- Naltrexone, acamprosate, disulfiram, and nalmefene (in Europe) are accepted treatments for reducing alcohol consumption. All have shown evidence for efficacy in some studies but the effect is not robust.

- Anticonvulsants including valproic acid, carbamazepine, gabapentin, and topiramate have been studied for both alcohol withdrawal and treatment of alcohol use disorders; evidence of efficacy of these agents is inconclusive.

- Other agents including baclofen, ondansetron, lithium, and selective serotonin reuptake inhibitors have been studied for decreasing alcohol consumption; evidence remains inconclusive regarding the efficacy of these agents.

- Acceptance and prescription of pharmacologic agents for treatment of alcohol use disorders is limited in clinical practice.

- Studies of all agents in patients with liver disease are lacking.

- Pharmacologic treatments should be combined with psychosocial treatment in a comprehensive rehabilitation program.

Introduction

Pharmacologic interventions to treat alcohol use disorders target both symptoms of alcohol withdrawal and alcohol consumption. Ethyl alcohol is a simple two-carbon molecule, which is rapidly absorbed from the stomach and duodenum. Consumption of ethyl alcohol produces the familiar effects of euphoria, relaxation, sedation, cognitive impairment, and motor slowing. Individuals who drink heavily may develop physiologic dependence and may experience symptoms of withdrawal. The majority of patients experience only mild–moderate withdrawal and may seek no treatment. Mild–moderate withdrawal is best treated by reassurance, reality orientation, appropriate nutrition, and hydration. Approximately 10% of patients will experience more severe withdrawal requiring pharmacologic intervention. Withdrawal symptoms include autonomic hyperactivity, anxiety, insomnia, and tremor. Seizures, agitation, and hallucinations occur less frequently. Release of inhibition of gamma-aminobutyric acid A (GABA-A) receptors and increased activity of the *N*-methyl-D-aspartic acid (NMDA) glutamate receptors have been implicated in the etiology of withdrawal

---

Alcohol Abuse and Liver Disease, First Edition. Edited by James Neuberger and Andrea DiMartini.
© 2015 John Wiley & Sons, Ltd. Published 2015 by John Wiley & Sons, Ltd.

symptoms. Symptoms of withdrawal are alleviated with administration of GABA-A agonists such as benzodiazepines. These medications appear to both alleviate symptoms of withdrawal and prevent complications such as alcohol withdrawal seizures and delirium tremens. Anticonvulsants, including carbamazepine, valproic acid (VPA), and gabapentin have shown efficacy for mild–moderate alcohol withdrawal. Other agents such as dexmedetomidine, propofol, and memantine have received increasing attention for treatment of alcohol withdrawal (see Chapter 17) [1].

The primary route of alcohol metabolism is initial oxidation by alcohol dehydrogenase to acetaldehyde. Acetaldehyde is subsequently metabolized to acetic acid, which is then broken down into carbon dioxide and water. The actions of ethyl alcohol in the central nervous system are complex and appear to be mediated by multiple neurotransmitters. GABA-A receptor activation may produce the anti-anxiety, motor, and sedative–hypnotic effects of alcohol. Serotonin, cannabinoid, nicotinic, and opioid actions may alter the reinforcing effects of alcohol. Pharmacologic interventions targeted at reducing alcohol consumption affect both alcohol metabolism and those neurotransmitters responsible for mediating the reward producing effects of alcohol [1]. Interventions that target alcohol consumption appear to have only modest effects in reducing alcohol consumption. It is highly recommended that patients also engage in a psychosocial rehabilitation program.

All patients should receive a thorough evaluation including history, physical examination, mental status examination, urine drug screening, and other appropriate laboratory studies prior to the initiation of pharmacologic treatments. Consultation with experts in addiction medicine and/or psychiatry is highly recommended in cases where the patient is medically compromised or has advanced liver disease.

Treatment of alcohol withdrawal

Benzodiazepines remain the mainstays of pharmacologic treatment for alcohol withdrawal. The GABA-A agonist activity of the benzodiazepines suppresses the autonomic hyperactivity seen in alcohol withdrawal. Long-acting benzodiazepines such as diazepam and chlordiazepoxide are often considered first line because breakthrough symptoms are avoided and the medications "self-taper"

over a number of days but any benzodiazepine can be used. Benzodiazepines are metabolized by the liver and many have long-acting active metabolites. In the face of significant liver disease, the half-life of benzodiazepines may be significantly prolonged and side effects such as sedation, cognitive impairment, falls, and delirium are problematic. In patients with mild hepatic impairment, long-acting benzodiazepines are generally tolerated. In patients with moderate to severe liver disease, use of short-acting benzodiazepines without active metabolites such as lorazepam or oxazepam are recommended.

Anticonvulsants have been studied extensively in recent years and are accepted alternatives to benzodiazepines in mild–moderate withdrawal. Carbamazepine, valproate, and gabapentin have been studied most extensively. These medications appear to decrease the symptoms of withdrawal, prevent alcohol withdrawal seizures, and prevent delirium tremens in these cases. Carbamazepine and valproate are hepatically metabolized and may cause hepatotoxicity. It is recommended that these be avoided in patients with liver disease. Gabapentin is not hepatically metabolized and is considered safe in patients with liver disease. It can be sedating and may impair cognition. It should be used with caution in patients at risk for hepatic encephalopathy. Carbamazepine, valproate, and gabapentin have all been shown to alleviate symptoms of the "post-acute withdrawal syndrome" and reduce the amount of heavy drinking and number of days of alcohol consumption after an episode of acute detoxification. Post-acute withdrawal syndrome is a constellation of symptoms that may last weeks to months after detoxification. Symptoms include irritability, cognitive problems, fatigue, disrupted sleep, depression, and anxiety. Studies of all of these agents in patients with liver disease are lacking.

Recent research has shown efficacy for the α2-adrenergic agonist, dexmedetomidine, as an adjunctive treatment in cases of complicated alcohol withdrawal. Use of this agent provides sedation, decreases delirium, and allows for use of lower doses of benzodiazepines in these cases. Propofol, a GABA-A agonist, has also been used as an adjunctive agent in these cases. NMDA antagonists such as memantine have also received interest in treating alcohol withdrawal as increased glutamate activity is thought to be contributing to the withdrawal state [1]. There are no studies of these agents in patients with liver disease.

Agents for reducing alcohol consumption

Disulfiram

Disulfiram was the first drug therapy approved by the FDA in 1951 for the treatment of alcohol dependence. Disulfiram exerts its action by interfering with the metabolism of alcohol. Figure 19.1 summarizes the major route of alcohol metabolism. Disulfiram irreversibly inhibits aldehyde dehydrogenase (ALDH), the second step in alcohol metabolism. ALDH converts acetaldehyde to acetate. Blocking this enzyme causes a buildup of acetaldehyde resulting in unpleasant effects such as nausea, flushing, diaphoresis, tremor, palpitations, dizziness, and headache. Disulfiram is an aversive therapy to prevent future use and has no significant effect in reducing alcohol craving.

Evidence for the efficacy of disulfiram is conflicting, largely because most of the research has lacked adequate control groups and blinding. To date, the US Veterans Administration Cooperative Study is the most cited randomized, controlled, blinded, multicenter study of disulfiram. In this study, 605 participants aged 60 and younger who met the National Council on Alcoholism diagnostic criteria for alcoholism received:

1 Disulfiram 250 mg/day with riboflavin 50 mg/day;
2 Disulfiram 1 mg/day with riboflavin 50 mg/day; or
3 No disulfiram with riboflavin 50 mg/day.

There was no difference between the groups in the rate of abstinence or time to first drink. However, participants receiving disulfiram 250 mg/day had fewer drinking days (49 ± 8.4) after relapse as compared with the other two groups (75.4 ± 11.9 in the 1 mg and 86.5 ± 13.6 in the no disulfiram groups, respectively). The strongest predictor of an effect of treatment was observed in those trials that administered disulfiram under supervision [2].

The FDA-recommended average daily maintenance dose is 250 mg, with a range of 125–500 mg (maximum daily dose). When disulfiram is taken in conjunction with alcohol it can induce aversive effects as noted above. However, serious cardiovascular effects (i.e. chest pain, tachyarrhythmias, hypertension, hypotension, and hemodynamic instability) have also been described when alcohol is consumed on disulfiram [3]. Side effects noted when taking disulfiram alone include optic neuritis, peripheral neuritis, and hepatotoxicity. Psychosis has been noted to occur with disulfiram when taken in high doses in patients predisposed to psychotic illness. Patient should be warned about the potential alcohol content of tonics, mouth washes, cough syrup, and other over-the-counter preparations. Use of these substances in conjunction with disulfiram may precipitate an aversive reaction. In addition, many liquid medications and some intravenous medications contain small amounts of alcohol and may precipitate a reaction. Patients should abstain from alcohol consumption for a minimum of 12 hours prior to the first dose of disulfiram and should be warned that aversive effects when combined with alcohol may occur for up to 14 days after discontinuation of disulfiram.

Severe and sometimes fatal hepatitis and/or hepatic failure have been associated with the use of disulfiram and may occur in patients with or without a prior

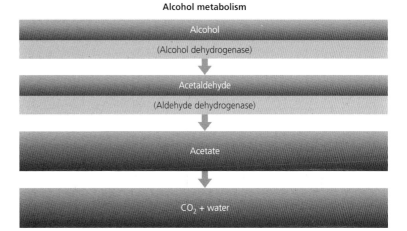

Alcohol metabolism

Alcohol
(Alcohol dehydrogenase)

Acetaldehyde
(Aldehyde dehydrogenase)

Acetate

CO_2 + water

Figure 19.1 Major pathway of alcohol metabolism. (Source: Adapted from Kranzler et al. 2005 [1])

history of abnormal hepatic functioning. No dosage adjustment is recommended with hepatic impairment, but the manufacturer's label warns of using disulfiram with extreme caution in hepatic cirrhosis or insufficiency. The true incidence of disulfiram hepatotoxicity is unclear and the mechanism behind disulfiram-induced hepatotoxicity is poorly understood. One hypothesis is that hepatotoxicity is caused by the production of toxic metabolites of the drug [4]. Disulfiram treatment is not indicated for pregnant women, patients with severe cardiovascular or cerebrovascular disease, organic brain syndrome, or those with significantly abnormal liver functioning. It should also be used with caution in patients with a history of diabetes mellitus, hypothyroidism, or seizures. Disulfiram is not recommended for liver transplant recipients because of possible serious side effects and significant interactions with drugs requiring CYP450 metabolism (e.g. post-transplant immunosuppressants) [3].

Oral naltrexone

The FDA approved naltrexone in 1994 for the treatment of alcohol dependence. Naltrexone is an opioid antagonist that is thought to decrease excessive drinking by reducing the positive reinforcing effects of alcohol and by suppressing cravings. Naltrexone is thought to exert its action by blocking opioid receptors on dopamine-containing neurons in the brain reward pathways. Naltrexone may be more effective for people with a family history of alcohol dependence. It does not cause dependency and does not make patients feel sick if they drink alcohol while taking it.

A meta-analysis of 64 randomized, placebo-controlled trials from 1970 to 2009 demonstrated naltrexone to be more efficacious in reducing heavy drinking and craving rather than maintaining abstinence. Naltrexone treatment was found to have a bigger effect size when abstinence was required prior to initiation of treatment [5]. A review article looking at 5997 alcohol-dependent patients from 1990 to 2006 demonstrated an advantage for naltrexone in "heavy or excessive drinking" over placebo in 19 (70%) of 27 clinical trials looking at this outcome, whereas only 9 (36%) of 25 clinical trials looking at abstinence or "any drinking" demonstrated an advantage for prescribing naltrexone over placebo [6]. The COMBINE Study showed that oral naltrexone with medical management without combined behavioral intervention was more effective than placebo in

increasing the percentage of days abstinent (80.6% and 75.1%, respectively) and in reducing the risk of a heavy drinking day (28% reduction in risk) after 16 weeks of treatment. Medical management consisted of manual guided education, brief advice, and discussion of medications but no specific behavioral therapy. In this study, specific behavioral therapy did not add to the benefit of naltrexone.

The FDA-recommended average daily maintenance dose of naltrexone is 50 mg, with a range of 50–100 mg (maximum daily dose). Common side effects include gastrointestinal upset, headache, and fatigue. There are no adequate studies of naltrexone in patients with alcoholic liver disease. To date, there are no reported cases of hepatic failure due to naltrexone administration at the recommended daily dosage of 50 mg. The primary evidence of hepatotoxicity has been reported with dosages of 100–300 mg/day, when administered to subjects with obesity or dementia. These patients had elevated transaminase levels, which returned to baseline in a matter of weeks after the drug was discontinued. However, because of evidence that naltrexone may be hepatotoxic, it is recommended that markers of liver function, including gamma-glutamyl transferase (GGT), aspartate aminotransferase, alanine aminotransferase, and bilirubin be monitored before and during treatment (at baseline, 1 month after starting treatment, and yearly thereafter). Naltrexone is an opioid antagonist and may precipitate opioid withdrawal and block the analgesic effects of opioids. Patients should be assessed for opioid use prior to initiation of naltrexone, and they should be counseled with regard to the effects of naltrexone if they are taking opioids. It is recommended that a urine drug screen be obtained prior to initiation of treatment with naltrexone. There are no adequate or well-controlled studies of naltrexone in pregnant women. Naltrexone should be discontinued 48–72 hours prior to procedures requiring opioids for anesthesia or management of postoperative pain. In the event of unexpected severe pain, effective analgesia may be difficult to obtain and initial use of nonopioids is recommended.

Extended-release naltrexone

Extended-release naltrexone was developed with the intent to reduce the fluctuations in plasma levels associated with oral intake and to increase medication adherence and efficacy. The FDA approved it in 2004 for the treatment of alcohol dependence. Extended-release naltrexone is formulated into polyactide-co-glycolide, small-diameter (<100 µm), injectable microspheres along with other proprietary active moieties that lead to its extended release over several weeks. Pharmacokinetic studies of extended-release naltrexone in humans have shown stable, pharmacologically relevant plasma levels of naltrexone in humans for at least 28 days [7].

Extended-release naltrexone is available in a once-monthly intramuscular injection at a dose of 380 mg. The most common side effects include injection site tenderness, nausea, headache, and fatigue. The intramuscular formulation may produce less hepatotoxicity than oral naltrexone because it does not undergo first-pass metabolism in the liver. A trial of oral naltrexone is recommended prior to initiation of the injectable formulation. Naltrexone, as with other drugs approved for alcohol dependence, is recommended with concurrent psychosocial interventions.

Nalmefene

Nalmefene is an opioid antagonist similar in structure to naltrexone with a longer half-life (8–10 hours), more effective binding to central opioid receptors, higher bioavailability, and no observed dose-dependent liver toxicity. Nalmefene was developed as an as-needed treatment to help patients remain abstinent or reduce their drinking by motivating them to actively engage in their own treatment. At present, it is only available in Europe for the treatment of alcohol dependence. The indications for its usage in the United States include management of known or suspected opioid overdose and for the complete or partial reversal of opioid drug effects, including respiratory depression, induced by either natural or synthetic opioids [7].

Nalmefene is available as 18-mg film-coated tablets. The maximum dose of nalmefene is one tablet per day. On each day the patient perceives a risk of drinking alcohol, they are instructed to take one tablet, preferably 1–2 hours prior to the anticipated time of drinking. Nalmefene is indicated for the reduction of alcohol consumption in adults with a high drinking risk who do not manifest physical withdrawal symptoms and who do not require immediate detoxification. High drinking risk is defined as use of >60 g/day pure alcohol for men and >40 g/day pure alcohol for women (equal to about 5–6 standard drinks of alcohol for men and 3–4 for women). In one European study of 667 patients, nalmefene taken as needed was superior to placebo in reducing heavy

drinking days (by 3.2 days per month) and total alcohol consumption (by 14.3 g/day) [8]. Nalmefene is recommended in conjunction with continuous psychosocial support. Common side effects with nalmefene include gastrointestinal side effects (nausea), dizziness, insomnia, and headache.

Acamprosate

Acamprosate has been available in Europe since 1989; it was approved by the FDA in 2004 for the treatment of alcohol dependence in the United States. Its mechanism of action is not completely understood, but it is an amino acid derivative that increases GABA neurotransmission and is thought to exert its therapeutic effects by modulating the excitatory glutamate amino acid system (NMDA) in the brain. Acamprosate is thought to reduce the rate of at which patients with alcohol use disorders return to drinking and to reduce the drinking among patients who relapse.

Evidence of the efficacy of acamprosate is strongest in trials conducted in Europe. Two trials in the United States, a 6-month multisite [9] and the COMBINE study failed to show any advantage for acamprosate over naltrexone alone or over placebo [10]. Reasons for the differences in effectiveness of acamprosate between European and US studies are unclear, but may be due to study design, severity of disease, typology of patients, and use of inpatient detoxification. Genetic factors may have a role in patient response to acamprosate. One study found that genetic variations in a gene for GATA-binding protein (GATA4) were significantly associated with relapse risk during a 90-day medical treatment period.

Acamprosate is available as 333-mg tablets. It is poorly absorbed and the recommended dosage is two 333-mg tablets three times per day. Efficacy appears to be best in patients who are abstinent from alcohol and who are receiving psychosocial treatment. Given the potential problem with adherence to three times daily dosing, pairing acamprosate with meals or bedtime is suggested. The most common side effect of acamprosate is diarrhea. Other common side effects include headache, dizziness, fatigue, nervousness, insomnia, and pruritus. Acamprosate is renally excreted and considered safe in patients with hepatic disease. It is recommended that baseline renal function be assessed prior to initiating acamprosate. There are no adequate or well-controlled studies of acamprosate in pregnant women (Table 19.1).

Table 19.1 FDA-approved medications for alcohol use disorders.

Medication	Regimen	Mechanism of action	Common side effects	Relative contraindications
Naltrexone	25–100 mg/day	Mu opioid antagonist blocks craving, stops reinforcing effects of alcohol	GI upset, headache, insomnia, fatigue, dizziness	Opioid use or opioid withdrawal, acute hepatitis or liver failure
Acamprosate	333–666 mg 3 times daily	GABA agonist/glutamate antagonist, helps modulate overactivity of glutamate after stopping chronic heavy alcohol use	Diarrhea	Severe renal impairment
Disulfiram	125–500 mg/day	Inhibits alcohol metabolism by accumulation of acetaldehyde which produces unpleasant symptoms	Nausea, vomiting, flushing, changes in HR and BP if taken concurrently with alcohol; drowsiness, lethargy, headache by itself	Cardiac and pulmonary disorders, liver disease, renal disorders, epilepsy, diabetes mellitus, psychosis, use of alcohol-containing products

Source: Adapted from [1–7,9–11].

BP, blood pressure; GABA, gamma-aminobutyric acid; GI, gastrointestinal; HR, heart rate.

Anticonvulsants

The anticonvulsants carbamazepine, VPA, gabapentin, and topiramate have been evaluated in clinical trials for their efficacy in alcohol withdrawal and dependence. Anticonvulsants are thought to decrease cravings by strengthening GABA-mediated neurotransmission, inhibiting the excitatory effects of glutamate receptors, suppressing glutamate release, calcium-blocking channels, and decreasing alcohol-induced dopamine release in the nucleus accumbens. A 2014 Cochrane Review found insufficient evidence for the efficacy of anticonvulsants in the treatment of alcohol use disorders based on the small number and only moderate quality of studies [12].

Carbamazepine

Carbamazepine is FDA approved for the treatment of epileptic seizures and trigeminal neuralgia, but has been used off-label for the treatment of mental illness, restless legs syndrome, alcohol withdrawal, and promoting abstinence from cocaine use. Carbamazepine has been shown to be helpful in the management of alcohol withdrawal and has been associated with improved short-term drinking outcomes post-detoxification. Severe alcohol use causes long-lasting neuronal and neurochemical changes in the brain that make individuals with alcohol dependence more vulnerable to the effects of alcohol over time. Subsequent drinking episodes become more severe and alcohol withdrawal symptoms may occur upon cessation of drinking. Carbamazepine does not prevent alcohol use or prolong the time to first drink but may reduce the adverse effects of each drinking episode and block the "kindling" effect associated with recurrent episodes of alcohol withdrawal [13].

To date, there are insufficient studies of carbamazepine use in alcohol dependence and liver disease. There have been rare reports of hepatic failure with the use of carbamazepine. The most significant side effects related to carbamazepine include blood dyscrasias and hypersensitivity reactions. Retrospective case–control studies have found a strong association between the risk of developing Stevens–Johnson syndrome and toxic epidermal necrolysis (SJS/TEN) with carbamazepine treatment and the presence of an inherited variant of the HLA-B gene, HLA-B*1502, which has been found in certain Asian populations. Carbamazepine has several drug–drug interactions and is an autoinducer of itself. Baseline complete blood count with differential, serum electrolytes, and liver function testing is recommended prior to initiating carbamazepine therapy. Patients with high-risk ancestry should also be tested for HLA-B*1502. A bone density scan and electrocardiogram are recommended for patients over age 45. Patients with a cardiac history should also receive an electrocardiogram. Patients with alcohol dependence considering carbamazepine therapy should be educated with regard to the potential for SJS/TEN [14]. Carbamazepine is teratogenic and not recommended for pregnant women because of its potential to cause neural tube defects.

Valproic acid

The exact mechanism of action of VPA is unknown but it is thought to increase brain GABA and serotonin levels. There are very few studies of VPA for the treatment of alcohol dependence but it has been shown to be helpful in both the treatment of alcohol withdrawal as well as in reducing relapse to heavy drinking [15]. It may also be helpful in the treatment of benzodiazepine withdrawal and may be particularly suitable for patients with a concurrent diagnosis of bipolar illness, which has the highest rate of co-occurring alcohol dependence compared with any other severe psychiatric disorder [16]. VPA is generally well tolerated and is available in different formulations. The enteric-coated derivative, divalproex sodium (Depakote) is better tolerated than VPA. The most common side effects associated with VPA include gastrointestinal side effects, tremor, drowsiness, hair loss, weight gain, asthenia, dizziness, benign thrombocytopenia, and headache. Severe side effects include pancreatitis, hepatitis, and encephalopathy. VPA is contraindicated in those with with severe liver impairment. It is teratogenic and may cause neural tube defects, thus it is not recommended for pregnant women. Baseline liver function tests should be obtained in patients considering VPA therapy. VPA should be discontinued if hepatic transaminase levels reach 2–3 times the upper limit of normal after initiation. In patients with mild–moderate liver disease, the risks of VPA therapy must be weighed against the potential benefits and patients receiving VPA therapy should be monitored closely for worsening liver function. It is suggested that alternatives with less potential for hepatotoxicity be considered prior to VPA in these patients.

Gabapentin

Gabapentin is FDA approved for the treatment of epileptic seizures and neuropathic pain, but has been used off-label for several indications, including chronic pain, mood, anxiety, and sleep problems. Gabapentin potentiates GABA activity indirectly by blocking voltage-gated calcium channels at selective presynaptic sites. It is thought to normalize the stress-induced GABA activation in the amygdala that is associated with alcohol dependence and to reduce alcohol-cued craving and disturbances in sleep and mood. Gabapentin is also thought to help with protracted alcohol withdrawal, which includes sleep difficulty, irritability, concentration problems, anxiety, and dysphoria.

There are several small studies showing the efficacy of gabapentin in the treatment of alcohol dependence. The first large, placebo-controlled trial assessing the effectiveness of gabapentin in the treatment of alcohol dependence was published by Mason et al. [17] in 2014. This study looked at rates of complete abstinence and no heavy drinking as primary outcomes and changes in mood, sleep, and craving as secondary outcomes over a 12-week period. The patients selected were outpatients with alcohol use disorders who were able to abstain from alcohol for several days prior to initiating gabapentin. The study found that gabapentin, particularly at a dosage of 1800 mg/day, was more effective in treating alcohol dependence and relapse-related symptoms of insomnia, dysphoria, and craving than placebo. Seventeen percent of patients receiving gabapentin 1800 mg were abstinent at 12 weeks compared with 4.1% in the placebo group. The rate of no heavy drinking was 22.5% in the placebo group compared with 44.7% in the gabapentin 1800 mg group [17].

Gabapentin is generally well tolerated and does not seem to have an abuse potential. Regimens of 1800 mg taken once daily appear to be most beneficial. Common side effects include headache, fatigue, sedation, insomnia, and dizziness, which are more likely to occur at higher doses. Dosing of gabapentin in the evening is recommended to avoid daytime sedation. Gabapentin is renally excreted and considered safe in patients with liver disease. Caution is advised when using gabapentin in patients at risk for hepatic encephalopathy and/or cognitive impairment from other causes as gabapentin may worsen those symptoms.

Topiramate

Topiramate is FDA approved for the treatment of migraines and pediatric epilepsy. Topiramate has a complicated mechanism of action including potentiation of GABA-mediated neuronal inhibition and antagonism of AMPA and kainate glutamate receptors. Through its multiple mechanisms of action, it is thought to decrease both craving and withdrawal symptoms related to alcohol use. More recent research has postulated that topiramate may alter the subjective effects of alcohol.

Two large, placebo-controlled trials support the efficacy of topiramate for the treatment of alcohol dependence. Topiramate was shown to decrease the percentage of heavy drinking days (mean of 8.44% fewer heavy drinking days), decrease the number of drinks per drinking day, increase the number of days abstinent per month, and reduce plasma GGT levels. It was also shown to reduce alcohol craving and obsessive drinking behavior. Topiramate appears to have efficacy in improving quality of life, decreasing the severity of alcohol dependence, and reducing the detrimental effects associated with heavy drinking. It has been recommended as a harm reduction strategy in patients with alcohol use disorders who cannot attain the goal of abstinence [18].

Topiramate is available as an oral tablet in doses of 25, 150, 100, and 200 mg or as a capsule in doses of 15 or 25 mg. Topiramate requires slow titration to prevent side effects. A starting dose of 25 mg/day with a 25 mg/week dose increase to reach a total dose of 300 mg/day is recommended. Topiramate 300 mg/day has been shown to significantly reduce drinks per drinking day in alcohol-dependent patients. Topiramate reduces appetite and may cause weight loss. Other side effects include cognitive impairment, transient paresthesias, sedation, renal acidosis, and kidney stones resulting from carbonic anhydrase inhibition. There are rare reports of spontaneous myopia, angle-closure glaucoma, increased intraocular pressure, ocular pain, and blurry vision. Patients taking topiramate should be counseled with regard to adequate hydration. Concomitant use of topiramate with VPA has been associated with the development of hyperammonemia with or without encephalopathy. Baseline and routine monitoring of serum bicarbonate levels is recommended to monitor for the rare but serious dose-related hyperchloremic, non-ion gap, metabolic acidosis that can occur. Topiramate is predominately excreted by the kidneys; up to 20% is hepatically metabolized. It has not been studied in patients with advanced liver disease.

Baclofen

The FDA originally approved baclofen in 1977 for the treatment of spasticity. Baclofen is a GABA-B receptor agonist. Baclofen may be helpful in reducing alcohol withdrawal-related anxiety and alcohol cravings. It may also be useful in promoting maintenance of alcohol abstinence. Baclofen is primarily eliminated by renal excretion and undergoes little liver metabolism (~15%). Preliminary studies indicate it is safe even when patients continue to consume alcohol or relapse to heavy drinking.

Baclofen is the only anticraving drug that has been studied in alcohol-dependent patients with liver cirrhosis. In this study, baclofen was effective in helping patients achieve abstinence and well tolerated (71% in baclofen group vs. 12% in placebo group achieved abstinence at 12 weeks) [10]. To date, there are only four randomized controlled trials that have been published examining the use of baclofen in the treatment of alcohol dependence. These studies excluded patients with medical or psychiatric comorbidities and as such may have limited external validity given the narrow inclusion and exclusion criteria. Baclofen was shown to be more effective than placebo at prolonging time to first drink, reducing overall drinking days, and maintaining alcohol abstinence in some of these studies. Patients treated with baclofen had improvements in anxiety but not depression scores.

Baclofen is available as an oral tablet in doses of 10 and 20 mg. Baclofen at 30–60 mg/day may be safe and effective for the treatment of alcohol dependence in patients with liver cirrhosis. Given the limited data available, caution should be used in those with impaired renal functioning (the manufacturer's label does not recommend renal dose adjustments for baclofen). Caution is also warranted in those with concurrent seizure disorders or psychiatric illness. The most commonly reported side effects include drowsiness, headache, nausea, and vertigo. Nausea can be minimized by gradual titration to target dose or taking baclofen with food [19]. There have been no negative sequelae noted to-date when baclofen has been discontinued in alcohol dependence studies. However, baclofen has been shown to cause rare but serious adverse effects when used for other indications including encephalopathy, seizures, and hyperammonemia. Discontinuation of baclofen may precipitate seizures and other neuropsychiatric symptoms including delirium, cognitive impairment, tremor, and hallucinations.

Ondansetron

Serotonin has been shown to have a role in regulating the severity of alcohol drinking [1]. Ondansetron is a serotonin receptor type 3 (5-HT3) antagonist and may be helpful in a subgroup of patients with early onset alcoholism. This is defined as age of onset less than 25, a strong family history of alcohol use disorders, and possessing the LL polymorphism in the serotonin transporter gene. It is hypothesized that serotonergic dysfunction may have a key role in alcohol dependence in these patients. In this subgroup of patients, ondansetron has been shown to reduce cravings, decrease intensity of alcohol intake, and increase total days abstinent. It is contraindicated with congenital long QT syndrome because of its association with QTc prolongation (which occurs primarily at higher doses). Ondansetron is primarily eliminated by hepatic metabolism. Patients with severe hepatic impairment (Child–Pugh score >9) should have their daily dose of ondansetron limited to 8 mg (or 0.15 mg/kg) [20].

Selective serotonin reuptake inhibitors

The most extensively studied selective serotonin reuptake inhibitors (SSRIs) for the treatment of alcohol dependence include fluoxetine, citalopram, and sertraline. The results of studies published to date are mixed and there are no studies that specifically look at SSRIs in the treatment of alcohol dependence with liver disease. It is possible that SSRIs are more efficacious in a subgroup of alcoholic patients, particularly those with late onset alcoholism who have a functional polymorphism in the gene encoding the serotonin transporter protein (5-HTT) [21].

Lithium

The evidence supporting lithium in the treatment of alcohol dependence has yet to be conclusively established. Lithium may be associated with improved early treatment adherence and sobriety. However, a large multicenter, double-blind, placebo-controlled trial in depressed and nondepressed alcohol-dependent veterans did not show any significant differences between the two groups with respect to number of drinking days, alcohol-related hospitalizations, and severity of depression. Lithium may be most helpful for those patients with co-occurring bipolar disorder. Lithium is not metabolized by the liver and therefore is safe in mild–moderate liver disease. However, as it is eliminated by renal excretion it should be used with caution in advanced liver disease when fluid–electrolyte balance and renal function may be impaired (Table 19.2) [1].

Conclusions

Pharmacologic treatment of alcohol use disorders in liver disease is limited to the treatment of withdrawal states and for reducing alcohol consumption. There are no pharmacologic treatments that are proven to "prevent alcohol use" or provide a "permanent cure" for alcohol use disorders. The use of pharmacologic treatments combined with concurrent psychosocial treatment is highly recommended.

Benzodiazepines remain the mainstay of treatment for moderate to severe alcohol withdrawal. "Social treatment" including appropriate nutrition, hydration, and supportive care is generally adequate for mild withdrawal states. Anticonvulsants have received much attention as alternatives and several other treatments are being investigated as alternatives to benzodiazepines. In mild–moderate liver disease, the practitioner must be mindful of the potential toxicities of the treatments they propose to use and carefully weigh the risk against potential benefits prior to choosing a treatment for withdrawal states. In severe liver disease, avoiding agents with hepatotoxic side effects and using agents that are not hepatically metabolized is highly recommended.

Many agents have been investigated for the treatment of heavy alcohol consumption and alcohol use disorders. There is evidence for the efficacy of some agents in reducing alcohol consumption and days of heavy drinking but no agent has shown robust results in producing abstinence in this population. Clinical use of these agents remains limited. Disulfiram, carbamazepine, and VPA have the potential for significant hepatotoxicity and caution is advised when using these agents in patients with liver disease, particularly severe liver disease.

Table 19.2 Off-label medications for treating alcohol use disorders.

Medication	Regimen	Mechanism of action	Common side effects	Relative contraindications/notes
Valproic acid	750–3000 mg/day in single or divided doses; maximum 60 mg/kg/day	Causes increased availability of GABA, an inhibitory neurotransmitter, to brain neurons or may enhance the action of GABA or mimic its action at postsynaptic receptor sites	Sedation, GI effects, asymptomatic hepatic transaminase elevation	Pregnancy, liver disease
Carbamazepine	300–1600 mg/day in single or divided doses	Blocks voltage-gated sodium channels in an activity and use-dependent manner	Sedation, tremor, menstrual disturbances	HLA-B*1502 in certain Asian populations, first trimester of pregnancy
Gabapentin	600–1800 mg/day	Acts to balance dysregulation of GABA/glutamate in early alcohol abstinence	Sedation, dizziness, fatigue, GI effects	
Topiramate	25 mg/day and increase by 25–50 mg/day at weekly intervals to a target of 300 mg/day in divided doses	Blocks neuronal voltage-dependent sodium channels, enhances GABA-A activity, antagonizes AMPA/kainate glutamate receptors, and weakly inhibits carbonic anhydrase	Impaired cognition, weight loss, paresthesias	Risk of acidosis
Baclofen	5 mg three times daily for 3 days, then 10 mg 3 times daily. May increase to 20 mg 3 times daily	GABA-B receptor antagonist	Nausea, fatigue, sedation, vertigo, abdominal pain	
Ondansetron	4 µg/kg 2 times daily	Serotonin receptor type 3 antagonist	GI effects, headache, fatigue, QT prolongation	
SSRIs	Fluoxetine, citalopram, and sertraline most extensively studied. Serotonin receptor antagonists at different receptor subtypes			
Lithium	400–1200 mg/day; dose is guided by plasma levels, maintain of 0.6–1.0 mmol/L	Exact mechanism of action unknown; may stabilize catecholamine receptors, alter calcium-mediated intracellular functions and increase GABA activity	Fatigue, tremor, weight gain, GI effects	Baseline CBC, CMP, TSH, T4, Ca, EKG for patients with cardiac problems, pregnancy test
Nalmefene	20–80 mg/day as needed	Opioid receptor antagonist in the CNS	Drowsiness, GI symptoms, dizziness, tachycardia, hypertension	Twice as potent as naltrexone. Only available in Europe for the treatment of alcohol dependence

Source: Adapted from [1,7,8,12–21].

Ca, calcium; CBC, complete blood count; CMP, comprehensive metabolic panel; CNS, central nervous system; EKG, electrocardiogram; GABA, gamma-aminobutyric acid; GI, gastrointestinal; HR, heart rate; SSRI, selective serotonin reuptake inhibitor; T4, thyroxine; TSH, thyroid-stimulating hormone.

References

[1] Kranzler HR, Ciraulo DA, Jaffe JH. *Clinical Manual of Addiction Psychopharmacology*. American Psychiatric Press, Washington, DC; 2005, 1–55.

[2] Su J, Pettinati HM, Kampman K, O'Brien C. The status of disulfiram a half century later. *J Clin Psychopharmacol* 2006; **26**(3): 290–302.

[3] Chick J. Safety sssues concerning the use of disulfiram in treating alcohol dependence. *Drug Saf* 1999; **20**(5): 427–435.

[4] Björnsson E, Nordlinder H, Olsson R. Clinical characteristics and prognostic markers in disulfiram-induced liver injury. *J Hepatol* 2006; **44**: 791–797.

[5] Maisel NC, Blodgett JC, Wilbourne PL, Humphreys K, Finney JW. Meta-analysis of naltrexone and acamprosate for treating alcohol use disorders: when are these medications most helpful? *Addiction* 2012; **108**(2): 275–293.

[6] Pettinati, HM, O'Brien, CP, Rabinowitz, AR, et al. The status of naltrexone in the treatment of alcohol dependence: specific effects on heavy drinking. *J Clin Psychopharmacol* 2006; **26**(6): 610–625.

[7] Franck J, Jayaram-Lindström N. Pharmacotherapy for alcohol dependence: status of current treatments. *Curr Opin Neurobiol* 2013; **23**: 692–699.

[8] Van den Brink W, Audin H, Bladstrom A, Torup L, Gual A, Mann K. Efficacy of as needed nalmefene in alcohol dependent patients with at least a high drinking risk level: results from a subgroup analysis of two randomized controlled 6 month studies. *Alcohol Alcohol* 2013; **48**: 570–578.

[9] Mason BJ, Goodman AM, ChabacS, Lehert P. Effect of oral acamprosate on abstinence in patients with alcohol dependence in a double-blind, placebo-controlled trial: the role of patient motivation. *J Psychiatric Res* 2006; **40**: 383–393.

[10] Addolorato G, Mirijello A, Leggio L, Ferrulli A, Landolfi R. Management of alcohol dependence in patients with liver disease. *CNS Drugs* 2013; **27**: 287–299.

[11] Witkiewitz K, Saville K, Hamreus K. Acamprosate for treatment of alcohol dependence: mechanisms, efficacy and clinical utility. *Ther Clin Risk Manag* 2012; **8**: 45–53.

[12] Pani PP, Trogu E, Pacini M, Maremmani I. Anticonvulsants for alcohol dependence. *Cochrane Database Syst Rev* 2014; **2**: CD008544.

[13] Mueller TI, Stout RL, Rudden S, et al. A double-blind, placebo-controlled pilot study of carbamazepine for the treatment of alcohol dependence. *Alcohol Clin Res* 1997; **21**: 86–92.

[14] Grover S, Kukreti R. HLA alleles and hypersensitivity to carbamazepine: an updated systematic review with meta-analysis. *Pharmacogenet Genom* 2014; **24**: 94–112.

[15] Brady KT, Myrick H, Henderson S, Coffery SF. The use of divalproex in alcohol relapse prevention: a pilot study. *Drug Alcohol Depend* 2002; **67**: 323–330.

[16] Le Fauve CE, Litten RZ, Randall CL, Moak DH, Salloum IM, Green AI. Pharmacological treatment of alcohol abuse/dependence with psychiatric comorbidity. *Alcohol Clin Res* 2004; **28**(2): 302–312.

[17] Mason BJ, Quello S, Goodell V, Shadan F, Kyle M, Begovic A. Gabapentin treatment for alcohol dependence a randomized clinical trial. *JAMA Intern Med* 2014; **174**(1): 70–77.

[18] Johnson BA, Rosenthal N, Capece JA, et al. Topiramate for treating alcohol dependence: a randomized controlled trial. *JAMA* 2007; **298**: 1641–1651.

[19] Brennan JL, Leung JG, Gagliardi JP, Rivelli SK, Muzyk AJ. Clinical effectiveness of baclofen in the treatment of alcohol dependence: a review. *Clin Pharmacol* 2013; **5**: 99–107.

[20] Figg WD, Dukes GE, Pritchard JF, et al. Pharmacokinetics of ondansetron in patients with hepatic insufficiency. *J Clin Pharmacol* 1996; **36**(3): 206–215.

[21] Enoch MA. Genetic influences on response to alcohol and response to pharmacotherapies for alcoholism. *Pharmacol Biochem Behav* 2014; **123**: 17–24.

CHAPTER 20

Treatment of extrahepatic manifestations of alcohol abuse

Joaquim Fernández-Solà

Alcohol Unit, Hospital Clínic, Institut d'Investigacions Biomèdiques August Pi i Sunyer (IDIBAPS), CIBEROBN Fisiopatología de la Obesidad y la Nutrición, Instituto de Salud Carlos III, University of Barcelona, Barcelona, Spain

---

KEY POINTS*

- Ethanol is a toxic substance with widespread toxic systemic effects. It diffuses widely through biologic membranes, is a sensitizing agent, a potent enzymatic inductor with active metabolites, and may also cause disturbances in second intracellular messengers and direct DNA damage. All these factors confer a high potential for toxic systemic damage.

- In addition to the systemic effects of alcohol, there are also organ-specific factors that confer propensity or protection against this toxic effect. The sum of the systemic plus the local effects explains the final differential organ damage.

- There is clear relationship between liver and systemic involvement in alcohol-induced organ damage. The greater the liver damage, the greater the systemic damage expected. Clinicians should evaluate both the type (acute, subacute, chronic) and degree of organ damage (transitory, initial, established reversible, established irreversible, end-stage organ damage).

- Treatment of global manifestations of alcohol abuse needs a multidisciplinary evaluation based on clinical suspicion and appropriate complementary studies. Therapeutic planning needs to consider possible interference or interactions between the different treatments administered.

Introduction

Ethanol (EtOH) is a very active toxic substance, with widespread diffusion throughout the body and with a high degree of interaction with biologic structures; this results in a significant potential for damage. It has been said that alcohol is a "perfect toxic" for the human body, as the damage is not usually so intense as to cause severe acute life-threatening damage but it induces progressive damage while giving some benefit.

---

*This work was supported by SGR-2013-1158 Generalitat de Catalunya, Spain and also by the research network CIBEROBN Fisiopatologia de la Obesidad y la Nutrición, Instituto de Salud Carlos III, Madrid, Spain.

Alcohol consumption is the world's third highest risk factor for disease and disability, and is the greatest risk factor in middle-income countries. Approximately 4.5% of the global burden of disease and injury is attributable to alcohol [1]. Alcohol misuse is linked both to the increase in incidence of disease and impairment of the course of many diseases [2].

Although the liver is the main target for alcohol toxicity because of its local high metabolic rate and active metabolites, almost all organs in the human body can be affected. The 2005 WHO report on excessive alcohol consumption [3] identified more than 60 diseases where alcohol is the main contributory factor; furthermore, alcohol consumption has been identified as a significant contributory factor in over 200 others. Box 20.1 summarizes this potential extensive systemic involvement.

Alcohol Abuse and Liver Disease, First Edition. Edited by James Neuberger and Andrea DiMartini.
© 2015 John Wiley & Sons, Ltd. Published 2015 by John Wiley & Sons, Ltd.

Box 20.1 Systemic damage associated with excessive alcohol use.

Central and peripheral nervous system

Increased risk of hemorrhagic stroke
Sensorimotor polyneuropathy
Autonomic neuropathy
Wernicke's encephalopathy and related diseases
Alcohol-related dementia
Alcohol withdrawal including seizures and delirium
Generalized brain atrophy
Cerebellar degeneration
Persisting cognitive effects
Behavioral effects

Heart and vascular system

Hypertension
Increased risk of ischemic peripheral vascular disease
Alcoholic cardiomyopathy:
• Subclinical
• Diastolic dysfunction
• Clinical (heart failure, arrhythmias)
Sudden death

Digestive tract

Esophagitis
Acute and chronic gastritis
Varices
Acute and chronic pancreatitis
Gastrointestinal bleeding

Bone and skeletal muscle

Osteoporosis
Skeletal myopathy
• Subclinical
• Clinical (muscle weakness, myalgia)

Nutritional status

Caloric malnutrition
Protein malnutrition
Vitamin, ionic and mineral deficiencies
Pellagra

Endocrine metabolic dysfunction

Disruption of gonadal axis
Hypertriglyceridemia, increased HDL cholesterol levels
Reduced insulin sensitivity
Plasma acidemia
Increased oxidative tissue stress
Fetal alcohol syndrome

Hepato-immune dysfunction

Lymphocyte dysfunction
Immunocomplex induction
Altered phagocytic activity
Bone marrow dysplasia
Disruption of platelet aggregation and fibrinolysis
(fibrinogen, plasminogen activator inhibitor)
Increased risk of infection (Gram-negative, mycobacterial)

Increased risk of cancer

Mouth
Larynx
Esophageal
Gastric
Colon–rectum
Liver
Kidney
Breast

Therefore, any therapeutic approach for the treatment of alcohol-induced organ damage must include consideration of this potential for associated extensive systemic damage. This approach requires clinical evaluation of a multidisciplinary scenario in which the liver and the other organs are clearly inter-related [4]. Indeed, in alcohol misuse there is a positive correlation between the presence of cirrhosis and extrahepatic manifestations (such as alcoholic cardiomyopathy) [5]. In any individual with alcohol abuse, the greater the hepatic involvement, the greater the expected systemic involvement. Thus, integral treatment in a subject with alcohol abuse should include this systemic overview within a multidisciplinary approach.

Reasons for the multisystemic effects of ethanol

Ethanol is a small-sized, highly interactive molecule, with hydrophilic and lypophilic properties that allow global diffusion throughout the human body.
• Alcohol may cross extra- and intracellular compartments interacting with subcellular organelles and target the same DNA molecules in the cell nuclei.
• Alcohol is a potent enzyme inducer, and its metabolism results in active metabolites (such as acetaldehyde acetate and fatty acid ethyl esters).

- It is also a powerful sensitizing agent interfering with many different cell structures (membranes, channels, pores).
- Ethanol may become integrated in the structure of the membranes themselves generating mixed complexes with phospholipids such as phosphatydyl-ethanol, and changing the membrane acting potential in excitable cells as well as the properties of membrane transport ion channels. Ethanol is able to disturb the main metabolic processes of protein synthesis and degradation and glucose and lipid metabolism. Ethanol induces protein interactions, generating ethanol-protein adducts, and active immunocomplexes.
- It has a proinflammatory effect, increasing local and systemic cytokine and interleukin production.
- Ethanol is able to interfere with most energy-generating processes mainly at a mitochondrial level and also disturbs endocrine regulation pathways [6].
- The disturbance in intracellular signal mechanisms such as calcium-mediated cell signaling induced by ethanol may activate cell apoptosis either through direct or mitochondrial caspase pathways resulting in direct DNA damage.

In addition, it should be remembered that these damaging effects by ethanol are not isolated, but there are different synchronic and synergic effects with other pathogenic mechanisms. Ethanol has been described to generate more than 30 synchronic effects in a single cell. Finally, ethanol is also able to increase or potentiate other pathogenic effects (such as those of hepatitis C virus, tobacco, cocaine) resulting in a different pattern of disease.

At a local organ level, ethanol is able to disturb the regulation of protective growth factor agents such as ghrelin, leptin, insulin-like growth factor 1, and myostatin, increasing the degree of organ damage. The type of action of these local protective factors varies between organs.

The effect that ethanol causes in each tissue mainly depends on the amount of ethanol itself and the characteristics of the relevant organ, with a balance between damaging and protective effects. The final effect is a result of this balance between the aggression mechanisms and the capacity of the cells to establish defensive mechanisms [4].

Evaluation of alcohol toxicity

In reference to the mechanisms of tissue damaging alcohol effects, consideration should be given to the duration of the toxic impact, the pattern of alcohol misuse, and organ sensitivity:

- Duration of toxic impact: acute, subacute, or chronic toxic effects.
- The consequences of alcohol misuse is related to:
  - Threshold range of ethanol for toxicity varies between different tissues;
  - Period of consumption (usually >10 years is required for chronic effects to become clinically apparent);
  - Heavy episodic drinking which may be especially toxic for tissue damage;
  - Type of alcoholic beverage (wine, beer, spirits). Organ damage is more often associated with beverages of higher alcohol concentrations, but this may simply reflect the fact that more alcohol is ingested on a volume-for-volume basis as it is the amount of alcohol consumed that is the major risk factor for organ damage. However, some degree of antioxidant protection is present in wine and beer.
  - Lifetime dosage of alcohol consumed (TLDA; kg EtOH/kg body weight).
- Organ sensitivity:
  - Ethanol may cause different types of damage according to the characteristics of the different cells in which the presence of the following should be considered:
    - specific factors (type of cell, enzymatic or metabolic factors); or
    - nonspecific factors (genetic predisposition, gender).

Organ-specific damage in alcohol abuse

Alcohol consumption produces not only global systemic effects, but may also cause local organ-specific effects and the resulting tissue damage is a combination of both [6]. In addition to the toxic-induced tissue damage, any organ exposed to alcohol will induces compensatory mechanisms to diminish or attenuate this damage. For instance, when alcohol induces muscle apoptosis and myocyte death, the hypertrophic influx of local growth

Box 20.2 Progressive categories of the effects of alcohol-induced organ damage.

1 Non detectable effects
2 Detectable but transitory effects (less than 3 months)
3 Subclinical dysfunction, initially without and later with clinical damage
4 Clinical effects with reversible structural damage
5 Advanced clinical effects with irreversible structural damage

factors and the regenerative response of myoblasts are able to partially compensate this cell loss.

These factors may be specific of the type of cell on which ethanol acts (such as epithelial, metabolically active, excitable, embryonic cells). In addition, each individual carries inherent propensities for protection against end-organ damage due to alcohol consumption. Recently, many previously unrecognized polymorphisms related to alcohol metabolism or enzyme activity have been reported to be influenced by alcohol or its metabolites [7]. This confers different levels of risk for alcohol-associated damage to specific organs. In addition, there is also genetic and gender predisposition to alcohol-induced organ damage, with women being more susceptible than men to develop alcohol-related organ damage at similar levels of alcohol consumption.

In this process of progressive organ damage, the duration of exposure to alcohol is important because the type of damage is usually progressive. Thus, there is commonly a transitory period when the damaging effects of ethanol are balanced by the local compensatory mechanisms without major organ damage. When these local compensatory mechanisms fail, the damage inflicted by ethanol becomes more apparent, with overt functional decline and establishment of detectable organic damage (Box 20.2).

The mechanisms whereby alcohol misuse results in specific organ-damage in any individual subject remain to be determined.

Baseline considerations for treatment

All treatment approaches in subjects with alcohol abuse should start with an attempt to stop alcohol intake and by a systematic evaluation of organ injury [4]. It is therefore necessary to establish a full alcohol history record, including evaluation of alcohol consumption in:
• Quantity: grams per day, number of standard drinks;
• Type of alcohol consumed: wine, beer, spirits;

Box 20.3 Threshold range for ethanol-mediated organ damage.

Cardiovascular
• Hypertension >40 g/day. RR 2 at >60 g/day
• Atherosclerosis >40 g/day
• Coronary disease RR >1 with 30 g/day women, 40 g/day men
• Arrhythmia sudden death (binge >5 drinks week or >100 g/day)
• Dilated cardiomyopathy: dose-dependent:
  ○ Diastolic dysfunction >5 kg/kg (33% affected)
  ○ Systolic dysfunction >9 kg/kg (13% affected)

Kidney
Albuminuria at >30 g/ day

Neurologic
• Cerebrovascular lesions:
  ○ Ischemic stroke RR 1.69 with >60 g/ day
  ○ Hemorrhagic stroke RR 2.18 with >60 g/day
• Alcoholic-induced brain impairment (alcoholic dementia) with >30 g/day
  ○ Cortical atrophy with >10 kg alcohol/kg in men, >5 kg alcohol/kg in women
• Alcoholic fetal syndrome >30 g/day
• Cerebellar degeneration: 30% alcohol misusers with >30 g/day
• Peripheral and autonomic neuropathies:
  ○ 40 g/day women and 60 g/day men x 10 years
  ○ Neuropathy (20% clinical, 70% subclinical by EMG)

Liver
Exponential ratio >30 g/day x 10 years. Starts with 1–2 kg alcohol/kg. Usually >4 kg alcohol/kg

Bone
Osteopenia with >20 g/day

Cancer
According to tumor type >4 kg alcohol/kg. >10 g/day breast, in combination with other factors

EMG, electromyogram; RR, relative rate.

• Frequency: acute, recent, and cumulated doses); and
• Extent of binge drinking.

One approach is to use the time-line follow-back method that considers anchor points in life events related to alcohol consumption and establish different periods of alcohol intake in quantity and mean dose. Most diseases from alcohol damage are related to the cumulated dose of alcohol consumed over a lifetime, defined as threshold doses for alcohol toxicity in specific organs (Box 20.3). If the individual exceeds this threshold dose, there is high likelihood of damage.

In addition to alcohol abuse, it is also necessary to consider other toxic dependences (especially other toxins such as tobacco, marijuana, cocaine, infections such as hepatitis C virus, other intrinsic liver diseases such as metabolic, genetic, or autoimmune liver diseases) that may interfere and potentiate the toxic effects of alcohol.

Another important point in extrahepatic manifestations of alcohol abuse is the consideration of the type of cell damaged, because alcohol does not induce the same pattern of damage in epithelial, metabolically active, excitable, and embryonic cells [6].

- Metabolically active cells (such as hepatocytes or acinar pancreatic cells) are prone to oxidative, energetic, and metabolic damage involving mitochondrial damage and disturbances in protein synthesis, carbohydrate, and lipid pathways.
- Excitable cells (i.e. neurons or myocytes) are prone to disturbances in membrane permeability, ion channels, and second-messenger transients that disturb excitability. Binge drinking is an especially damaging for excitable cells (such as neurons and myocytes). Epithelial and embryonic cells may develop direct DNA damage and apoptosis.

Other common systemic effects of alcohol involve enzymatic and hormonal disturbances, oxidative damage, immunologic, nutritional, vitamin and/or mineral deficiencies, and energetic disturbances.

After considering the impact of alcohol itself and other specific or nonspecific factors of organ damage, a comprehensive plan to evaluate organ damage should be implemented [4]. Box 20.4 shows the main usual procedures with complementary procedures to evaluate this systemic alcohol-related organ damage.

Treatment of systemic organ damage in alcohol abuse

Basic points

- Treatment should be aimed at complete abstinence of alcohol intake and control or abstinence of other substance dependences with potential synergic effects.
- Evaluate the degree of systemic organ involvement.
- Evaluate the type (acute, subacute, chronic) and degree (transitory, initial, established reversible, established irreversible) of organ damage (Box 20.2).
- Establish a plan for treatment.

Box 20.4 The usual main complementary procedures to evaluate systemic ethanol-related organ damage.

Cardiovascular system	ECG, chest X-ray, echosonography
Central neurologic system	Cognitive evaluation, brain CT, MRI
Peripheral neurologic system	Osteotendinous reflexes, electromyography
Muscle	Electromyography, serum muscle enzymes, muscle biopsy
Bone	Skeletal X-ray, densitometry, bone scintigraphy
Oxidative damage	Serum superoxide dismutase, malondialdehyde, tissue antioxidant status
Nutritional damage	Anthropometric evaluation. Weight, BMI, serum proteins: total protein, albumin, pre-albumin, retinol- binding protein, transferrin, lymphocyte count, hemoglobin

Specific points of treatment of organ damage
Mortality and morbidity

The hazardous and harmful use of alcohol is a major global contributing factor to death. Almost 4% of all deaths worldwide are attributed to alcohol, more than caused by HIV/AIDS, violence, or tuberculosis. The harmful use of alcohol is a particularly serious threat to men and is the leading risk factor for death in males aged 15–59 years, mainly due to injuries, violence, and cardiovascular diseases. Of all male deaths, 6.2% are globally attributable to alcohol, compared with 1.1% of female deaths [8]. Harmful drinking can also be very costly to communities and societies. Alcohol is also associated with many serious social issues, including violence, child neglect and abuse, and absenteeism in the workplace [1]. Lower socioeconomic status and educational levels result in a greater risk of alcohol-related death, disease, and injury, a social determinant that is greater for men than women.

Cardiovascular damage

Low doses of alcohol consumption are associated with a lower risk of cardiovascular death but this protective effect disappears at doses above 40 g/day for men and

30 g/day for women [9]. This effect is likely to occur because coronary risk improves with low dose of alcohol consumption in relation to the increase of high-density lipoprotein (HDL) cholesterol and other hemostatic factors.

Arrhythmias Ethanol consumption can induce a diversity of acute or chronic cardiac rhythm disturbances. Atrial extrasystoles and atrial fibrillation are the most frequent abnormalities in the context of binge drinking in the so-called "holiday heart syndrome," but ventricular extrasystoles and ventricular tachycardia are more dangerous and can result in sudden death. These arrhythmias are more frequent after acute binge drinking, in situations of alcohol abstinence or delirium, in the presence of malnutrition and ionic disturbances, and in subjects with previous alcohol cardiomyopathy.

It is necessary to evaluate and control the frequent ionic disturbances (sodium, potassium, magnesium, phosphorus) that may induce and maintain the development of arrhythmias. Ethanol cessation helps to control the persistence of arrhythmias. Antiarrhythmic drugs such as digoxin, amiodarone, beta-blockers, and calcium-channel blockers (verapamil, diltiazem) are the most useful drugs for the treatment of the acute phase of arrhythmias. In this acute phase the patient should be medically controlled and this usually requires intensive care unit (ICU) admission and electrocardiographic (ECG) monitoring because of the possibility of developing cardiac arrest. 24-hour Holter monitoring may help to detect clinically nonapparent arrhythmias.

Antithrombotic prophylaxis should be considered, balancing the risks and benefits because alcohol misusers, especially those with cirrhosis, are prone to bleeding and are also more likely to fall and develop trauma.

Cardiomyopathy Development of heart failure in alcoholic cardiomyopathy is dose-dependent and is reported in around 13% of alcohol misusers. This cardiomyopathy is manifested by exertional dyspnea, orthopnea, and peripheral edema. The main diagnostic procedures are chest X-ray and cardiac echosonograpy. Left ventricular diastolic dysfunction precedes systolic dysfunction in alcoholic cardiomyopathy.

Management of alcoholic cardiomyopathy is similar to idiopathic dilated cardiomyopathy with oxygen supply, diuretic (furosemide, spironolactone) and renin–angiotensin–aldosterone (RAA) inhibitors. Heart transplantation may be necessary in end-stage dilated

cardiomyopathy in prolonged abstainers without any other major systemic organic damage (dementia, cancer, cirrhosis).

Hypertension Alcohol-related arterial hypertension is dose-dependent, and may develop with the daily alcohol consumption of 40 g and usually improves with abstinence. When necessary, vasodilators (RAA inhibitors, β or α1-adrenergic blockers) are the treatment of choice.

Neurologic damage

Alcohol-induced neurologic damage may be central or peripheral and is usually multifactorial [10]. The main related pathogenic factors are:

• Direct effects of alcohol on neural tissue;
• Thiamine deficiency; and
• Malnutrition.

Protein supplementation and long-term thiamine treatment are recommended.

Alcohol withdrawal syndrome The alcohol withdrawal syndrome, which, as its name implies, arises soon after the cessation of drinking, varies from a mild disorder of autonomic hyperactivity to a severe life-threatening medical condition manifested by systemic hypertension, tachycardia, tremors, hyperreflexia, irritability, anxiety, headache, nausea, and vomiting. These symptoms may progress to delirium tremens, seizures, coma, cardiac arrest, and death.

Delirium tremens Alcohol abstinence-associated delirium requires prevention and treatment with benzodiazepines or clomethiazole. The recent guidelines of the European Association for the Study of the Liver state that benzodiazepines are the treatment of choice in patients with acute withdrawal syndrome and alcoholic liver disease (ALD) [4].

Seizures These can occur during alcohol withdrawal and require treatment with clonazepam or a similar benzodiazepine. After recovery from seizures, maintenance antiepileptic drugs are not required.

Encephalopathy Wernicke's encephalopathy is a medical emergency and is characterized by:

• Changes in mental status;
• Ocular abnormalities;
• Motor problems, such as gait disturbances and ataxia.

A high level of suspicion is necessary to detect the presence of subclinical situations involving the appearance of some of the symptoms of thiamine deficiency. It may be difficult to differentiate Wernicke's encephalopathy from hepatic encephalopathy (HE) and the two may coexist. HE is associated with varying degrees of drowsiness and tends to fluctuate in severity. The features of HE may be subclinical. The diagnosis may be confirmed by the characteristic liver flap but the presence of fetor is unreliable. The use of electroencephalography (EEG) or critical flicker sensitivity may help with the diagnosis of HE but in Wernicke's encephalopathy, EEG may be within normal limits in the early stage but shows nonspecific slowing of the dominant rhythm in the later stages.

Some studies have suggested that in those alcohol abusers with Wernicke's encephalopathy, the thiamine-dependent enzyme transketolase has a higher affinity for thiamine; others have reported variants in the thiamine transporter gene. Assessment of thiamine status is difficult and is most commonly detected measuring red cell thiamine transketolase activity before and after addition of thiamine pyrophosphate or by measuring serum thiamine directly with chromatography.

Treatment of Wernicke's encephalopathy requires high-dose thiamine supplementation with a minimum infusion of 500 mg thiamine hydrochloride (dissolved in 100 mL 0.9% saline) over 30 minutes, three times a day for 2–3 days. In the absence of a response, supplementation may be discontinued after 2–3 days. In the case of response, intravenous or intramuscular infusion of 250 mg/day thiamine for 3–5 days or until clinical improvement ceases should be maintained. Prolonged thiamine supplementation is recommended with an oral dose of 50 mg /day. On suspicion of the presence of Wernicke's encephalopathy, thiamine must be administered before or concomitantly with intravenous administration of glucose because glucose alone can precipitate the disorder in thiamine-deficient individuals.

Brain damage Brain damage and atrophy may be clinically suspected by cognitive impairment and confirmed by computed tomography, nuclear magnetic resonance, and cognitive tests. However, these features are nonspecific and may be difficult to distinguish from the effects of age and other factors.

Peripheral neuropathy This is suspected with the presence of distal weakness or dysesthesia and a decrease in osteotendinous reflexes and is confirmed by electroneurography.

These abnormalities may partially respond to treatment and prolonged supplementation with thiamine, cobalamine, pyridoxine, and folate in addition to physiotherapy. Prophylactic treatment with the intramuscular administration of 250 mg thiamine once daily for 3–5 consecutive days should be used in all patients with severe alcohol withdrawal, poor nourishment, and those with a poor diet and signs of malnutrition to prevent irreversible neurologic damage.

Digestive tract damage

Esophageal problems Gastroesophageal reflux and esophagitis are frequent in patients with alcohol misuse because alcohol induces gastric acid secretion and inhibits the gastroesophageal sphincter tone. The treatment of these disorders requires dietary and postural measures as well as maintained pharmacologic treatment with gastric proton pump inhibitors (such as omeprazole or pantoprazole) in addition to mucosal protectors such as carbenoxolone which must be used in caution because of the potential effects on electrolytes.

Gastric problems Chronic gastritis is also frequent and usually requires treatment that is similar to that for reflux. In addition, infection with *Helicobacter pylori* should be looked for and treated appropriately.

Gastrointestinal bleeding Both esophagitis and gastritis may be related to episodes of gastrointestinal bleeding and chronic anemia. In the presence of chronic anemia, prolonged iron and folate supplementation is usually necessary.

Episodes of upper digestive tract bleeding are frequent in alcohol misusers, especially in those with cirrhosis. The main causes of hemorrhage:
- Mallory–Weiss syndrome (suspected after repeated vomiting in binge drinking), gastric peptic ulcers;
- Portal hypertension gastropathy; or
- Varices.

Endoscopy is usually necessary for diagnosis (and treatment in the case of variceal bleeding). Admission to an ICU is usually required as management usually requires hemodynamic monitoring, control of bleeding, blood or blood product transfusion, and monitoring for infection, encephalopathy, renal impairment, and withdrawal symptoms. Specific pharmacologic treatment with proton pump inhibitors in gastric ulcers and terlipressin or octreotide infusion combined with endoscopic sclerotherapy or band ligation to control acute esophageal variceal bleeding may be needed. Antibiotics should be given to all those with acute gastrointestinal bleeding.

Prolonged iron supplementation may be required following hemodynamic stabilization of digestive tract bleeding, including blood transfusion and management of anemia.

Prevention of esophageal variceal bleeding or rebleeding involves repeated sclerotherapy or variceal ligation in addition to pharmacologic treatment with nonselective beta-blockers such as propranolol or carvedilol.

Pancreas Acute pancreatitis is frequent in alcohol abusers and requires dietary control, analgesia, and intravenous fluid therapy, usually with hospital admission. Frequent acute complications such as kidney failure and sepsis require ICU management. The presence of pancreatic abscesses or cysts may require surgery.

Chronic pancreatitis may cause maldigestion and malabsorption with steatorrhea and weight loss. Pancreatic insufficiency may be suspected in the presence of steatorrhea and progressive weight loss but may be corrected with diet and pancreatic enzyme administration before meals. Chronic abdominal pain syndromes attributed to alcoholic pancreatitis are often untreatable despite pancreatic enzyme replacement and require multimodal analgesia combining paracetamol, anti-inflammatory drugs, and gabapentine although nonsteroidal anti-inflammatory drugs must be used with caution because of renal and gastric toxicity; paracetamol, up to 3 g/day is usually well tolerated. If opiates are required, care must be taken to avoid constipation that may result in encephalopathy.

There is a dual relationship between alcohol consumption and diabetes mellitus. Light to moderate drinking may be beneficial to metabolic control while heavy drinking is detrimental.

Bowel Functional diarrhea is frequent in alcoholic patients with visceral dysautonomia. Dietary measures with fractioned astringent diet and anticholinergic drugs such as loperamide may be useful.

Nutrition and metabolism

Caloric and protein malnutrition are common in chronic alcohol abusers. Indeed, alcohol misuse is the main cause of malnutrition in western countries as a consequence of poor dietary intake, malabsorption, and protein and carbohydrate disturbances. The presence of malnutrition interferes with immunity and metabolism and increases systemic organ damage, especially cardiovascular, neurologic, musculoskeletal, and immunologic. The deleterious effects of ethanol are synergistic with the coexistence of malnutrition in many tissues making it necessary to correct malnutrition to improve dysfunction and organ damage.

Evaluation of caloric malnutrition requires anthropometric measurements including body mass index (relevant if <18 kg/cm^2), evaluation of triceps skinfold, and lean body mass. Protein malnutrition should be suspected when there are significant reductions in serum proteins (total protein, albumin, pre-albumin, retinol binding protein, and transferrin) and hematologic parameters (total lymphocyte count, prothrombin, and hemoglobin).

Malnutrition can be corrected with oral or parenteral dietary supplementation according to the clinical condition of the patient. Vitamin (folate, E, B1, B3, B6) and mineral deficiencies (Mg, Ca, P) and excess iron and copper are frequently seen in the context of malnutrition and require specific supplementation, sometimes over prolonged periods. Especially in patients awaiting liver transplantation, correction of malnutrition is more important than concerns about high protein diets triggering encephalopathy.

Lipids Lipid levels are often abnormal and high levels of serum triglycerides are seen which resolve with abstinence. Ethanol causes organ toxicity with involvement of a number of genes encoding functional proteins involved in nucleic acid binding, transcription, and signal transduction. These ethanol-responsive genes are also correlated with other biologic pathways, such as inflammation, angiogenesis, and the integrin signaling pathway. These findings provide some insight into the molecular targets of alcohol-induced toxicity and how genetic mutation affects the toxicity phenotype [7].

Nutritional support and oxidative damage Oxidative tissue damage is a frequent cause of direct tissue damage in alcohol misuse [6]. The direct toxic effect of alcohol on tissues is increased in the presence of free radicals and oxidative stress. It is important to consider this situation with evaluation of plasmatic or tissue oxidative status. This evaluation involves multiple parameters, the most useful being serum measurements of malondialdehyde, superoxide dismutase, and glutathione.

Oxidative damage may be corrected with antioxidant therapy (tocopherol, selenium, beta-carotenes, *N*-acetylcysteine, or ascorbic acid), although there is little evidence of their beneficial effect. Some dietary control such as the Mediterranean diet have been shown to improve the oxidative status and decrease long-term organ damage.

Endocrine disturbances

In addition to diabetes mellitus, alcohol toxicity may be associated with other endocrine disturbances including gonadal dysfunction. Interactions are complex as ethanol may act in one or more ways including a direct impact on endocrine cells resulting in decreased hormone secretion. Furthermore, in those with liver disease, there may be alterations in hormone binding, decreased hormone production, or activation by the liver or nonendocrine tissues and alterations in target tissue response.

Bone and skeletal damage

Alcohol misuse is a main factor in the induction of osteopenia and osteoporosis in both sexes. In western countries, up to one-third of alcohol misusers develop osteoporosis. The mechanism of the production of alcohol-associated osteopenia appears to be a direct effect of alcohol on bone cells, suppressing the function of osteoblasts, and an indirect or modulating effect through mineral regulating hormones such as vitamin D metabolites, parathyroid hormone, and calcitonin. There is a dose-dependent effect, starting at a daily alcohol intake of 20 g. The presence of liver disease, malnutrition, hypogonadism, and vitamin D deficiency impairs the course of osteopenia. Secondary hyperparathyroidism is usually related to chronic vitamin D deficiency.

Clinical suspicion should be raised by the presence of pathologic fractures, especially of the hip. Diagnosis should be confirmed by bone densitometry. The presence of malnutrition and cirrhosis makes improvement difficult. Treatment should include protein replacement, calcium, and vitamin D supplementation and the administration of bisphosphonates, active weight-bearing exercise, and avoidance of smoking. Alcoholic men are prone to avoid pharmacologic treatments for osteopenia.

Skeletal myopathy is present in one-third of chronic alcohol misusers [9]. The acute form presents with muscle swelling and rhabdomyolysis that may cause kidney failure. Chronic skeletal myopathy may be suspected with the presence of proximal weakness, pain, and muscle atrophy. Myometry may be useful to corroborate the loss of muscle strength. Serum muscle enzymes (creatine kinase, aldolase) usually rise in acute phases of skeletal myopathy. Clinical suspicion may be confirmed by electromyography and muscle biopsy. Correction of malnutrition and electrolyte disturbances, rest, analgesia, and the prevention of renal failure with fluid therapy are useful in acute phases. Physiotherapy is recommended during the recovery period to improve the clinical course of the disease.

Inflammation

Ethanol has a dual effect on inflammatory response with a clear anti-inflammatory effect at low doses while reverting to a proinflammatory effect at high doses. The presence of systemic inflammation increases cardiovascular risk and also impairs the course of other systemic inflammatory diseases such as sepsis, chronic hepatitis C, or HIV infection. The mechanisms of alcohol-induced inflammation are diverse, including a rise in serum interleukins, cytokines, tumor necrosis factor α (TNF-α), C-reactive protein, NADPH, activation of lipid peroxidation and oxidative stress, depletion of gutathione and superoxide dismutase, an increase of endothelial nitric oxide (NO) synthase, development of endothelial dysfunction by vascular cell adhesion molecule (VCAM) or intercellular adhesion molecule 1 (ICAM-1) activation, and disturbances in monocyte adhesion to the endothelium. Other than alcohol abstinence, no single medical intervention has been described to be useful to correct alcohol-related systemic inflammation. Specific anti-inflammatory treatment has yet to demonstrate any beneficial effect. Antioxidant therapy, treatment of concomitant infectious and inflammatory processes, and dietary control such as the Mediterranean diet have been shown to improve the oxidative status and decrease long-term inflammatory organ damage.

Infections

Patients with alcohol misuse, especially those with established liver disease, are more susceptible to infections. The WHO 2011 report provided new evidence pointing to a causal link between alcohol and infectious diseases [1]. Alcohol consumption weakens the immune system, thereby facilitating infection by pathogens causing pneumonia and tuberculosis. This effect is markedly more pronounced with heavy drinking, and there may be a threshold effect.

Pneumonia is the main infection in this clinical setting, especially if the alcoholic misusers are also smokers. Soft tissue infection and sepsis are also more prevalent in these subjects. Overall, alcohol misusers are more prone to infections with Gram-negative bacilli, anaerobes, mycobacteria, fungi, and *Listeria* than nonalcoholic subjects.

A strong association has been found between alcohol consumption, HIV infection, and sexually transmitted diseases. There is a clear causal effect of alcohol consumption on the adherence of HIV/AIDS patients to antiretroviral treatment. There should be a high degree of clinical suspicion, especially if there is fever; there should be a low threshold for treatment with broad-spectrum antibiotics, which should be started before the results of cultures and sensitivities are available.

Malignancy

The development of different types of cancer (ear, nose, and throat, oropharynx, esophagus, liver, colon, breast) should be considered in any alcoholic subject. The higher the consumption of alcohol, the greater the risk for these cancers. Even the consumption of two drinks per day causes an increased risk for some cancers, such as breast cancer. Many of these cancers are also related to cigarette smoking which is frequently associated with alcohol excess.

Thus, there should be a low threshold for screening for cancer. Cessation of smoking and alcohol consumption are key elements in the treatment plan of any patient with alcohol misuse with the risk of cancer.

Pharmacologic interactions

In the global evaluation of alcohol misusers, the potential for alcohol to interact with prescribed medications should be considered. Chronic ingestion of excessive amounts of alcohol may lead to the induction of the metabolizing enzyme CYP2E1 with consequences for adrenergic, analgesic, anesthetic, antibiotic, and antiepileptic drugs.

Future treatments to prevent systemic organ damage by alcohol will combine classic approaches while also taking into account the use of new antiapoptotic factors, specific antioxidants, and tissue-specific growth factors such as insulin-like growth factor-1, ghrelin, myostatin inhibitors to decrease alcohol-mediated organ damage and favor tissue regeneration [4]. A better understanding of the relationship between genotype and phenotype of ethanol-responsive genes will provide useful approaches for further research on alcohol-induced toxicity and potential therapy [7].

References

[1] World Health Organization. *Global Status Report on Alcohol and Health*. WM 274. World Health Organization, Geneva, Switzerland; 2011, 1–286.

[2] National Clinical Guideline Centre (UK). *Alcohol Use Disorders: Diagnosis and Clinical Management of Alcohol-Related Physical Complications [Internet]*. Royal College of Physicians (UK), National Institute for Health and Clinical Excellence Guidance, London; 2010.

[3] World Health Organization. *Public Health Problems Caused by Harmful Use of Alcohol*. Fifty-Eighth World Health Assembly, Geneva, 25 May 2005. Resolution WHA58.26.

[4] Fernández-Solà J. Management of extrahepatic manifestations of alcoholic liver diseases. *Clin Liver Dis* 2013; **2**(2): 89–91.

[5] Estruch R, Fernández-Solà J, Sacanella E, Paré C, Rubin E, Urbano-Márquez A. Relationship between cardiomyopathy and liver disease in chronic alcoholism. *Hepatology* 1995; **22**: 532–538.

[6] Molina PE, Hoek JB, Nelson S, et al. Mechanisms of alcohol-induced tissue injury. *Alcohol Clin Exp Res* 2003; **27**(3): 563–575.

[7] Zakhari S. Alcohol metabolism and epigenetics changes. *Alcohol Res* 2013; **35**(1): 6–16.

[8] Rehm J, Mathers C, Popova S, Thavorncharoensap M, Teerawattananon Y, Patra J. Global burden of disease and injury and economic cost attributable to alcohol use and alcohol-use disorders. *Lancet* 2009; **373**: 2223–2233.

[9] Urbano-Márquez A, Fernández-Solà J. The effects of alcohol on skeletal and cardiac muscle. *Muscle Nerve* 2004; **30**: 689–707.

[10] de la Monte SM, Kril JJ. Human alcohol-related neuropathology. *Acta Neuropathol* 2014; **27**(1): 71–90.

CHAPTER 21

Treatment of liver disease

James Neuberger

Liver Unit, Queen Elizabeth Hospital Birmingham, Birmingham and Organ Donation and Transplantation, NHS Blood and Transplant, Bristol, UK

KEY POINTS

- Patients with chronic alcohol-associated liver disease need regular follow-up in clinic.

- Patients should be monitored for alcohol and other substance abuse and offered support to become or remain abstinent.

- Patients should also be monitored for other effects of alcohol use and offered appropriate support (general and nutritional health, reproductive health, bone health).

- Liver function usually improves with abstinence.

- Decompensation is characterized by the development of jaundice, ascites, and encephalopathy.

- There are many causes of decompensation including infection (bacterial, viral, or protozoal), electrolyte disturbance, drugs and toxins (including alcohol), bleeding, venous thrombosis (portal or hepatic), hepatocellular carcinoma development, and constipation.

- The onset of new symptoms should lead to a search for precipitating factors and consideration of referral for transplant assessment.

- Those with cirrhosis should be monitored for complications, especially for esophageal and gastric varices and liver cell cancer, so appropriate prophylaxis or treatment can be offered.

Introduction

The treatment of the patient with alcohol-related liver disease (ALD) is aimed at maintaining health, supporting abstinence, improving liver function, and early detection and treatment of complications of established liver disease. Liver function may improve over 12 months following abstinence

Follow-up

Most patients with ALD should be followed up in a clinic in order to encourage abstinence, offer support for relapse, assess liver and other organ damage, and for general and nutritional advice and support. Patients should be offered history, examination, routine blood tests and, where cirrhosis is present,

---

Alcohol Abuse and Liver Disease, First Edition. Edited by James Neuberger and Andrea DiMartini.

© 2015 John Wiley & Sons, Ltd. Published 2015 by John Wiley & Sons, Ltd.

regular follow-up and surveillance for varices and liver cell cancer.

It should be remembered that the so-called liver function tests are neither liver-specific nor measure liver function. For example, both an elevated serum bilirubin and raised mean cell volume (MCV) may be seen in liver disease and in hemolysis, both of which are associated with alcohol and many other factors. It is often helpful to measure specific markers of alcohol and substance abuse but this should be done with informed patient consent. Those with cirrhosis or advanced liver disease should be monitored for decompensation and transplant consideration.

Various scores have been developed to help assess prognosis (such as the Child–Pugh and Model for end-stage liver disease (MELD) scores). These are useful aids but must not be used a substitute for clinical judgment.

General health

Patients should be encouraged to maintain a healthy lifestyle with a normal balanced diet, avoidance of smoking and other toxins, and continued abstinence from alcohol. In many cases, alcohol-associated damage may coexist with other causes of liver disease and these may require specific management.

Medication As discussed in Chapter 10, most patients, even with advanced liver disease, tolerate medication well and treatment should be given in normal doses. Drugs that should be used with caution include the following:

- Nonsteroidal anti-inflammatory drugs, because they may precipitate renal failure;
- Sedatives (such as benzodiazepines), because they may produce encephalopathy; and
- Drugs that cause constipation as they may precipitate encephalopathy.

Nutrition High salt diets should be avoided in those with cirrhosis. There is no need to avoid fat unless the patient is intolerant and symptomatic. Even in those with encephalopathy, dietary protein should not be restricted. Many advocate the use of thiamine and vitamin B supplementation. Replacement of fat soluble vitamins (A, D, E, and K) should be considered in those with cholestasis.

Bone health ALD may be associated with osteoporosis so those at risk should be offered advice (stop smoking,

healthy diet, regular weight-bearing exercise), screening with dual-energy X-ray absorptiometry (DEXA) scanning every 3–5 years, and intervention as appropriate.

Reproductive health
Females

Contraception Many patients with advanced liver disease have reduced fertility. The risks of contraception must be balanced against the benefits. Oral contraceptives may be associated with an increased risk of vascular thrombosis and mechanical devices may be associated with an increased risk of sepsis and heavier bleeding.

Pregnancy While women with significant liver disease are less fertile, pregnancy may occur. Risks are greater in the first trimester when the increase in vascular volume may be associated with an increased risk of variceal bleeding. The delivery should be carefully monitored and the interventions considered early. Raising of portal pressure should be avoided as far as possible. Ideally, women should be given prepregnancy counseling and review so medication can be reviewed and revised and nutritional deficiencies identified and corrected.

Males

There is an increased risk of erectile dysfunction; drugs such as Viagra are usually well-tolerated, even in those with varices.

Immunization

While responses may be less in those with cirrhosis, there is no reason not to give immunizations if indicated although care should be taken with intramuscular injections in those with prolonged clotting or low platelets. Those taking immunosuppressive agents should not have live or attenuated vaccines.

Cirrhosis

While cirrhosis is a histologic diagnosis, its likely presence is suggested by one or more of several tests:
- Blood tests
  - General, such the aspartate aminotransferase to platelet ratio index (APRI) score;
  - Fibrosis markers:
    – procollagen peptide 3;
    – hyaluronic acid;

Box 21.1 Some causes of hepatic decompensation.

- Return to alcohol
- Use of illicit substances
- Other drugs (especially sedatives)
- Infection
- Bleeding
- Renal failure or electrolyte disturbance
- Constipation
- Portal vein thrombosis
- Hepatocellular carcinoma development

Box 21.2 Management for prevention of bleeding from varices.

- If no varices are present and there is no evidence of hepatic decompensation, then endoscopy should be repeated in 3 years
- If no varices and hepatic decompensation are present, endoscopy should be repeated annually
- If small varices are present with signs of decompensation and red wale spots, treatment with beta-blockers should be offered
- If small varices with no signs of decompenation and spots, endoscopy should be repeated annually
- If medium or large varices are present, treatment should be offered with pharmacotherapy, band ligation or sclerotherapy. Nitrates should not be used

- matrix metalloptotein-2;
- Fibrotest;
- ActiTest.
- Imaging
  - Ultrasound;
  - CT;
  - MRI;
  - Fibroscan.

Patients with cirrhosis may show decompensation and precipitating factors should be looked for. Some of the more common precipitating factors for decompensation are shown in Box 21.1. The onset of such symptoms should raise consideration for liver transplantation.

Detection and management of complications of portal hypertension

Patients with alcoholic liver disease are at risk of the complications of portal hypertension and this may occur before the onset of cirrhosis because of the perisinusoidal and bridging fibrosis. The two main complications are the development of varices and its consequences, and of ascites.

Varices

Portal pressure rises as a consequence of increased intrahepatic resistance and vasoconstriction, and so leads to the development of portosystemic collateral formation. Esophageal and gastric varices are the most important complications but varices may present anywhere in the gastrointestinal tract and form when the wedged hepatic venous pressure exceeds 10 mmHg. In those with cirrhosis, varices develop in about 8% per year and are present in about 50% of those with cirrhosis. Variceal bleeding occurs in 10–15% per year, and

of those who bleed, 20% will be dead within 6 weeks and 60% will rebleed within 2 years. Thus, detection and prevention of variceal bleeding is important.

Prophylaxis of variceal bleeding

Primary prophylaxis Once cirrhosis is suspected, patients should undergo upper gastrointestinal endoscopy to look for varices. The approach to prophylaxis is well established and outlined in Box 21.2. For pharmacologic prophylaxis, propranolol, nadolol, or carvedilol should be used. Nitrates are not indicated.

Secondary prophylaxis If the patient has bled, then long-term prophylaxis with either pharmacotherapy or band ligation should be offered. Shunt (TIPS or surgical) may be indicated for those with recurrent bleeding despite adequate therapy or those who are intolerant of treatment. Once patients have bled from varices, they should be offered treatment as for large varices.

Management of acute bleeding varices

Acute bleeding varices are a medical emergency and patients require immediate resuscitation, intravenous terlipressin, antibiotics, and early endoscopy for diagnosis and band ligation or variceal injection where possible. Failure to control bleeding should lead to urgent consideration of a shunt (see Shunt section). Sengstaken tubes are useful in those rare cases where immediate control of variceal bleeding is required and as a temporary measure. Most patients who require a Sengstaken tube will need to be offered anesthesia and ventilation.

Box 21.3 Causes of ascites.

Liver disease:
- Parenchymal disease
- Portal vein thrombosis
- Budd–Chiari syndrome
- Sinusoidal obstruction

Right heart failure

Pancreatitis

Nephrotic syndrome

Infection:
- Bacterial
- Mycobacterial

Malignancy

Myxedema

Box 21.4 Treatment of hepatic ascites.

First line
- General treatment (avoid inappropriate medications)
- Sodium restriction
- Diuretics (furosemide and spironolactone)

Second line
- Paracentesis
- Shunt
- Transplantation

Ascites

Around half of patients with compensated cirrhosis develop ascites within 10 years; once ascites develops, 15% will die within 1 year and over 40% in 5 years. Although hepatic fibrosis is the most likely cause of ascites in the context of alcohol excess, other causes must be considered (Box 21.3). Patients with ascites usually present with abdominal distension which may extend into the thorax (hydrothorax). Occasionally, hydrothorax may be the sole manifestation of ascites.

The diagnosis can be made on the basis of history and examination but imaging is more sensitive and reliable than clinical examination, especially in those with small amounts of ascites. The development or sudden exacerbation of ascites should prompt review of precipitating factors as in Box 21.3.

Diagnostic paracentesis may be required when there is uncertainty as to the cause of the ascites or if the patient in unwell, to exclude infection. The procedure is often performed under ultrasound guidance and replacement of clotting factors and platelet support are usually not required. This is done using a 15 or 22 G needle, inserted either in the midline, between the pubis and umbilicus or left or right lower quadrant. Ascitic fluid should be tested for cell count, microscopy, and culture; some units also measure albumin, protein, lactate, cholesterol, glucose, amylase, and other analytes depending on the clinical situation. Some offer routine antibiotic prophylaxis to those with ascetic protein concentration of <15 g/L.

Treatment of ascites

There should be a stepped approach to the treatment of ascites (Box 21.4).

First line treatment

This is primarily with diet modification and diuretics. The patient should be put on a sodium-restricted diet (aiming for a maximum intake of 80–120 mmol/day – including medications and intravenous fluids) and diuretics. The commonly used diuretics include a combination of furosemide (40–80 mg/day) and spironolactone (100 mg/day increasing up to 800 mg/day). Amiloride is a possible substitute for those who develop problems such as gynecomastia, with spironolactone. The ascites may take several days to show a response and diuretics increased gradually with carful monitoring of weight and renal function. The patient should lose no more than 0.5 kg/day (unless there is peripheral edema). More rapid weight loss should be avoided as this may precipitate intravascular volume depletion and lead to renal failure. The urea, creatinine, and electrolytes should be monitored and medication adjusted if there is evidence of renal impairment or electrolyte disturbance. Measurement of renal sodium excretion is helpful especially when the response is slow and may indicate noncompliance with dietary restriction.

Unless there is evidence of hyponatremia (serum sodium <130 mEq/L), there is no need to limit water intake. Equally, there is no evidence to suggest that bed-rest or treatment with vaptans are effective in the treatment of ascites although the latter may be effective for hyponatremia.

Second line treatment

If the patient fails to respond, it is important to review the diagnosis and ensure the patient is compliant with diet and medication. Midodrine can be considered.

Paracentesis is effective both in relieving ascites and as a regular treatment. A large-bore needle is inserted into the ascites and fluid drained rapidly. Some units use a pump to increase the rate of drainage. When significant volumes of ascites are removed (>5 L), it is usual practice to administer colloid, with 6–8 g albumin for 1 L of ascites removed.

Shunt

A transjugular intrahepatic shunt (TIPS) is usually inserted by an interventional radiologist under local anesthesia and a beneficial effect seen in over 75%. Complications of shunt are uncommon but include immediate problems such as bleeding and infection, shunt thrombosis or stenosis, hemobilia, encephalopathy, and hepatic deterioration and displacement. Late complications include shunt thrombosis or stenosis; these complications can sometimes be treated by interventional radiology. Currently used shunts are coated and usually remain patent for many years. Contraindications to TIPS include encephalopathy and advanced liver disease. Other shunts, such as the peritoneovenous shunts have largely fallen into disuse.

TIPS or paracentesis? There is little difference in outcomes in patients between fortnightly paracentesis and TIPS but most patients find a shunt preferable.

Renal impairment and hyponatremia

Renal impairment may be a consequence of overuse of diuretics, because of intrinsic renal disease, or may be a sign of hepatorenal syndrome (HRS). It should be remembered that serum urea and creatinine are often low in those with advanced cirrhosis so a value in the normal range may indicate renal impairment in this situation.

HRS is a form of functional renal failure without identifiable renal pathology and is characterized by increased intrarenal vascular resistance and disturbance of the arterial circulation. HRS carries a poor prognosis. Treatment includes the use of intravenous albumin and systemic vasoconstrictors as terlipressin, midodrine, or octreotide. TIPS has also been effective in some patients.

Hyponatremia (serum sodium <130 mEq/L) may also be a sign of diuretic excess or be dilutional due to water overload. Diuretics should be stopped and water intake restricted to 1 L/day. Vaptans may be helpful in this situation.

Spontaneous bacterial peritonitis

Spontaneous bacterial peritonitis (SBP) is defined as infection of the ascites and is often spontaneous, although it often follows interventions such as endoscopy. Presentation varies from severe abdominal pain and fever to asymptomatic decompensation. It is important to have a low threshold for diagnosis and early treatment needs to be instituted before micobiologic results are available. The diagnosis is made by diagnostic paracentesis and finding a polymorphonuclear count >250/mL. Cultures are often negative but common organisms include *Escherichia coli, Streptococcus viridans, Staphylococcus aureus*, and enterococci. Treatment should be with broad-spectrum antibiotics and modified in the light of bacterial sensitivities.

As recurrence is common, those who have had SBP should be offered long-term antibiotic prophylaxis with drugs such as norfloxacin 400 mg/day or ciprofloxacin 250 mg/day.

Hepatocellular carcinoma

Patients with cirrhosis, especially males and those with hepatitis C virus infection, are at risk of developing hepatocellular carcinoma (HCC). As treatments now are much more effective, screening and surveillance are recommended.

Once cirrhosis is identified, patients should be offered an ultrasound examination, repeated every 6 months. While a progressive rise in serum α-fetoprotein (AFP) is strongly suggestive of HCC, its use in surveillance is no longer recommended although many clinicians still use this every 3 months. There are many causes for a raised AFP and not all HCCs are associated with a rise in AFP.

If a lesion is seen on ultrasound that is suspicious of HCC, then a further imaging modality is required, such as CT or MR with angiography showing intense arterial uptake followed by washout in the delayed phases is usually diagnostic.

There are several effective treatment options: percutanous ethanol injection, radiofrequency ablation, resection (unlikely in those with cirrhosis), chemembolization, chemotherapy (not very effective although agents such as sorafenib have been used), and transplantation. The most appropriate therapy should be discussed by the multidisciplinary team.

Hepatic encephalopathy

Hepatic encephalopathy (HE) may be overt or subclinical and difficult to detect. Clinically, HE may present as slight confusion, dyspraxia, sleep disturbance, and day–night sleep reversal, somnolence, and coma. It may be difficult to distinguish from other causes of confusion, including vascular dementia.

HE tends to fluctuate in severity. Diagnostic pointers include the "hepatic flap" and dyspraxia. Long track signs may be present. Hepatic fetor is an unreliable sign. Blood ammonia levels correlate poorly with HE. EEG may show the characteristic triphasic waves but these are usually seen only in advanced stages. Other neurologic tests include the use of visual, auditory or somatosensory evoked potentials. Treatment is to look for and treat any underlying precipitating factor. Drug therapy: lactulose should be given to maintain 2–3 soft bowel motions per day. Nonabsorbable antimicrobials such as neomycin may be useful, at least in the short term. There are concerns about oral absorption with consequence risk of deafness. More recently, rifaximin has been found to be effective. Although dietary protein restriction has been advocated it should not be advised because the side effects of poor nutrition outweigh any benefits.

Cardiorespiratory problems

Shortness of breath is not uncommon in patients with cirrhosis and has many causes (Box 21.5). The onset of shortness of breath requires full evaluation.

Conclusions

Patients with ALD require careful monitoring in the clinic. With abstinence, liver function usually improves but those with cirrhosis require ongoing monitoring

Box 21.5 Causes of shortness of breath in patients with cirrhosis.

Complications of cirrhosis
- Hepatopulmonary syndrome
- Portopulmonary syndrome
- Hepatic hydrothorax
- Hepatic cardiomyopathy

Conditions associated with liver disease
- Alcoholic cardiomyopathy
- α1-antitrypsin deficiency
- Fibrosing alveolitis

Conditions unrelated to cirrhosis

to look for complications. These require appropriate interventions.

Further reading

European Association for the Study of the Liver (EASL). EASL clinical practice guidelines on the management of ascites, spontaneous bacterial peritonitis and hepatorenal syndrome in cirrhosis. *J Hepatol* 2010; **53**: 397–417.

Garcia-Tsao G, Sanyal AJ, Grace ND, Carey W. Practice Guidelines Committee of the American Association for the Study of Liver Disease, the Practice Parameters Committee of the American College of Gastroenterology. Prevention and management of gastroesophageal varices and variceal hemorrhage in cirrhosis. *Hepatology* 2007; **46**: 922–938.

Runyon B. Management of adult patients with ascites due to cirrhosis: Update 2012. *Hepatology* 2013; 1–37.

Sherman M, Bruix J, Poryako M, Tran T. AASLD Practice Guidelines Committee. Screening for hepatocellular carcinoma: the rationale for the American Association for the Study of Liver Diseases recommendations. *Hepatology* 2012; **56**: 793–796.

CHAPTER 22

Treatment of alcoholic hepatitis

Mark Thursz and Stephen Atkinson

Department of Medicine, Imperial College London, London, UK

KEY POINTS

- Alcoholic hepatitis (AH) is a clinical syndrome characterized by onset of jaundice less than 3 months in duration in actively drinking patients.

- The need for liver biopsy to diagnose the condition is controversial but with compatible clinical history and biochemistry, and, in the absence of other causes of liver disease, compatible clinical history, and biochemistry, the diagnosis can be often be made without recourse to biopsy.

- Numerous clinical scoring systems attempt to predict outcome in AH. The modified Maddrey's discriminant function (mDF) with a cutoff ≥32 or hepatic encephalopathy at presentation identifies a group of patients with a high risk of death at 1 month with good sensitivity but low specificity. These criteria currently define severe AH.

- Irrespective of severity, treatment of AH involves counseling for and measures to achieve abstinence from alcohol, nutritional assessment and support, management of alcohol withdrawal, and aggressive screening and treatment of infection.

- General measures are adequate therapy in patients with nonsevere disease. Short-term survival in this group is 95–100% with supportive measures. Patients with severe disease have high mortality (approximately 35% at 1 month) and specific treatment is warranted.

- Currently, the choice of specific therapy is between corticosteroids and pentoxifylline. Controversy surrounds their efficacy and relative benefit. Current guidelines advocate consideration of either for patients with severe disease with the ultimate choice guided by consideration of contraindications to steroid use and local policy.

- Liver transplantation for AH has favorable outcomes in highly selected patients with AH refractory to treatment. Wider use of transplantation in this setting requires further study, evaluation of longer term outcomes, and consideration of ethical and resource issues.

Diagnosis of alcoholic hepatitis

AH is a clinical syndrome characterized by the recent onset of jaundice in patients with a history of heavy alcohol misuse. Patients are either actively drinking or only recently abstinent; many cease alcohol consumption because of symptoms arising from the physical illness. Despite the often sudden and florid presentation, the condition represents an exacerbation of underlying chronic liver disease. Around 50–70% of patients presenting with AH also have cirrhosis. Consequently, the term "acute AH" is a misnomer and its use not recommended.

Clinically, patients are recently jaundiced (onset less than 3 months) and may demonstrate other features of hepatic decompensation. AH is considered one of the

---

Alcohol Abuse and Liver Disease, First Edition. Edited by James Neuberger and Andrea DiMartini.
© 2015 John Wiley & Sons, Ltd. Published 2015 by John Wiley & Sons, Ltd.

Box 22.1 Laboratory features of alcoholic hepatitis.

> Leucocytosis
> Raised bilirubin
> Modestly raised transaminases with AST : ALT >2 : 1
> Prolonged prothrombin time
> Other:
> • Raised MCV
> • Raised GGT
> • Raised immunoglobulin (especially IgA)
> • Increased cholesterol and triglycerides
> • Raised serum ferritin

main causes of acute-on-chronic liver failure. Fever, anorexia, and right upper quadrant pain are common. Examination may reveal tender hepatomegaly or a hepatic bruit; signs of chronic liver disease may be present.

Laboratory tests may demonstrate leucocytosis and elevated C-reactive protein levels as the condition is inflammatory (Box 22.1). Serum bilirubin is elevated and the prothrombin time typically prolonged. Liver biochemistry will show only moderate elevations of aspartate and alanine transaminases (AST and ALT) – typically less than 300 IU/mL with an AST : ALT ratio >2 : 1. Levels greater than 500 IU/mL should trigger consideration of an alternative or concomitant diagnosis. Biochemistry may also reveal abnormalities attributable to excess alcohol consumption (e.g. elevated gamma-glutamyl transferase (GGT), raised mean corpuscular volume (MCV), thrombocytopenia) (Figure 22.1) [1,2].

Many experts argue that in cases where patients with a long history (>20 years) of heavy alcohol use (>100 g/day) present with recent onset jaundice (>5 mg/dL or 80 μmol/L), compatible liver biochemistry, and prothrombin time prolongation AH can be diagnosed clinically. Other causes of acute or chronic liver disease (viral hepatitides, veno-occlusive disease, or biliary obstruction) should be excluded. In patients with chronic liver disease, especially if the etiology is not solely alcohol, AH must be distinguished from alternative diagnoses, particularly decompensated cirrhosis. Liver biopsy is usually required for this [3].

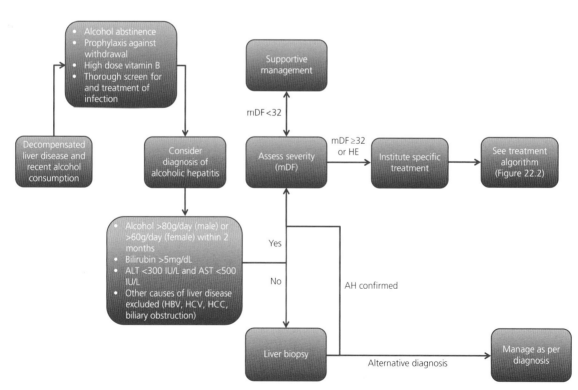

Figure 22.1 Diagnosis and management of alcoholic hepatitis.

Role of liver biopsy

It is important to distinguish between the clinical syndrome of AH and the histologic features of alcoholic steatohepatitis (ASH) – the latter may be present on biopsy without the former. Histologic features of ASH are well established – fatty change, hepatocyte damage (necrosis, ballooning), and neutrophilic infiltrates. Features such as Mallory–Denk bodies, periportal fibrosis, megamitochondria, bile duct proliferation, and canalicular cholestasis may also be present. Despite recognition of these features there is no consensus view as to the minimum combination and quantification of histologic features required to make a diagnosis of ASH.

The role of liver biopsy in the diagnosis and management of AH is controversial. Advocates argue that histologic confirmation is necessary as clinical diagnostic criteria are insufficient. Estimates of the accuracy of clinical criteria in predicting histologic ASH vary widely. Some studies have reported liver biopsy confirmed clinically suspected AH in only half of cases. In contrast, an analysis of 11 trials in severe AH with biopsy-proven disease as an inclusion criteria demonstrated histologic confirmation of the clinical diagnosis in 96% of patients when a minimum threshold for bilirubin of 80 μmol/L (~5 mg/dL) was applied [3].

Ultimately, the decision to perform liver biopsy is dependent upon the comparative risks of biopsy and treatment alongside the probability of an alternative diagnosis and the likelihood that histology will alter management. Practical considerations must also be taken into account. Liver biopsy in this group of patients is often problematic due to coagulopathy and ascites. This necessitates the transjugular approach which is typically not available outside of specialist centers. Delay in obtaining histology may lead to diagnostic inaccuracy. Current guidance from the American Association for the Study of Liver Diseases (AASLD) advocates the use of liver biopsy where there is uncertainty regarding the diagnosis or medical treatment is being considered [1].

Determination of disease severity

Patients with AH demonstrate significant heterogeneity in clinical progress after initial presentation. While some patients recover rapidly following cessation of alcohol intake, others deteriorate, developing complications of liver failure. Accurate prognostication is key to determining when the risk–benefit calculation favors prescription of medications with potentially serious side effects [1]. Most prognostic scores estimate the risk of mortality at 1 month, recognizing that longer term mortality is determined largely by recidivism.

Maddrey's discriminant function

Maddrey's discriminant function was the first prognostic score to be developed in AH. It was derived from attempts to predict patients who would benefit from corticosteroid treatment due to high risk of mortality. The analysis identified serum bilirubin, prothrombin time (PT), and encephalopathy as the main factors discriminating between survivors and nonsurvivors. After modification, the current formula used to calculate the DF is:

$$mDF = 4.6 * \left[PT(patient) - PT(control) \right] + Bilirubin(mg/dL)$$

Prospective studies have demonstrated that when the mDF is ≥32 the risk of mortality from untreated AH at 28 days is 35–50%. Where the mDF does not reach this threshold spontaneous survival rates at 28 days are 90–100%. Using a cutoff of 32, the mDF has a high sensitivity for early mortality (~85%) but specificity is comparatively low (50–60%). Despite this the mDF is the most widely employed scoring system for determining severity in AH and forms the basis for the conventional definition of severe AH when the mDF is ≥32 or there is evidence of encephalopathy [4,5].

Model for end-stage liver disease

Originally described as a means of predicting outcome after transjugular intrahepatic portosystemic shunt placement, use of the model for end-stage liver disease (MELD) scoring system has been extended to prediction of prognosis in cirrhosis and selection for liver transplantation. In addition to measures of hepatic synthetic function (bilirubin, PT), the MELD score also incorporates renal function (creatinine). Studies comparing the performance of the two systems demonstrate similar performance in prediction of mortality. The optimal cutoff point for use of the MELD score to predict mortality in this setting is unclear. The AASLD advocates using a cutoff ≥18 to define severe AH [1].

Table 22.1 Components of the Glasgow Alcoholic Hepatitis score.

Parameter	Score given		
	1	2	3
Age	<50	≥50	–
White cell count (10⁹/L)	<15	≥15	–
Urea (mmol/L)	<5	≥5	–
PT ratio (INR)	<1.5	1.5–2.0	>2.1
Bilirubin (μmol/L)	<125	125–250	>250

INR, international normalized ratio; PT, prothrombin time.

Glasgow AH score

The Glasgow alcoholic hepatitis score (GAHS) was derived form a cohort of patients with symptomatic AH presenting to hospital services in Glasgow and validated in a cohort of patients from Birmingham, London, and Newcastle. Diagnosis was made clinically, patients were included only where the bilirubin exceeded 4.7 mg/dL. Logistic regression analysis identified age, bilirubin, urea, PT, and peripheral white cell count as independently associated with outcome and these parameters were incorporated into a scoring system (Table 22.1). A GAHS above 9 was noted to correspond with a stepwise increment in mortality at 28 and 84 days. Comparison of the GAHS (≥9) with mDF (≥32) demonstrated greater overall accuracy (81% and 49% for 28-day mortality) but higher specificity (89% and 39%, respectively) came at the cost of lower sensitivity (54% and 82%, respectively). The score compared favorably to MELD in its ability to predict 28 and 84-day mortality. Advocates of the score cite its easy calculation, accuracy, and use of the same cutoff to predict 28 and 84-day outcomes as advantages over alternative systems; however, the score has not yet been validated outside of a UK population [4,5].

Age, bilirubin, INR, and creatinine score

The age, bilirubin, international normalized ratio (INR), and creatinine (ABIC) score was proposed following analysis of factors predicting survival at 90 days in a group of patients with biopsy-proven AH. Those with mDF ≥32 were treated with steroids. The final score was derived using the formula:

$$\text{ABIC} = (0.1 \times \text{age, years}) + (0.08 \times \text{bilirubin, mg/dL})$$
$$+ (0.3 \times \text{serum creatinine, mg/dL}) + (0.8 \times \text{INR})$$

Cutoffs were chosen to identify populations at low (cutoff <6.71, 100% 90-day survival), moderate (6.71–8.99, 70%), and high (≥9, 25%) risk of death. Interestingly, the authors of this study found that in their validation cohort the ABIC score remained predictive for mortality at 1 year in contrast to mDF, GAHS, and MELD, which were not.

Histologic scoring

While efforts to derive scoring systems has predominantly focused on the use of clinical parameters, groups have tried to develop schemes based upon histologic features. Perhaps counterintuitively, both a more marked neutrophil infiltrate and the formation of megamitochondria (a feature of intracellular oxidative stress) have been associated with a more favorable outcome in patients with severe AH (mDF ≥32). In contrast, features of bilirubinostasis appear to confer a worse prognosis and increased risk of infection. The relationship between the degree of fibrosis and outcome is unclear. Two studies have examined this and found variously that worsening fibrosis predicts death or failed to demonstrate an association. Two histologic scoring systems have been developed: the AH histologic score (AHHS) and the steatohepatitis score. Both systems appear comparable to each other and clinical scoring systems to predict outcome though only the former has been validated. The AHHS has recently been published and there may be a role for its combination with clinical data and scores either in series or parallel.

Summary

Few conditions boast as wide a range of scoring systems as AH. Additional scoring systems have been developed with the aim of determining response to treatment. We recommend the use of mDF with a cutoff of ≥32 to define severe disease and trigger evaluation for treatment. Additional scoring systems may be used to define the subgroup of patients with severe disease at highest risk of death.

General considerations

Abstinence from alcohol

Abstinence from alcohol is the central tenet of the management of AH and has a significant impact on medium and long-term survival. Consequently, management of the condition requires appropriate detoxification strategies with treatment of withdrawal if this occurs. These topics are discussed in earlier chapters in this book. However, abstinence is insufficient to ensure recovery from liver injury and prevent progression of AH, hence the search for specific treatments.

Management of nutrition and fluid status

Malnutrition and micronutrient deficiencies are common amongst the cohort of patients presenting with AH. Protein-calorie malnutrition is often present and is associated with complications of cirrhosis and adverse outcomes. In a series of patients with severe AH, 100% of 363 patients were assessed as having calorie or combined protein-calorie malnutrition.

Several studies have examined the role of enteral and parenteral nutritional support as a treatment for AH. Many of these studies suffer from small sample size. Overall, studies suggest enteral nutritional supplementation improves liver function. However, a significant impact on short-term survival has not been conclusively proven. One study compared the efficacy of total enteral nutrition (2000 kcal/day) with prednisolone 40 mg/day for 7 days. Results indicated no statistically significant difference in overall mortality but there was a different time-course to the occurrence of deaths between the two groups. Mortality occurred earlier in the enterally fed group while the group treated with prednisolone demonstrated an excess of deaths, mainly attributable to infection, during the 1-year follow-up period. Studies have examined the role of parenteral nutritional supplementation in the management of AH but failed to demonstrate any clear benefit on relevant clinical outcomes [6].

It is recommended patients with AH should have formal nutritional assessment and monitoring of oral intake during their inpatient stay. Replacement of thiamine using high dose, parenteral vitamin B complex is recommended as prophylaxis against Wernicke's encephalopathy. Replacement of lipid-soluble vitamins is also often necessary. Vitamin K deficiency may artificially prolong the PT and parenteral replacement upon admission is advised. Total enteral nutrition should be provided with the use of oral nutritional supplementation as necessary. Dietary protein appears well tolerated in AH. Hepatic encephalopathy, or the risk thereof, does not provide grounds to restrict protein intake and a diet containing 1.5 g protein/kg/day is recommended [2].

Patients with AH often have issues related to fluid status. Development of acute renal failure, typically resulting from acute tubular necrosis or type 1 hepatorenal syndrome, is not uncommon and confers a worse prognosis. Appropriate fluid replacement and management is important as a consequence.

Screening and treatment of infection

The prevalence of infection at presentation in patients with severe AH is high and reported as 25.6% in a study of 246 patients. Studies indicate this may be attributable to defects in cellular immunity. Vigilance is required as the underlying condition gives rise to clinical features of a systemic inflammatory response including fever, leucocytosis, and elevation of biochemical markers of inflammation. Patients admitted with severe AH should undergo comprehensive screening for infection on admission with prompt administration of antibiotics [2].

Specific treatments

AH is characterized by marked inflammation and, in those with adverse outcomes, delayed or absent recompensation of hepatic function. The search for treatments for AH has therefore centered upon compounds with anti-inflammatory or hepatotrophic properties. The two most widely known treatments for AH are corticosteroids and pentoxifylline – their efficacy in the treatment of the condition is the source of intense debate.

Corticosteroids

Steroids are used in a wide range of inflammatory disorders; Porter et al. [7] first conceived their use in AH on this basis in 1971. Since this time there have been many trials of their usage and several meta-analyses. Despite this extensive investigation controversies remain as to the exact role that corticosteroids should have in the management of AH. Early studies were hampered by small sample sizes, variable eligibility criteria, and heterogeneous study populations. It is unsurprising that early meta-analyses based upon such studies failed to demonstrate a survival benefit from the use of steroids in the treatment of AH. The development of mDF permitted some standardization of trials in the field. In 2003, a Cochrane meta-analysis of 15 trials (721 patients) concluded that when all data were combined no statistically significant beneficial effect of steroids

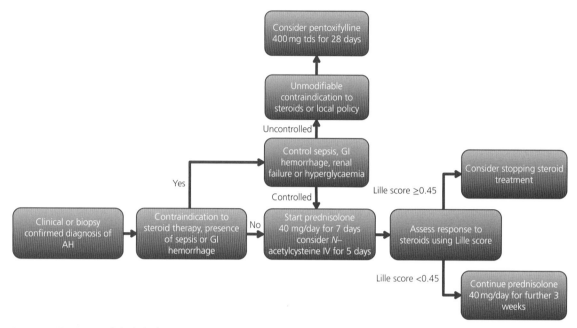

Figure 22.2 Treatment of alcoholic hepatitis.

could be discerned [8]. A subgroup analysis evaluating trials that only included patients with mDF ≥32 or with spontaneous hepatic encephalopathy did show a statistically significant reduction in 28-day mortality in patients treated with corticosteroids. However, there was substantial and significant heterogeneity between the trials and consequently no firm conclusion could be drawn. In an attempt to overcome this limitation a meta-analysis was performed in 2002 using individual patient data from three randomized controlled trials evaluating the use of steroids in AH. Patients included for randomization in these trials with mDF ≥32 or hepatic encephalopathy were retrospectively identified and their data collated for analysis (n = 215). The primary endpoint used was 28-day mortality and a statistically significant survival benefit for steroid treatment was observed (85% and 65%; $p = 0.001$). A further meta-analysis using a similar methodology, but including a further two trials comparing corticosteroids to therapies of unproven benefit (antioxidants and nutrition), produced similar results [9].

In the group of patients with severe disease it seems there is a tendency towards benefit from steroids. On this basis current guidelines recommend consideration of

steroid therapy in patients with mDF ≥32. Steroid usage is potentially associated with adverse physiologic effects including increased susceptibility to infection and gastrointestinal hemorrhage. This has led to efforts to define the groups of patients who will benefit from steroids to minimize steroid exposure in cases where they will be ineffective and, simultaneously, define a population of patients for whom novel treatments are required [1,2].

Assessment and prediction of steroid responsiveness

Initial efforts to design a scheme capable of assessing response to steroids focused on early changes in bilirubin. Mathurin et al. [10] analyzed biochemical data and clinical outcomes from 209 patients with AH and mDF ≥32 treated with steroids. They defined an early change in bilirubin level (ECBL) as a serum bilirubin concentration lower on day 7 than day 1. Survival analysis demonstrated significantly divergent curves – at 6 months 83% of patients who had an ECBL were still alive. In stark contrast only 23% of those without an ECBL survived to 6 months. Further analysis of the data identified age, mDF, and creatinine as further independent prognostic variables.

The Lille model combines age, creatinine, albumin, prothrombin time, bilirubin on day 0 and bilirubin at day 7 using the following equation:

$$\text{Lille score} = 3.19 - 0.101 * (\text{age, years})$$
$$+ 0.147 * (\text{albumin day 1, g/L})$$
$$+ 0.0165 * (\text{day 0 bilirubin}$$
$$- \text{day 7 bilirubin, } \mu mol/L)$$
$$- 0.206 * (\text{renal insufficiency})$$
$$- 0.0065 * (\text{bilirubin day 0 in } \mu mol/L)$$
$$- 0.0096 * (\text{prothrombin time, s})$$

Renal insufficiency was defined as a creatinine >1.3 mg/dL (115 μmol/L) and for the purposes of calculation rated 0 if absent and 1 if present.

The score was initially derived in a cohort of patients with severe AH treated with steroids and validated in a separate group of patients meeting the same criteria. Using an endpoint of mortality at 6 months, receiver operated characteristic (ROC) analysis demonstrated that the area under the curve was 0.85 in the validation group, significantly higher than mDF, MELD, or GAHS. Survival probability at 6 months of patients with a Lille score above 0.45 (nonresponders) is about 25%. In contrast, those with a Lille score below this (responders) have a predicted 6-month survival of 85%. Subsequent work on the score has sought to enhance its value by subdividing patients into complete responders (Lille score ≤0.16), partial responders (0.16–0.56), and null responders (≥0.56). Overall 28-day survival (treated and untreated) differs significantly between the three groups: 91%, 79%, and 53%, respectively. Interestingly, the impact of steroid treatment on 28-day survival appears greatest in those designated complete responders (96% steroid treated and 81% nonsteroid treated; $p = 0.005$) with virtually no impact in those classified as null responders [9].

While the Lille score purports to assess steroid response after 7 days of treatment, proponents of the GAHS argue it is able to predict whether patients will benefit from steroids. An analysis of data from patients with mDF ≥32 suggested that when the GAHS was <9 treatment with steroids had no impact on 28 or 84-day survival. Where the GAHS was ≥9 there was a significant improvement in survival at 28 (78% and 52%; $p = 0.002$) and 84 days (59% and 38%; $p = 0.02$). Analysis of treatment and patient outcomes in the validation

cohort used for the ABIC score found that patients with a high risk of death did not appear to derive a survival benefit from treatment with corticosteroids [4].

It has also been argued that certain histologic features may predict response to steroid treatment. Increasing neutrophil infiltration has been associated with steroid responsiveness though this finding was not replicated in a more recent study looking to develop a histologic scoring system for use in AH.

Steroids for AH – to use or not to use?

The available evidence indicates patients with nonsevere AH (mDF <32, no encephalopathy) do not benefit from treatment with corticosteroids. This is unsurprising given the natural history of mild to moderate disease. Consequently, these patients should receive standard medical care only. Those who demonstrate an improvement in their bilirubin and PT over the course of the first week following presentation will likely recover with abstinence from alcohol and appropriate medical support. Those who deteriorate and reach the criteria for severe disease should have their treatment re-evaluated and be managed in the same manner as those with severe disease at presentation.

In patients with severe AH there is a heterogeneous response to steroids. Prediction of treatment response is, currently, an inexact science. However, assessment of treatment response seems more accurate. International guidelines recommend considering steroid treatment in patients presenting with AH and mDF ≥32 and/or encephalopathy. Current European Association for the Study of the Liver (EASL) guidelines recommend considering steroid treatment in patients with severe AH and potentially discontinuing steroids in those with a poor or null response to steroids (defined as Lille score >0.45 or ≥0.56, respectively) [1]. At present no recommendation can be made to withhold treatment with steroids from patients with severe AH based upon a score generated at presentation. STOPAH (STeroids Or Pentoxifylline for AH) is the largest trial in AH to date with 1103 participants [11]. The trial reported that treatment with steroids was associated with a reduction in 28-day mortality that did not reach statistical significance (odds ratio 0.72, 95% CI 0.51-1.01, p = 0.056). Logistic regression analysis accounting for baseline factors independently associated with 28-day mortality indicated treatment with steroids was associated with a significant reduction in the risk of death at 28 days (OR 0.61, 95% CI 0.41-0.90, p = 0.014). Any benefit from steroid treatment did not persist beyond 28 days.

Unlike many previous trials patients presenting with renal failure, gastrointestinal haemorrhage or infection were recruited to STOPAH. Patients were enrolled once these factors had been judged controlled by the attending physician. No interaction was identified between patients with these presentations, prednisolone treatment and mortality. STOPAH confirmed that as long as a prompt and aggressive policy of screening and treating infection at presentation is followed steroids can be given without negatively impacting survival. However STOPAH data did indicate that treatment with prednisolone did confer an increased risk of developing a new infective episode (13.5% and 7.9% in groups treated with or without prednisolone respectively).

The data from STOPAH indicate no overall clinical benefit from treatment with prednisolone on short-term mortality. However post-hoc analysis indicates a subset of patients are likely to derive benefit from steroid treatment. An excess of subsequent infective episodes in the prednisolone treated group emphasise the importance of considering discontinuing treatment in non-responders, as previously discussed, and raise questions regarding whether the 4 week treatment course is too long. We recommend that patients with severe AH should receive steroid treatment in accordance with the algorithm outlined in Figure 22.2.

Pentoxifylline

Pentoxifylline is a competitive nonselective phosphodiesterase inhibitor with a weak anti-TNF effect. The latter action led to suggestions that it might be efficacious in the treatment of AH. Its potential use was attractive because of concerns of infection and gastrointestinal hemorrhage with steroid therapy.

Following an initial pilot study Akriviadis et al. [12] undertook a randomized, double-blind, placebo-controlled trial in 101 patients with severe AH (mDF ≥32 or encephalopathy). They described reduced mortality in the pentoxifylline treated group (24.5% and 46.1%; *p* = 0.037), making particular mention of a decrease in mortality associated with development of hepatorenal syndrome in the treated arm. A similar study in patients with decompensated cirrhosis (Child–Pugh C) failed to demonstrate any

impact on survival but did demonstrate a reduction in complications associated with cirrhosis including hepatorenal syndrome. The authors performed a subgroup analysis on the patients with AH at enrolment and found no significant impact of pentoxifylline upon survival. Smaller trials have demonstrated a tendency towards improved short-term survival in patients with severe AH treated with pentoxifylline but have failed to reach statistical significance.

A Cochrane meta-analysis was performed using data from 336 patients enrolled in five trials [13]. Although initial analysis indicated pentoxifylline improved short-term mortality and reduced the risk of hepatorenal syndrome this was not supported by subsequent analysis designed to account for multiple testing on accumulating data. Subsequent trials have sought to compare pentoxifylline with corticosteroids or determine whether there is incremental benefit when the two are combined.

A systematic review was published in 2013 aiming to answer questions relating to the role of pentoxifylline in the treatment of severe AH. The data were drawn from 10 trials and covered 884 participants. It concluded that, compared with placebo, pentoxifylline significantly reduced the risk of fatal hepatorenal syndrome but no significant evidence existed to support its superiority over steroids or an advantage to combined treatment [14].

Pentoxifylline does not appear to be an effective rescue therapy in steroid nonresponders. Conclusive evidence that pentoxifylline is an effective treatment for severe AH is lacking. Given its relatively favorable side effect profile it is often deployed where there are clinical concerns regarding the administration of steroids. Currently published guidelines support the use of pentoxifylline in the treatment of severe AH and advise using clinical features such as severe sepsis, active gastrointestinal bleeding, or the presence of early renal failure, in combination with local guidelines, to determine whether this agent is chosen in preference to steroids [1,2]. Data from STOPAH [11] demonstrated no clinical benefit from treatment with pentoxifylline, on this basis its use for the treatment of severe AH, certainly as an alternative to steroids, is difficult to justify.

Antitumor necrosis factor biologic therapies

Observations that pentoxifylline appeared to confer some benefit when used in the treatment of severe AH and increasing evidence for tumor necrosis factor (TNF) in the pathogenesis of liver injury in severe AH led to trials of anti-TNFα biologics. An initial evaluation of the safety of combining infliximab with steroid treatment demonstrated, in a small number of patients, no excess of adverse events and a significant improvement in mDF over 28 days in the treated group. Significantly, an upper limit of 55 was applied to the mDF. This, combined with a more aggressive dosing regimen, may explain why a subsequent trial using infliximab in combination with steroids, which did not apply an upper limit to the mDF, had to be terminated prematurely. Interim data analysis demonstrated an excess of infections (72% and 17%; $p = 0.002$) and infection related deaths (39% and 18%, not statistically significant) in the infliximab treated arm.

Etanercept, another anti-TNF agent, has also been trialled in severe AH. Unlike infliximab it has been trialled without concomitant steroids. Despite this, results from a trial in 48 patients with moderate to severe AH (MELD ≥15) still demonstrated an excess of both infection-related serious adverse events and 6-month mortality in the treated group.

The available evidence suggests anti-TNF therapy results in excessive immunosuppression in a group of patients already vulnerable to infection. This leads to unacceptable risks of serious infection and detrimentally impacts mortality and morbidity. Mechanistic studies examining hepatic regeneration also indicate that TNF-α is important in this process and may provide further reasons to view its inhibition in this clinical context as undesirable. The use of anti-TNFα agents in severe AH cannot be recommended and it seems unlikely that further evaluation of this class of drugs will be undertaken or, indeed, would be appropriate [1,2].

Insulin and glucagon

A significant proportion of patients with severe AH exhibit a clinical course of their illness over which there is either delayed or absent recompensation of hepatic function. During this time they remain vulnerable to infection and development of complications of liver failure. These clinical observations led to trials of agents with hepatotrophic effects in attempts to find therapy to promote hepatic regeneration.

Insulin and glucagon are the two hepatotrophic agents most extensively studied and their use has been trialled in four separate studies between the early 1980s and 1990s. Initial investigations suggested more rapid improvement in liver biochemical parameters and an improvement in short-term mortality in patients treated with insulin and glucagon when compared with patients receiving a placebo infusion of 5% dextrose. Subsequent studies in slightly larger cohorts of patients failed to show any demonstrable clinical benefit to insulin and glucagon therapy. Hypoglycemic adverse events were described in treated groups. The available evidence does not support a role for insulin and glucagon therapy in the management of severe AH.

Anabolic steroids

Observations of protein-energy malnutrition and catabolism in patients with AH led to trials of anabolic steroids, both alone and in combination with steroids and/or nutritional supplementation. Initial observations were mixed but a randomized controlled trial carried out by the Veterans Affairs cooperative in 263 patients with AH appeared to demonstrate that oxandrolone improved long-term survival. Significantly, the trial included patients with moderate and severe disease and failed to show any benefit from prednisolone therapy. A further study with a total of four arms took patients with AH (Child–Pugh B, n = 11; Child–Pugh C, n = 28) and compared the efficacy of oxandrolone alone and in combination with nutritional therapy with no treatment and nutritional therapy alone. Nutritional therapy consisted of intermittent infusions of crystalline amino acids. Groups treated with oxandrolone or nutritional therapy showed greater improvements in galactose and antipyrine metabolism (used as markers of hepatic function) but no significant changes in relevant clinical endpoints. Subsequently, the Veterans Affairs group carried out a further trial using oxandralone and nutritional supplementation. Their results indicated a survival benefit from oxandralone therapy in those with moderate protein-energy malnutrition which was greatest in those receiving adequate calorific intake. Any benefit from oxandralone therapy appeared to be abrogated by inadequate calorie consumption or severe protein-energy malnutrition.

Testosterone replacement has also been evaluated as a treatment for alcoholic liver disease – primarily in the context of cirrhosis but these trials also included a proportion of patients with AH. None demonstrated any significant impact on clinically relevant endpoints. These findings were upheld by a Cochrane analysis of the available data relating to the treatment of alcoholic liver disease with androgenic anabolic steroids. The analysis concluded that no benefit from the treatment of alcoholic liver disease with anabolic steroids could be discerned, including the subgroup of patients with AH. The weight of evidence indicates that anabolic steroids are ineffective in the treatment of AH and their use cannot be recommended.

N-acetylcysteine and antioxidants

The generation of reactive oxygen species and consequent oxidative stress have been identified as prominent features of alcohol-induced steatohepatitis and have been consistently implicated in the pathogenesis of AH. Disruption of metabolic pathways known to have a role in mitigating the damage caused by reactive oxygen species is also a feature and provided further justification for trials of antioxidants in the treatment of AH.

A study investigating the efficacy of vitamin E together with selenium and zinc appeared to show a significant 1-month survival benefit to antioxidant treatment. Conversely, a subsequent trial using vitamin E alone failed to show any effect on short-term mortality. Groups have sought to maximize the potential of antioxidant therapy through the simultaneous combination of multiple agents. A "cocktail" of antioxidants including N-acetylcysteine (alongside β-carotene, vitamins C and E, selenium, methionine, allopurinol, and desferrioxamine) compared unfavorably to corticosteroids in a randomized trial. A statistically significant excess of deaths was noted in the antioxidant treated group (46% and 30% at 1 month; $p = 0.05$). A subsequent study attempted to determine whether antioxidants offered a survival advantage when combined with steroids or in patients in whom steroids were contraindicated – none was found. Both trials have been criticized however – the former because of its inclusion of patients with non-severe disease and the latter because of stratification of patients prior to randomization, a lack of clarity regarding the contraindications to steroids, and pooling of study groups for analysis.

A French group sought to determine whether any benefit could be derived from the addition of N-acetylcysteine alone (5 days of therapy) to corticosteroids in the treatment of severe AH. Their study enrolled a total of 174 patients and examined mortality at 1, 3, and 6 months. Analysis demonstrated a significant decrease in mortality at 1 month in the N-acetylcysteine treated group (8% and 24%). N-acetylcysteine treatment was also accompanied by a reduction in infective complications and deaths from hepatorenal failure. The mortality benefit observed was not sustained at 3 or 6 months and, in multivariate analysis, treatment with N-acetylcysteine was not associated with 6-month survival.

Routine use of antioxidant therapies is not recommended based upon the available evidence. A possible synergy exists between N-acetylcysteine and corticosteroid therapy; however, independent confirmation of effect is required before its use can be recommended [2].

Other agents

A number of other treatments have been trialled at some point in the treatment of AH: calcium channel blockers, propylthiouracil, colchicine, milk thistle (silamarin), and penicillamine. A number of these agents showed promise as therapy for alcoholic cirrhosis, though none has become accepted therapy. Their evaluation in AH has failed to yield any positive findings [1,2].

Liver transplantation

Liver transplantation is an accepted and effective treatment in patients with decompensated cirrhosis resulting from alcohol. Until recently liver transplantation was not countenanced in actively drinking patients making AH an automatic contraindication. Much of the reluctance to transplant individuals who have not yet demonstrated their ability to abstain from alcohol stems from concerns regarding recidivist drinking. A period of 6 months' abstinence is usually quoted; however, this is not universal and the evidence upon which it is based is controversial. The studies cited to support it are small and plagued by the difficulty of obtaining accurate information regarding drinking habits. Other concerns that are raised include the fact that a proportion of patients will recover without the need for transplantation and that the condition of AH itself may predispose to poorer outcomes [15].

In light of the dismal prognosis in patients who unresponsive to steroids (30% survival at 6 months), a group of European hepatologists proposed automatic denial of liver transplantation to these patients was unethical and warranted an assessment of feasibility and outcomes. They successfully negotiated to undertake a limited number of liver transplants in carefully selected patients with severe AH refractory to steroid treatment (Lille score >0.45). Those put forward for early liver transplantation had their current illness as their first presentation of liver disease, underwent careful psychiatric and psychologic evaluation, had a supportive family, and agreed to lifelong abstinence from alcohol [16].

The study reported 6-month survival of 77% in transplanted patients compared with 24% in a set of matched controls (90% of deaths in the control group occurred within 2 months). Liver transplantation conferred a prognosis approximating that of patients responding to steroid treatment. Significantly, 3 of 26 patients transplanted had returned to drinking at the time of publication. Relapses occurred late (720–1140 days post-transplantation) and despite aggressive support none of the patients achieved abstinence again. These data were supported by a subsequent study by the United Network of Organ Sharing (UNOS). Patients transplanted for alcoholic liver disease whose explants demonstrated a histological diagnosis of ASH had comparable outcomes to those with decompensated cirrhosis.

These studies present challenges to the widely held belief, and often-stated policy, that AH is an absolute contraindication to liver transplantation. Long-term follow-up data are lacking; however, adequate data exist to support further evaluation.

Widespread adoption of a transplantation policy as laid out in the French study would add to the demand for donor organs, which are already in short supply. During the study period transplants undertaken for AH accounted for approximately 3% of all operations at the seven centers involved. Before this can happen, however, a frank debate involving the public and policymakers will be required – hepatologists will have a key role in leading and informing discussion [17].

Future therapeutic directions

While current treatment options are somewhat limited, a number of promising therapeutic strategies are in development particularly in the group of individuals with apparent steroid-resistance and a very poor prognosis.

A strategy that has been adopted is to attempt to overcome steroid resistance through the use of "sensitization treatments." Using *ex vivo* assays on mononuclear cells isolated from peripheral blood (PBMCs), a group of researchers in Newcastle demonstrated greater resistance to steroids in lymphocytes from patients with AH compared with controls which could be reversed by theophylline. Steroid resistance appeared greater in those "resistant" to steroids clinically and seemed to decrease with resolution of AH in survivors. As yet no clinical trials have been undertaken to investigate the potential role for theophylline in patients with AH not responding to steroids but further exploration is warranted. A similar study has used the IL-2 receptor blocker basiliximab (anti-CD-25) to successfully reverse *in vitro* steroid resistance in steroid nonresponders.

Previously documented experiences with anti-TNF therapy have not prevented further consideration of manipulation of pro- and anti-inflammatory cytokine pathways. The NIH has recently granted funding to a trial seeking to explore the use of an IL-1 receptor antagonist (anakinra) in the treatment of moderate and severe AH. IL-22 is a member of the IL-10 superfamily of cytokines and has a number of actions including anti-inflammatory, antimicrobial, and antisteatotic actions in addition to proproliferative and antiapoptotic functions. Its expression on only epithelial cells such as hepatocytes makes it a tempting molecular target in the treatment of AH. IL-22 treatment in animal models has shown promising results. Recent data (albeit in a limited number of patients simultaneously treated with pentoxifylline) suggest that those patients who deteriorated had lower numbers of circulating IL-22 producing T cells. IL-22 seems a promising molecular target and clinical studies should be considered.

Further molecular targets that may be suitable for manipulation in AH include IL-8 (reduce neutrophil recruitment without affecting function), IL-10 (anti-inflammatory), hepatocyte growth factor (to augment regenerative responses), anti-IL-17A (reduce recruitment and activation of pro-inflammatory Th17 T cells), and bile acids (modify inflammatory and regenerative responses). The data relating to steroid resistance and initial trials of IL-8 inhibition suggest that manipulation of a single aspect of the inflammatory response may be ineffective and combination therapies required [18].

References

[1] O'Shea RS, Dasarathy S, McCullough AJ, Practice Guideline Committee of the American Association for the Study of Liver Diseases and the Practice Parameters Committee of

the American College of Gastroenterology. AASLD Practice Guideline – Alcoholic Liver Disease. *Hepatology* 2010; **51**(1): 307–328.

[2] European Association for Study of the Liver (EASL). EASL Clinical Practical Guidelines – Management of Alcoholic Liver Disease. *J Hepatol* 2012; **57**(2): 399–420.

[3] Dhanda AD, Collins PL, McCune CA. Is liver biopsy necessary in the management of alcoholic hepatitis? *World J Gastroenterol* 2013; **19**(44): 7825–7829.

[4] Lafferty H, Stanley AJ, Forrest EH. The management of alcoholic hepatitis: a prospective comparison of scoring systems. *Aliment Pharmacol Ther* 2013; **38**(6): 603–610.

[5] Mathurin P, Lucey MR. Management of alcoholic hepatitis. *J Hepatol* 2012; **56**(Suppl 1): S39–S45.

[6] Stickel F, Hoehn B, Schuppan D, Seitz HK. Nutritional therapy in alcoholic liver disease. *Aliment Pharmacol Ther* 2003; **18**(4): 357–373.

[7] Porter HP, Simon FR, Pope CE, Volwiler W, Fenster LF. Corticosteroid therapy in severe alcoholic hepatitis. A double-blind drug trial. *New England Journal of Medicine* 1971; **284**(24):1350–1355.

[8] Rambaldi A, Saconato HH, Christensen E, Thorlund K, Wettersley J, Gluud C. Systematic review: glucocorticoids for alcoholic hepatitis: a Cochrane hepato-biliary systematic review with meta-analyses and trial sequential analyses of randomized clinical trials. *Aliment Pharmacol Ther* 2008; **27**(12): 1167–1178.

[9] Mathurin P, O'Grady J, Carithers RL, et al. Corticosteroids improve short-term survival in patients with severe alcoholic hepatitis: meta-analysis of individual patient data. *Gut* 2011; **60**(2): 255–260.

[10] Mathurin P, Abdelnour M, Ramond MJ, et al. Early change in bilirubin levels is an important prognostic factor in severe alcoholic hepatitis treated with prednisolone. *Hepatology* 2003; **38**(6):1363–1369.

[11] Thursz MR, Richardson P, Allison M, et al. Steroids or pentoxifylline for severe alcoholic hepatitis. *New England Journal of Medicine* 2015 (in publication).

[12] Akriviadis E, Botla R, Briggs W, Han S, Reynolds T, Shakil O. Pentoxifylline improves short-term survival in severe acute alcoholic hepatitis: a double-blind, placebo-controlled trial. *Gastroenterology* 2000; **119**(6): 1637–1648.

[13] Whitfield K, Rambaldi A, Wettersley J, Gluud C. Pentoxifylline for alcoholic hepatitis. *Cochrane Database Syst Rev* 2009; **7**(4): CD007339.

[14] Parker R, Armstrong MJ, Corbett C, Rowe IA, Houlihan DD. Systematic review: pentoxifylline for the treatment of severe alcoholic hepatitis. *Aliment Pharmacol Ther* 2013; **37**(9): 845–854.

[15] Dureja P, Lucey MR. The place of transplantation in the treatment of severe alcoholic hepatitis. *J Hepatol* 2010; **52**(5): 759–764.

[16] Mathurin P, Moreno C, Samuel D, et al. Early liver transplantation for severe alcoholic hepatitis. *N Engl J Med* 2011; **365**(19): 1790–1800.

[17] Burrough AK. Liver transplantation for severe alcoholic hepatitis saves lives. *J Hepatol* 2012; **57**(2): 451–452.

[18] Gao B, Bataller R. Alcoholic liver disease: pathogenesis and new therapeutic targets. *Gastroenterology* 2011; **141**(5): 1572–1585.

CHAPTER 23

Liver transplantation in people with alcohol-related liver disease

Santiago Tomé[1] and Michael R. Lucey[2]

[1] *Hepatology Unit, Internal Medicine Department, Hospital Universitario de Santiago de Compostela, Santiago de Compostela, Spain*
[2] *Department of Medicine, Division of Gastroenterology and Hepatology, University of Wisconsin School of Medicine and Public Health, Madison, WI, USA*

KEY POINTS

- Alcoholic liver disease (ALD) is a major indication for liver transplantation accounting in some series for up to 30% cases yet the use of deceased donor organs is not always supported by the public.

- Outcomes after liver transplantation for ALD are at least as good as for other indications although there is a greater risk of *de novo* malignancy.

- Pretransplant assessment by a multidisciplinary team is essential to identify those patients who will remain abstinent and how the team can support abstinence.

- There is little evidence that supports a fixed 6-month period of abstinence.

- Patients should be abstinent before and after transplant.

- Up to 15% patients will return to heavy alcohol consumption after transplantation and graft loss can occur.

- The role of liver replacement in those who present for the first time with alcoholic hepatitis is controversial yet good outcomes can be achieved in highly selected cases.

Introduction

Alcohol liver disease (ALD) is a major cause of end-stage liver cirrhosis and consequently a leading indication for liver transplantation. According with the latest data reported dealing with the global burden of alcoholic liver diseases, liver cirrhosis was responsible for 1,030,800 deaths annually worldwide [1]. From those deaths, 493,300 were related to alcoholic cirrhosis (47% of all cirrhosis deaths). In addition, liver cancer attributable to alcohol consumption was responsible of 80,600 deaths during the same period.

The frequency of liver transplantation for ALD mirrors the global impact of ALD, albeit with much lower absolute numbers. The two largest registries of liver transplant recipients (European Liver Transplantation Registry and the Scientific Registry of Transplant Recipients; see www.eltr.org and SRTR.org) indicate that ALD, either alone or in combination with hepatitis C virus (HCV) infection, was the most common indication for liver transplantation in Europe and the United States during the period 1988–2012. These data are in contrast to the prediction made in 1984 that not many patients with ALD would be chosen for liver transplantation. Indeed, the provision of liver transplantation for patients with a history of alcohol addiction continues to be controversial both among the general public and within the medical profession. In this chapter we review the

---

Alcohol Abuse and Liver Disease, First Edition. Edited by James Neuberger and Andrea DiMartini.
© 2015 John Wiley & Sons, Ltd. Published 2015 by John Wiley & Sons, Ltd.

process of assessing a patient who drinks in excess for liver transplantation. We address specific topics, such as the place of liver transplantation in the treatment of patients with severe alcoholic hepatitis, how to respond when a patient relapses either while awaiting or after transplantation, and we review the clinical outcomes after liver transplantation.

Spectrum of alcoholic liver disease

The spectrum of liver damage caused by alcohol is not uniform. For descriptive purposes, three main histologic stages are described as if they constitute separate and definitive lesions: steatosis, alcoholic hepatitis, and cirrhosis. In reality, these entities overlap, and it is difficult to find them isolated in their pure histopathologic form. Steatosis is a predictable histologic abnormality which develops in many heavy drinkers. It results from the redox imbalance generated by the metabolism of ethanol to acetate. Alcoholic steatosis completely reverses within several weeks of discontinuation of alcohol intake [2]. Alcoholic hepatitis is characterized by hepatocellular injury with associated inflammation and fibrosis. Like steatosis, alcoholic hepatitis usually improves with abstinence. When alcohol use continues unabated, inflammation triggers fibrogenesis and, over time, collagen is deposited in a characteristic perivenular and pericellular distribution. Approximately 40% of patients with this lesion (zone 3 fibrosis extending in a lattice-like perihepatocyte network) will develop cirrhosis within 5 years.

Importance of abstinence in recovery from ALD

The prognosis of ALD is strikingly related to abstinence. The deterioration in patients with ALD, manifesting as sepsis, bleeding for varices, ascites or hepatorenal syndrome, is often related to recent alcohol consumption. The 5-year survival of patients with clinically compensated alcoholic cirrhosis is about 90%, but declines to 70% if the patient continues to drink. When a patient with decompensated cirrhosis continues drinking, the chance of living 5 years is 30% at best. Additionally, abstinence has an important role in the reversibility of steatosis, alcoholic hepatitis, lipid peroxidation, inflammation, and

collagen deposition. In practice, understanding the addiction is the key to understanding the continuum from alcoholic fatty liver to alcoholic cirrhosis. Furthermore, abstinence leads to resolution of alcoholic fatty liver and alcoholic hepatitis, and, as shown by the classic studies of Powell and Klatskin [2], is associated with improved survival in alcoholic cirrhotic patients with decompensated liver function. Consequently, abstinence from alcohol is a cornerstone of the many different approaches to therapy.

A justification of the required abstinence period (usually 6 months) before liver transplantation has been to allow patients with severe alcoholic hepatitis and decompensated ALD the opportunity to recover with medical management. Unfortunately, rigid application of this abstinence period will also force some patients who would have a low risk of alcohol relapse to wait unnecessarily. For some of them this delay could be hazardous. Well-designed studies of alcoholic patients with long-term follow-up have shown that the rate of return to ever drinking is high among patients who had entered in transplantation with abstinence greater than 6 months, and return to hazardous drinking, referred to as a relapse, occurs in about 20% of this highly selected cohort. Yates et al. have reported through a mathematical model that strict application of the 6-month rule would exclude many alcoholic patients who are in need of transplantation but who are at no greater risk of relapse (see review in [3]).

Referral of the patient with ALD for liver transplantation

Once the alcoholic patient with liver disease has been admitted into an ongoing program of care, the medical professionals must then assess whether and when the patient should be referred to a transplant center. This assessment is not easy. It is complicated by the protean behavior of ALD in which the potential for recovery with maintenance of abstinence from alcohol is counteracted by the frequency of relapse to alcohol use which is the natural history of alcohol addiction.

Alcoholic patients at transplant centers form a highly selected sample. Indeed, we are uncertain of the true denominator of suitable candidates with ALD. For example, Davies et al. [4] retrospectively surveyed patients with liver diagnoses in a community hospital in

South Wales and found many patients who were not referred to a regional transplant center whom they would have considered suitable transplant candidates. ALD was most prevalent diagnosis among the group left to die or recover without a transplant referral. There appear to be societal prejudices against offering liver transplantation to patients with ALD. An opinion survey in the United Kingdom comprising members of the lay public, family medicine practitioners, and hospital-based specialists tested such preferences by asking respondents to allocate four donor livers among eight clinical scenarios. The authors found that both the lay public and the general practitioners placed a low priority on alcoholic candidates, even when the outcome after transplantation for the alternative patients was less favorable than that for the alcoholics [5]. More recently, Julapalli et al. (reviewed in [3]) retrospectively reviewed 199 ALD patients at a Veterans Affairs' hospital who met American Association for the Study of Liver Diseases (AASLD) guidelines for liver transplantation, and found that liver transplantation was recorded as having been discussed with the patient in only 59 (20%) of the 300 meetings with a health provider. Older age, ALD, and African American ethnicity were independently associated with an absence of any reference to liver transplantation. These data point out that the process of selection starts before the patient is considered by a transplant center.

However, the selection process may be more complex than simply one of lack of access to referral, or refusal of community physicians to send alcoholic patients to transplant centers. We should also consider the impact of the addictive state on the potential candidate. Weinrieb et al. found that ALD subjects with end-stage liver disease under consideration for liver transplantation had a different pattern of drinking than alcoholics without liver disease: few of the ALD cirrhosis patients admitted any recent alcohol use, or craving for alcohol. Weinrieb et al. speculated that the selection process had identified a cohort of alcoholics who had successfully eliminated their additive behavior. An additional explanation would be that the pattern of addiction that most facilitates the development of cirrhosis is one where the drinker does not experience withdrawal symptoms during intervals of abstinence. This pathophysiologic pattern would tend to keep the alcoholic away from medical attention until features of liver failure ensue, and may explain some of the differences described by Weinrieb et al. (reviewed by [6]).

Timing for liver transplantation and the concept of survival benefit

According with the guidelines of both the AASLD and the European Association for the Study of the Liver (EASL), patients should be referred for liver transplantation evaluation as soon as they develop evidence of hepatic dysfunction: Child–Turcotte–Pugh score more than 7 points and the model for end-stage liver disease (MELD) score more than 10 or when they develop their first major complication such as ascites, variceal bleeding, or hepatic encephalopathy. The first two criteria may appear too lenient, and should probably be when the MELD score is at least 15.

The ideal time for transplantation of patients with ALD is based on a balance of outcome from medical management compared with the outcome of liver transplantation. The minimal criteria designed in 1997 for use in the United States only required candidate patients to be in Child–Pugh Class B to order to be placed on the list. Poynard et al. (reviewed in [3]) have studied the efficacy of liver transplantation for alcoholic cirrhosis using matched and simulated controls. There was a significant benefit among patients with advanced cirrhosis (Child Class C; 11–15 points on the Child–Pugh scoring system) only. In patients with medium risk (Class B; 8–10 in the Child–Pugh score) there was no significant survival difference in comparison with controls. Poynard et al.'s data would suggest that liver transplantation should be confined to patients with advanced alcoholic liver failure.

Survival benefit considers outcome of transplantation by "starting the clock" at the time of placement on the waiting list, and encompasses events in the pretransplant waiting list time interval, the peritransplant, and post-transplant long-term follow-up. A retrospective review reported by Lucey et al. [6] of the United Network for Organ Sharing (UNOS) database showed that a favorable survival benefit for patients with ALD was first observed at the fairly low MELD score of 12–15. Despite this, in the United States, the adoption of regional sharing has made it all but impossible to transplant at these levels, other than with a live donor.

A benefit of a required interval of abstinence prior to liver transplantation is that it allows some patients to recover and avoid the need for transplantation. It is an as yet unanswered question as to how long this interval should be. Veldt et al. have shown that failure to recover from decompenstated ALD within 3 months of initiation of abstinence from alcohol carries a poor prognosis for spontaneous recovery. Likewise, those with alcoholic hepatitis without improvement after 7 days of corticosteroid therapy will be at risk of death if liver transplantation is not performed [3]. In light of the recently introduced donor organ sharing arrangements in the United States (colloquially known as "share 35"), it is very unlikely that patients with MELD scores less than 20, or even less than 30, will be offered a deceased donor liver. This leads to the paradoxical situation that the system will favor patients with severe alcoholic hepatitis, because they frequently have kidney and liver failure and high MELD scores, but will disadvantage abstinent ALD patients with MELD scores of 15–25, in whom the survival benefit is considerable.

Contrasting perspectives of addiction and transplant medicine

Addiction medicine specialists consider alcoholism to be a chronic disorder of remission and relapse, in which abstinence should be considered in quantitative terms and not as a categorical variable (yes/no). This point of view is well described by Fuller: "in alcoholism, as in diabetes a substantial partial response is better than no response" in other words, euglycemia 80% of time is better than euglycemia 20% of time (reviewed in [7]). In this formulation of alcohol use disorder, addiction specialists distinguish between a slip and a relapse. A slip is a temporary return to drinking, which is recognized by the patient as potentially harmful, and leads to renewed efforts toward abstinence. A relapse suggests a more sustained resumption of drinking. These events are sometimes characterized as "harmful," "abusive," or "addictive drinking," whereas the term "recidivism" is abjured on account of its pejorative connotations. In contrast, most transplant programs have adopted, at least in part, an absolutist view of drinking by alcoholics and characterize any drinking as a relapse. This mirrors the practices of insurance companies and third party payers who require a fixed period of abstinence for approval of transplantation. In contrast, in place of a fixed interval of sobriety to predict future abstinence, Beresford proposed that patients should be assessed by an expert in addiction medicine. He codified an overlapping patchwork of clinical features associated with

establishing sobriety: the patient´s acknowledgement of their problem with addiction, social support (particularly a spouse or life companion), paid employment, a home and four indicators of social integration: activities to replace drinking in the patient´s daily life, the support of a rehabilitation relationship, a source of improved self-esteem or of hope for the future, and the acknowledgement by the patient of negative consequences of returning to drinking. Beresford [8] highlighted the idea that there is no one ideal prognostic factor, "the range among the various factors is too wide to justify using any one as a strict inclusion or exclusion criteria."

Treatment of addiction is directed at establishing and maintaining abstinence from the addictive behavior. Although continuing drinking that is less frequent or of reduced amounts is less than ideal, it is better than continuing harmful drinking. In contrast, in the world of transplant hepatology, absolute abstinence is considered the only acceptable outcome, and any slip is judged to be a treatment failure. Many addiction specialists think that this is an unreasonable and unrealistic standard. Furthermore, some specialists believe that this preoccupation with complete abstinence works against the best interests of the alcoholic patient with liver failure, because the patient may be frightened to seek help when he or she experiences a slip. Recent long-term follow-up data suggest that relapse to harmful drinking affects the integrity of the allograft and survival after transplantation, whereas a slip alone does not, further emphasizing the importance of this clinical distinction.

How should abstinence be assessed and maintained?

The assessment of abstinence includes current drinking status and the likelihood to being abstinent before and after liver transplantation. Current drinking status relies on the patient's history and the corroboration of family. In this, there is an inherent risk of under-reporting, not least for fear of jeopardizing the opportunity for transplantation. The utility of biomarkers of alcohol use such as ethyl glucuronide, ethyl sulfate, and phosphatidyl ethanol has not been clearly established. There is no consensus among transplant professionals in North America or Europe on the appropriate response to discovered drinking. We would advocate a flexible approach which distinguishes between "slips" and "relapses" in those patients who have a history of chronic alcohol use and have resumed drinking before or after liver transplantation (see discussion in Contrasting perspectives of addiction and transplant medicine section).

Regarding predicting future drinking, prospective and retrospective studies have shown that 6 months' abstinence is a weak marker of drinking prognosis. Despite of this, the 6-month abstinence period has been incorporated into the routine assessment of alcohol candidates not only in the United States, but also in Europe. Addiction specialists have proposed that several social factors are associated with future sobriety. We advocate that the transplant team incorporates the addiction specialist into the team and that their report is an important part of the assessment of the alcoholic candidate.

Outcome of liver transplantation in patients with ALD

A recent analysis of the UNOS database (n = 38 899) with a median follow-up of 1.8 years compared transplant recipients with ALD with those patients with HCV infection. The presence of ALD did not influence mortality whereas survival after liver transplantation in patients with HCV infection was lower than in those patients without HCV. The European Transplant database has shown survival rates of 84%, 78%, 73%, and 58% at 1, 3, 5, and 10 years, respectively [9]. Similar figures have been shown from the UNOS database (www.unos.org). While there is no difference in post-transplantation survival between patients transplanted for ALD and those who were transplanted for other indications, these data are limited by inadequate information of drinking practices after liver transplantation. There is emerging evidence that patients who have drinking relapses have reduced survival, more progressive liver injury, and episodes of alcoholic hepatitis. Cuadrado et al. have found the 5-year survival rate to be similar between relapsers and nonrelapsers (92.9% and 92.4%, respectively) but, after 10 years, the survival rate decreased significantly in the relapse patients (45.1% and 85.5%; reviewed in [3]).

The cause of death among ALD liver transplant recipients is over-represented with cancers of the aerodigestive tract. This is most likely a consequence of the prevalence of cigarette smoking among ALD patients who receive a liver transplant. DiMartini et al. have

shown that ALD liver transplant recipients tend to resume smoking at high consumption rates soon after transplantation.

Relapse to alcohol use before or after liver transplantation

Despite the selection policies described, it is unequivocal that ALD patients return to alcohol use both before and after liver transplantation. Studies of pretransplant patients with ALD show a return to some alcohol use in approximately 25%. These data are confounded by the difficulty of obtaining accurate data when it is not in the best interest of the patient to admit drinking, and by the failure of some studies to distinguish between slips and relapses. After liver transplantation the use of alcohol ranges 8–22% for the first post-transplant year with cumulative rates reaching 30–50% by 5 years following transplantation. An analysis of a prospective, longitudinal cohort of patients who underwent transplantation for ALD by DiMartini et al. analyzed patterns of alcohol use after transplantation (Figure 23.1). Approximately 80% of the cohort either did not drink or consumed only small amounts occasionally. Conversely, among the remaining patients (approximately 20%), there were three patterns of harmful drinking. The patterns varied according to the time to relapse and whether the patients demonstrated sustained heavy use or subsequently modified drinking [10]. Similar results were found at the British single center cohort where 16% of patients had shown harmful drinking (reviewed in [3]). Patients reassuming alcohol intake after liver transplantation are at risk of developing medical problems often seen in the nontransplant setting such as pancreatitis, alcohol hepatitis, infections, and neurologic consequences of alcohol abuse. Patients who relapse (resume harmful drinking) have more rapid progression of liver fibrosis, and after 10 years show reduced survival. In addition, patients having relapses are more likely not to adhere to taking immunosuppression.

Specific work-up for ALD candidate

Alcoholic damage is not confined to the liver and evidence of other organ damage must be considered. All patients should be assessed for common comorbid liver conditions such as hepatocellular carcinoma and chronic viral hepatitis. It is mandatory in accurate cardiopulmonary

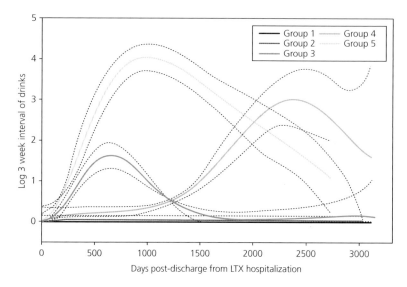

Figure 23.1 Trajectories of alcohol use after liver transplantation. Fifty-four percent of patients had no alcohol consumption. The majority (group 2) drank low quantities infrequently. An early onset consumption that diminished over time was identified in group 3, later onset moderate consumption that increased over time (group 4), and early onset heavy increasing pattern of use (group 5). (Source: DiMartini et al. 2010 [10]. Reproduced with permission of American Society of Transplantation and the American Society of Transplant Surgeons)

assessment. It is common practice to evaluate cardiac function by echocardiography and stress testing. Cardiac catheterization is recommended in those patients who have added risk factors such as diabetes, hypertension, or chronic smoking.

Chronic alcohol intake might be injurious for neurologic and hematologic systems and specific work-up to rule out neuropathy and Wernicke's encephalopathy should be performed. Chronic alcohol consumption is associated with impaired lymphocyte recruitment which may explain the increased morbidity and mortality of pulmonary infections in alcoholic subjects. Tuberculosis is a risk in all ALD candidates, and assessment for TB is mandatory in this population.

Post-transplant there is a higher incidence of malignancy, especially of the head and neck and esophagus. An oto-rhino-laryngology and lung evaluation, as well as a gastrointestinal endoscopy may be performed, in selected candidates, to rule out early cancers in these areas. Encouraging patients to stop smoking and not to resume after transplantation is key to reducing the burden of aerodigestive cancers after transplantation.

Role of liver transplantation in alcoholic hepatitis

Alcoholic hepatitis [11] "is a clinical syndrome of liver inflammation, hepatocyte injury, and fibrosis that occurs in the setting of recent consumption of large amounts of alcohol." Severe acute alcoholic hepatitis has a poor outcome with standard supportive management. Data from combined treatment studies of severe alcoholic hepatitis have shown a 28-day mortality of 34% in patients not receiving corticosteroids. These data highlight the high short-term mortality of patients admitted to hospital with alcoholic hepatitis. Until recently, patients with severe alcoholic hepatitis have been precluded from liver transplantation on account of recent alcohol. Nevertheless, EASL guidelines published in 2012 did not make a specific interval of abstinence a prerequisite for transplantation in patients with ALD. Therefore, there may be an opportunity for these patients with alcoholic hepatitis for access to liver transplantation

There are few data on the actual outcomes when patients with the clinical syndrome of severe alcoholic hepatitis receive liver transplants, and these are limited by retrospective case identification and small numbers. Two single center retrospective reviews have reported that when alcoholic hepatitis *defined in pathologic terms* is superimposed on cirrhosis the outcome of liver transplantation is similar to that in patients with alcoholic cirrhosis alone. A recent retrospective review of the UNOS database 2004–2010 found 130 patients with a diagnosis of alcoholic hepatitis had been listed for transplantation. Both graft and patient survival were similar to the cohort of patients without history of chronic excessive alcohol use (reviewed in [3]). A prospective pilot multicenter Franco-Belgian study involving seven liver transplantation centers performed early liver transplantation in patients with severe alcoholic hepatitis who failed to respond to 7 days of medical therapy. Selection for liver transplantation required that this was their first episode of liver disease, absolute consensus of paramedical and medical staff, no comorbidities, acceptable social integration, and supportive family members. This case-controlled study showed an unequivocal improvement of survival in patients who received early transplantation. In addition, only three participants reassumed alcohol after liver transplantation at 720, 740, and 1140 days. The highly selective nature of the study group is shown by the fact that the patients with alcoholic hepatitis receiving liver transplantation represented only of 2.8% of transplants performed in these seven centers during the period of the study. We view this landmark paper as a proof of concept study that demonstrates that the 6-month abstinence rule is not paramount, and that these results support future evaluation of liver transplant in a carefully selected subgroup of patients with severe alcoholic hepatitis who are failing to respond to medical therapy [11].

Treatment of addiction

The treatment of alcoholism can be considered under three overlapping headings: prevention of hazardous drinking, psychosocial treatment interventions, and pharmacologic interventions. Few studies have assessed the alcohol use before and after liver transplantation. Several reasons explain this lack of studies. The ALD population is heterogeneous regarding drinking history, including some patients who have been abstinent for years. In addition, some deny whereas others acknowledge the craving for alcohol. Finally, many in the transplant ALD population deny any interest in receiving treatment for alcoholism. Indeed, this surprising phenomenon was one of the causes of the failure of a trial of naltrexone among liver transplant recipients with alcoholism. An additional impediment in that study was that liver transplant recipients were unwilling to take a potentially hepatotoxic medication such as naltrexone. In contrast, Bjornsson et al. introduced a structured management program for alcoholism after liver transplantation, which comprised an assessment by a psychiatrist skilled in the care of alcoholics, the initiation of treatment in patients who had not been

treated in the past, encouragement to participate in motivational enhancement, and the use of an abstinence contract. The protocol was started before transplantation and continued after transplantation with interviews at 3 months and at 1, 3, and 5 years. In consecutive patients, they observed a reduction in the prevalence of alcohol use in comparison with a matched historical control group (48% and 22%), although they did not report their data in terms of harmful drinking. Future treatment initiatives should be targeted to the subcohort of ALD patients with persistent cravings, and the goal should be the prevention of harmful drinking (reviewed in [3]). In addition, all ALD liver transplant recipients should be encouraged to stop smoking.

Finally, some researchers have found that depression, anxiety, medication adherence, job counseling, family therapy, and financial counseling are also important areas of intervention in end-stage liver disease patients with alcohol use disorders. The importance of maintaining stability in these areas of a patient's life to their addiction recovery cannot be overstated.

Quality of life

Many studies in the medical literature have dealt with quality of life (QOL) in liver transplantation but lack of uniform design and the variety of instruments utilized to assess QOL represent a significant drawback. The majority of the studies have shown striking impairment before liver transplant, which improves significantly afterwards. Alcoholic patients appear to return to society to lead active and productive lives, despite the fact that they seem less likely to be involved in structured social activities than patients transplanted for nonalcoholic liver disease. The recipients continue to have many deficits compared with age-matched control populations. Additionally, some concern exists regarding the durability of such improvements. A deterioration of physical findings, fatigue, and well-being have been reported in a 12-year follow-up study (reviewed in [3]).

References

[1] Rehm J, Samokhvalov AV, Shield KD. Global burden of alcoholic liver diseases. *J Hepatol* 2013; **59**(1): 160–168.
[2] Powell WJ Jr, Klatskin G. Duration of survival in patients with Laënnec's cirrhosis: influence of alcohol withdrawal,

and possible effects of recent changes in general management of the disease. *Am J Med* 1968; **44**(3): 406–420.

[3] Lucey MR. Liver transplantation for alcoholic liver disease. *Nat Rev Gastroenterol Hepatol* 2014; **11**: 300–307.

[4] Davies MH, Langman MJ, Elias E, Neuberger JM. Liver disease in a district hospital remote from a transplant centre: a study of admissions and deaths. *Gut* 1992; **33**: 1397–1399.

[5] Neuberger J, Adams D, MacMaster P, Maidment A, Speed M. Assessing priorities for allocation of donor liver grafts: survey of public and clinicians. *BMJ* 1998; **317**: 172–175.

[6] Lucey MR, Schaubel DE, Guidinger MK, Tome S, Merion RM. Effects of alcoholic liver disease and hepatitis C infection on waiting list and posttransplant mortality and transplant survival benefit. *Hepatology* 2009; **50**: 400–406.

[7] Tome S, Lucey MR. Timing of liver transplantation in alcoholic cirrhosis. *J Hepatol* 2003; **39**: 302–307.

[8] Beresford TP. Psychiatric assessment of alcoholic candidates for liver transplantation. In: Lucey MR, Merion RM, Beresford TP, eds. *Liver Transplantation and the Alcoholic Patient*. Cambridge University Press, Cambridge, UK; 1994: 29–49.

[9] Burra P, Senzolo M, Adam R, et al; for ELITA and ELTR Liver Transplant Centers. Liver transplantation for alcoholic liver disease in Europe: a study from the ELTR (European Liver Transplant Registry). *Am J Transplant* 2010; **10**: 138–148.

[10] DiMartini A, Dew MA, Day N, et al. Trajectories of alcohol consumption following liver transplantation. *Am J Transplant* 2010; **10**: 2305–2312.

[11] Mathurin P, Moreno C, Samuel D, et al. Early liver transplantation for severe alcoholic hepatitis. *N Engl J Med* 2011; **365**(19): 1790–1800.

CHAPTER 24

Future directions: the need for early identification and intervention for patients with excessive alcohol use

Andrea DiMartini,[1] Shari Rogal,[2] and Stephen Potts[3]

[1] *Starzl Transplant Institute, University of Pittsburgh Medical Center, Pittsburgh, PA, USA*
[2] *Center for Health Equity Research and Promotion, VA Pittsburgh Healthcare System, Pittsburgh, PA, USA*
[3] *Department of Psychological Medicine, Royal Infirmary of Edinburgh, Edinburgh, UK*

KEY POINTS

- Effective screening and brief interventions exist for alcohol misuse.
- Preventative measures to avert alcohol-related psychiatric or medical outcomes are underutilized.
- Without a national strategy or policies, implementation of screening and intervention in primary care settings has been poor.
- When ambiguous recommendations on alcohol consumption are given patients may tailor information to suit their wishes.
- Secondary or tertiary interventions require coordination of care at the medical and psychiatric clinic levels.
- Ongoing care through consistent care providers who can monitor and follow up on adherence to medical advice is needed.

In the preceding chapters of this book we have reviewed the consequences of alcohol-induced diseases from the medical sequelae, specifically alcohol-related liver disease (ALD), to the psychiatric disorder of alcohol dependence that nearly always precedes it. We have learned about the natural history of both alcoholic liver disease and alcohol dependence and also that millions of individuals suffer and die from these disorders worldwide. As a conclusion to this scholarly compilation we will draw on the knowledge from the prior chapters (Figure 24.1) to propose future directions for clinical work and research in caring for these complex patients. There is a need to improve our strategies continually regarding the care of patients with alcohol-related disease as no strategies to date have substantially decreased the rates of alcohol use disorders (AUD) or related liver disease. We introduce various obstacles surrounding the

delivery of care to these patients and propose potential solutions. In this future directions chapter we address the potential points of intervention, optimal strategies for intervention, and challenges in the implementation of these interventions. Virtually all of the proposed future direction interventions specific to our defined ALD population could be adapted for potential research. Beyond brief interventions, which have been extensively studied, secondary and tertiary interventions have been rarely studied and mostly involve single center descriptive cohort studies. Additionally, we suggest coordinated care through multidisciplinary teams including liver and mental health specialists may be required to address the complex needs of these patients.

The population of individuals with excessive alcohol consumption is complex and may suffer from two distinct but potentially comorbid disorders: ALD and AUD,

---

Alcohol Abuse and Liver Disease, First Edition. Edited by James Neuberger and Andrea DiMartini.

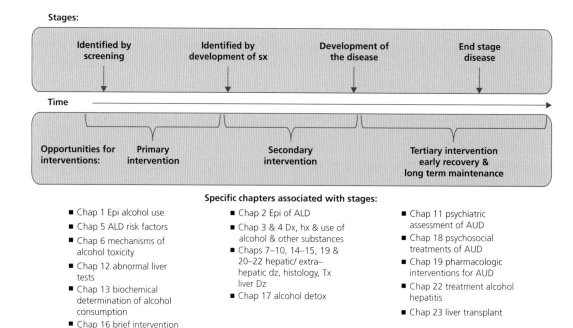

Figure 24.1 Considerations for optimizing outcomes across the spectrum of alcohol-related diseases with reference to specific chapters in this book.

which is a psychiatric diagnosis. While most individuals with ALD will additionally have an AUD, there are many individuals who meet criteria for an AUD but never develop liver disease. Conversely, some individuals drink modestly and develop end-stage ALD but do not meet criteria for moderate to serious AUD [1,2]. Exposure to alcohol alone, even in substantial quantities, does not necessarily result in the development of an addiction disorder or ALD. Both physical and psychiatric disorders need to be considered and formally diagnosed (see Figure 24.1 for reference to specific chapters that review diagnosis and treatment of these disorders). Identification and treatment of these consequences of excessive alcohol use is necessary but the most impactful approach from a public health perspective is primary prevention or early identification of at-risk individuals in order to prevent AUD and ALD before they occur.

Primary intervention strategies

In the United States and United Kingdom, an estimated 30% of the population is affected by alcohol misuse with most engaged in risky use, as defined in Table 24.1 (see also Chapter 1 for epidemiology of alcohol use) [3–5].

Table 24.1 Definitions of risky drinking by daily and weekly limits[a].

	Men	**Women**
On any single day	>4 standard[b] drinks in US or >3–4 units in UK[c]	>3 standard drinks or >2–3 units
Per week	>14 standard drinks or >21 units	>7 standard drinks or >14 units

[a]Only 2 in 100 who drink within these limits have an alcohol use disorder.

[b]To be comparable, standard drinks or units require conversion to grams of pure alcohol. A US standard drink equals 0.6 fluid ounces or 14 g of pure alcohol (e.g. a 12-oz 5% beer or 1.5 oz of 80 proof liquor).

[c]In the UK, one unit of alcohol is defined as 10 mL (7.9 g of pure alcohol). In other European countries units differ in size, ranging from 8 to 14 g of pure alcohol.

Even those who drink within safe limits can have problems if they drink too quickly or already have health problems (e.g. ALD). The term alcohol misuse encompasses the spectrum of unhealthy alcohol use including AUD, problem drinking (drinking despite consequences), and risky or hazardous drinking (amounts above recommended limits that increase the risk of health consequences) (Table 24.1) [6,7].

As discussed in Chapter 4, many individuals who eventually develop an AUD begin with risky patterns of consumption. Though excessive alcohol consumption patterns may be underway by early adulthood, less than 25% of individuals seek or receive treatment [8]. The difficulty is knowing who among the pool of individuals with excessive alcohol use will develop AUDs because, as the Institutes of Medicine report emphasizes, most individuals with unhealthy or risky alcohol use do not become alcohol dependent and would therefore benefit from a brief intervention [7].

Screening, through self-report instruments, and brief intervention may be useful in this group of high-risk individuals to define and intervene to avert the development of future problems (both ALD and AUD). Non-AUD individuals who are drinking at unhealthy levels are possibly unaware of the health risks of their consumption or have not experienced untoward consequences. This type of individual, although not seeking treatment, may be amenable to education and brief intervention (see Chapter 16 for brief interventions) [9]. A meta-analysis showed strong evidence that screening in primary care settings can accurately identify patients whose levels or patterns of alcohol consumption do not meet criteria for an AUD, but place them at risk for increased morbidity and mortality. Behavioral counseling interventions in these risky drinking adults has been shown to reduce overall alcohol consumption and heavy drinking episodes, with sustained effects for up to several years [3,4]. Notably, multi-contact interventions were most effective whereas single episode interventions appeared to be ineffective [3,4]. In this meta-analysis there was insufficient evidence to demonstrate the effect of a brief intervention in reducing alcohol-related liver disease although data was only available for 12-month outcomes [4].

Clinician training manuals for brief interventions and screening tools are available on the National Institute on Alcohol Abuse and Alcoholism website (www.niaaa. nih.gov/publications). While a number of screening measures exist, some designed for use in special populations, the Alcohol Use Disorders Identification Test (AUDIT) is the most widely studied and commonly used self-report screening instrument in primary care and identifies both excessive risky consumption patterns as well as those likely to have an AUD. Screening of risky

alcohol use will inevitably also uncover those with an AUD or perhaps those at risk for ALD and these patients would require referral to a specialty clinic for appropriate treatment rather than brief intervention (see Chapters 18 and 19 for treatments of AUD and Chapters 15, 21, and 22 for treatment of ALD). Biologic markers can be used to corroborate results of screening instruments (see Chapter 13) but they are generally less sensitive and specific than self-report instruments and should not be used as the sole screening method to identify excessive alcohol use. For example, the liver enzyme gamma-glutamyl transferase is a commonly used marker of liver disease but has poor sensitivity in nonmedical populations for identifying alcohol use and poor specificity in medically ill populations. Carbohydrate deficient transferrin is a marker of heavy sustained alcohol use but is costly and not widely available.

Despite the confirmed efficacy of brief alcohol counseling in reducing alcohol consumption among general outpatients [3,4], the translation of these strategies into clinical practice has been disappointing [6]. Providers in primary care practice face multiple competing demands on their time including diagnosing and treating a wide variety of acute and chronic diseases, providing preventative measures, and developing treatment plans. Ambitious efforts in primary care medicine to implement routine screening for AUD and provide brief counseling have not generally succeeded [10]. These challenges, in addition to lack of training on either guidelines for risky alcohol consumption or brief counseling interventions can result in ambiguous alcohol recommendations.

Trials throughout Europe and the multinational WHO study have tried a variety of education, coaching, incentives, and marketing approaches to promote adoption of screening and brief interventions, unfortunately with low implementation rates [6]. Even when rates of screening and brief intervention were acceptable, these rates were not sustained after the research study that supported these efforts concluded [6]. In the United States the Veteran Administration (VA) hospital system decided to implement a system-wide alcohol screening and brief intervention procedure. This effort was supported by a commitment from the highest levels of the administration and backed by performance measures and incentives and facilitated using computer-assisted technology (reminders and electronic medical record system that provided screening measures) [6]. Screening was only the first step and subsequent brief intervention completion was still low. However, awareness of those at risk is the first necessary step and documentation in the medical record could facilitate appropriate intervention at a future medical contact. While successful in a large VA system, whether this type of screening could be implemented on a national level might require further electronic medical record data management at a hospital system, insurance provider, or national level. Changes in the new ICD-11 codes to include harmful alcohol use and changes to the United States and other countries' medical services procedure coding systems to include alcohol screening and brief interventions may facilitate the use of these strategies in actual clinical care [6,11]. A possible solution would include incentivizing providers directly, perhaps by including alcohol cessation as a pay-for-performance measure on a system-wide level. This approach was successful in the United Kingdom for smoking cessation [12]. In the United Kingdom and European Union, the National Institute for Health and Care Excellence public guidance report additionally recommends consideration of policy measures such as alcohol pricing, availability, licensing, and marketing to reduce or prevent harmful alcohol consumption [13]. In some countries, protecting the public's health has been made part of the licensing objectives [13].

Some health care systems are unified in a way that facilitates achieving such targets, set at the national level but delivered locally. An example is Scotland, which in 2008, as part of a national alcohol strategy [14], established a high profile target to deliver standardized brief interventions in three priority settings (primary care, antenatal care, and the emergency department) [15]. Performance has substantially exceeded the targets, as measured in numbers of interventions delivered [16], though the outcomes in terms of reduced consumption and associated morbidity are less clear-cut.

Secondary intervention strategies

As noted in Chapter 8, the course of ALD tends to progress in a predictable fashion with discrete stages. In the absence of successful primary prevention, individuals may not present for medical care until they develop ALD. Secondary prevention is after the disease has occurred, but may still be in an early or preclinical phase where disease progression can be controlled or perhaps cured. Secondary prevention commonly occurs in the primary care settings or in specialty clinics such as gastroenterology.

The future of secondary interventions will require simple and accurate diagnostic tools. Currently, the ability to diagnose ALD is based on the patient's report of a significant history of alcohol consumption and clinical and laboratory evidence supporting ALD. Medical care providers may hope that serologic, radiographic, and examination findings will provide all the data required for diagnosis of ALD. However, alcohol exposure information is essential and requires asking the patient detailed questions (see Chapter 11). The ability to obtain an accurate consumption history is constrained by patient and physician factors including denial and under-reporting by the patient and lack of or inadequate questioning or underestimation of alcohol-related problems by the physician. Using a structured set of questions asking detailed information on quantity and frequency of alcohol consumption (e.g. AUDIT) could provide consistency in data gathering. However, these instruments target only recent consumption and additional questions on the complete history of alcohol use should be asked to capture estimates of patients' total exposure. The Skinner Lifetime Drinking History [17] is used in research settings for this purpose but is time-consuming and requires training to administer, making it difficult to use in clinical settings.

In addition to providing essential data for the identification of excessive alcohol use, screening instruments can provide other critical prognostic data. In an outpatient general medical clinic setting through seven large VA systems 31 311 men were surveyed using the AUDIT and CAGE surveys [18]. Higher scores on both measures significantly predicted those who would be hospitalized for alcohol-related gastrointestinal problems (liver disease, upper gastrointestinal bleeding, or pancreatitis) over the median 3.75 years of follow-up [18]. The authors concluded that, beyond screening, these tools can predict medical outcomes and can be used as surrogate markers of alcohol-related health risk in clinical practice [18]. They also suggest screening tools can provide important feedback to patients, risk stratification for physicians, and increased provider acceptance of the importance of brief screening [18]. Increasing identification of candidates for secondary prevention interventions will require simple tools with high sensitivity and specificity for identification that are acceptable to primary care providers.

Improved secondary prevention also requires interdisciplinary coordination of care. Unfortunately, in primary care clinics, few patients are even asked about alcohol use, advice provided about alcohol use is vague, and there is a lack of adequate follow-up care for those identified as having an AUD [19]. In addition to underestimating alcohol-related problems, physicians often fail to make specific recommendations for addiction treatment. In a large US national sample of primary care outpatients (n = 7371) only 48% of problem drinkers received any follow-up, with most being merely told to "stop drinking" [19]. Even in specialty clinics such as gastroenterology, where the volume of patients with health harmful alcohol consumption is expected to be higher, screening and brief intervention are not routine practice. Furthermore, screening in specialty medical settings is more likely to identify patients with AUD, a group for whom the efficacy of a brief intervention is not established. Two meta-analyses have found no evidence for brief behavioral interventions in primary care settings for individuals with alcohol dependence [4,20]. Thus, by the time an individual reaches the gastroenterologist clinic and is diagnosed with ALD, just recommending they stop alcohol use and employing a brief intervention or briefly educating them on the dangers of continued use will likely not be effective in stopping or reducing alcohol consumption. For these patients referral for formal addiction evaluation and counseling is best (see Chapter 18).

Conversely, in psychiatric clinical settings, while screening for AUD is routine, screening for comorbid alcohol-related medical disorders is not. Mental health providers should consider referral to primary care providers for evaluation of liver, if not overall health consequences, when excessive alcohol consumption patterns are identified (see Chapters 7–10). Some mental health clinicians may perform basic biochemical liver enzyme screening if medication administration is to be considered but a history of excessive alcohol exposure should prompt at least a case discussion with the primary care provider. Unfortunately, the sub-specialization of medicine lends to clinical providers focusing on their defined area in the limited time they have with a patient. In this traditional model each discipline plans care often in partial or total isolation from the others. This does not facilitate a comprehensive view or approach to patient care. Thus, comprehensive care of patients with AUDs likely requires an interdisciplinary team approach.

Identification of excessive alcohol use, ALD, or AUD does not guarantee patient acceptance of medical recommendations for abstinence or treatment. In medical disorders for which alcohol consumption is contraindicated, including liver disease, patients generally have difficulty following such advice especially if behavioral changes do not appear to have immediate benefits. Some patients who do not follow the advice immediately later reduce or discontinue use when physical symptoms emerge or they begin to experience side effects as a result of drinking [21,22]. Others may "tailor" the advice to suit their beliefs, either cutting or reducing consumption with the expectation this will reduce harm, only drinking on special occasions, or monitoring physical symptoms to see if they are experiencing harm [21,22]. Still others discount the medical advice or the actual risks to themselves or have personal motivations for their risk–benefit decision-making (immediate benefits of drinking such as reduction of stress and enhancement of social situations or celebration outweighs long-term risks) (see Chapter 18 for discussion of how to address these issues) [21]. For these patients, receiving multiple or ambiguous messages about alcohol consumption from a single provider or across providers may encourage or contribute to the "tailoring" of advice about alcohol consumption and encourage patients to pick the advice that best fits their intentions [10]. Appropriate and consistent presentation of specific advice, better training of physicians, and consultation with gastroenterology providers would improve provider knowledge and care delivery [10].

To avoid misinformation and "tailoring" of medical recommendations, ALD patients should receive ongoing care through consistent care providers who can monitor their condition and follow-up on adherence to advice given. Perhaps the optimal comprehensive treatment of patients with ALD would entail merging the treatment plans of two highly specialized medical disciplines: gastroenterology and addiction medicine. Gastroenterology clinics that deal with significant number of ALD patients should consider either partnering with mental health professionals or addiction clinics or at minimum having ready access to such referral sources. Establishing the initial contact for the patient may facilitate acceptance and follow-through with the referral. Collaborative care models are increasingly used to address complex comorbid medical disorders and ALD and AUD patients could be benefitted by such a treatment approach. One such model of a joint gastroenterology–psychiatry team addresses a range of alcohol and liver disease problems in a single setting. This multidisciplinary team provides a joint clinic ensuring that the medical, psychiatric, and counseling needs of the ALD patient are met at one clinic attendance [23]. In addition to providing comprehensive care to the patient, this team found that in a 2-year period after program inception referral rates to their clinic increased dramatically (>600%). Additionally, in their medical system, staff and professional provider identification and documentation of alcohol misuse and problems was improved as was knowledge about and referral for adequate alcohol treatment [23].

Tertiary intervention strategies

At tertiary prevention stage, interventions are aimed at reducing or slowing disease progression, minimizing complications, and optimizing quality of life and long-term outcomes. The future of tertiary interventions requires a focus on appropriate and effective referral for addiction counseling at all points of contact, improved coordination of care, using technology for monitoring, and the development of accurate predictive models and effective treatment models for post-transplant recidivism.

There are few studies examining the numbers of individuals who require addiction treatment and are first accessing medical treatment for end-stage liver disease (ESLD) or even the success of addiction referral when offered at these points. A single center inpatient–outpatient VA sample of 199 patients with liver disease meeting criteria for liver transplant referral through 300 medical encounters identified that 46% of patients were actively drinking. While 27% of patients were already in addiction rehabilitation, the medical record did not document a treatment referral for addiction counseling for 41% of these actively drinking patients with ESLD [24]. Given that access to mental health care through the VA system should not be an obstacle, the numbers of unreferred or untreated patients with ESLD outside of the VA may be even higher. While treating immediate medical issues such as medical stabilization may have been the focus of care, this cohort did include stable outpatients as well as inpatients. The discontinuity of inpatient and outpatient care can lead to situations where an immediate issue is dealt with while the underlying alcohol addiction that resulted in the need for medical care is not addressed.

Similarly, the numbers of individuals arriving at liver transplant evaluation with end-stage ALD without any prior addiction rehabilitation experience (nearly 50% in some studies) is discouraging [1,25]. Whether this suggests these individuals are not being encouraged to pursue addiction treatment, are resistant to treatment, or are not accessing the medical system until they become symptomatic in the later stages of liver disease is unknown. However, anecdotal reports by patients reveal many had medical encounters earlier in their liver disease course when they were counseled about the consequences of their drinking. As pointed out earlier in the chapter, when ambiguous recommendations on alcohol consumption are given patients may tailor information to suit their wishes. While some ALD liver transplant candidates report being recommended to stop drinking completely, others recall being told to "just cut down" on their drinking. Few recall being advised to attend addiction rehabilitation. Whether such accounts are accurate to the events is unknown but many of these individuals additionally claim to have stopped or cut down for a while and, experiencing no further problems, resumed drinking again (see Chapter 3). These are obviously missed opportunities to engage patients in addiction counseling at these critical points and also to continue long-term monitoring for continued abstinence. In these cases screening does not need to be performed as the individual has already been identified as having a significant alcohol problem. These patients will not likely respond to brief counseling which is not intensive enough to treat an alcohol addiction. If ongoing medical follow-up had been provided they might have received additional counseling against resuming drinking. Whether this would have effectively stopped their alcohol use or maintained abstinence is unknown. However, a medical system where the focus of care is crisis-oriented is not suited to the long-term management and monitoring needs of these patients. Perhaps a solution would include system-wide discharge planning that requires referral for addiction counseling for all patients with alcohol-related admissions, although this carries the risk of rapidly overwhelming addiction services with referrals of reluctant patients. A clear and consistent presentation of information at all points of contact with the medical system is needed to increase the efficacy of a tertiary intervention. It also serves to counterbalance patients' retrospective – and potentially inaccurate – accounts of the advice they received. Some transplant candidates report never having been advised to stop drinking, even by referring medical teams. If there is good documentation that they were in fact repeatedly and unequivocally advised to become abstinent, with offers of referral to assist in this, the discrepancy is evidence of a degree of denial that is relevant in assessing risk of post-transplant relapse and therefore candidacy.

Future interventions need to be created for extraordinary treatments such as liver transplantation which still lack precise predictive and treatment models for post-transplant recidivism. Perhaps by design the liver transplant evaluation necessarily focuses on the suitability of the candidate at that point and making predictions about future behaviors and is less about preparation and prevention. Because of the severity of the candidates' condition or their rate of medical decline there may be limited time to render an opinion (or even request additional steps such as completing addiction counseling). In this context there can be significant emphasis on the ability to predict future alcohol use for AUD and ALD individuals from their existing pretransplant characteristics. For example, pretransplant length of sobriety of 6 months or greater is a commonly used period of abstinence required of liver transplant candidates and some transplant programs will not consider individuals for referral until this period of abstinence is achieved. However, in the natural history of alcohol-dependent individuals while nearly 60% are able to achieve 6 months of sobriety at some point, nearly all of these will relapse, many back to heavy alcohol consumption [26]. In a meta-analysis of alcohol use following liver transplantation short length of sobriety was one of the most consistent predictors of future alcohol use [27], not of abstinence stability. In both liver transplant populations and studies of the natural history of alcohol-dependent individuals it is shown that longer periods of abstinence predict less likelihood to drink [1,26] but that stable abstinence is measured not in months but, like cancer remission, in years [26]. In addition, transplant candidates are by definition physically unwell, often to a degree requiring prolonged or repeated hospitalizations, when alcohol is unavailable to them or physically aversive in its effects. The predictive value of a period of abstinence spent in hospital or when physically unwell

at home is clearly lower than a similar period spent in good health and while exposed to temptations to drink.

Predictive factors in general have limited ability to determine those least likely to drink. Beyond length of sobriety other factors such as poor social support, a family history of an AUD [27], multiple failed addiction rehabilitations, and other substance use can have cumulative but small effect sizes [27]. Though a diagnosis of alcohol dependence is one of the strongest predictors of post-transplant alcohol use, conferring nearly three times greater likelihood to drink, less than half of such individuals actually drank following transplantation [1]. Thus, while the role of the liver transplant evaluation is to determine suitability for transplantation and there is an emphasis on predicting recidivism, from a mental health or addiction perspective, maintenance treatment to support long-term abstinence is the appropriate therapeutic approach. Patients' acceptance of their addiction and the contribution of alcohol to their health problems, and their approach to addiction rehabilitation may be most informative. It might be assumed that patients who are willing to participate, engage in, and derive benefit from addictions counseling would potentially be more easily encouraged to resume such therapy if and when alcohol use occurs following transplant. In fact, the psychosocial or mental health assessment may result in recommendations for initiation or continuation of addiction treatment before a final determination of transplant candidacy can be made.

At the point of liver transplant evaluation ALD/AUD patients may be requested to attend addiction rehabilitation, typically within a mental health system external to the transplant program by mental health or addiction specialists in the community. In the United States this largely depends on the individual's health insurance and the addiction or mental health treatment programs with which their insurance is contracted. In these scenarios the transplant team relies on the quality and intensity of the treatment provided outside of their purview. Additionally, feedback to the transplant team is typically limited except to confirm that the individual is attending the addiction treatment program and achieving treatment goals. In other countries, the funding and organizational arrangements differ, but the effect is the same – a separation of addiction treatment from pretransplant assessment or post-transplant follow-up, in cases where integration is required.

A well-designed solution which is equivalent to a collaborative care model at a tertiary level is to create an addiction treatment program that is embedded within the liver transplant unit. One such successful program demonstrated the feasibility of an addiction treatment program integrated within the liver transplant program providing close monitoring and ongoing treatment for waitlisted ALD candidates [28]. Addolorato et al. [28] found such a program could reduce post-transplant alcohol use compared with prior treatment model of addictions treatment external to the liver transplant program [28]. In this new embedded model the alcohol addiction clinician participated in the weekly liver transplant team meetings and assisted in determinations of both listing and delisting liver transplant candidates [28]. Interestingly, Addolorato et al. [28] found that in addition to lower rates of post-transplant alcohol use there was an increase in the number of liver transplants for ALD individuals, suggesting that the availability of professional input from the addictions treatment team may have reduced the transplant surgeons' reluctance to transplant ALD patients [28]. Additionally, establishing such a collaborative relationship may allow the liver transplant team to accept the mental health professional as an expert in the area of addictions and make use of addiction treatment recommendations for the patient. However, in Addolorato et al's model it is not clear whether the improved outcomes resulted from improved selection of candidates or were a result of the intervention itself. Whether this created greater accountability to the liver transplant team or oversight by the combined addictions liver transplant team that aided in the maintenance of abstinence is unknown.

A distinction needs to be drawn between collaborative *assessment*, which should the model for ALD/AUD liver transplant *candidates*, and collaborative *treatment* of transplant *recipients*, which is probably beyond the resources of most transplant services. Transplant units serve populations measured in millions, often with a wide geographic spread. Most units assess several hundred patients per year, and will build up, over time, a post-transplant population measured in thousands. Assessment can be intense, centralized within the unit, and undertaken on manageable numbers; ongoing treatment, after the early postoperative period, is necessarily much less intense, more widely dispersed, and relevant to many more patients. (For example, the Scottish Liver Transplant Unit in Edinburgh, UK, which serves the whole of Scotland, explicitly established collaborative assessment of transplant candidates at foundation in 1992. Other than a subset of local patients, ongoing treatment falls to separated, dispersed services close to their homes.)

Such comprehensive coordination of the aspects of their medical and mental health care will undoubtedly improve the overall quality of care and promote the likelihood of follow through with addictions maintenance therapy even following liver transplant. As liver transplant teams are invested in the long-term care of ALD/AUD recipients, mental health treatment should be an integral part of this long-term management. In an ideal setting, this type of collaborative care would occur not at the last minute as rescue therapy as the individual is pursuing liver transplant but substantially in advance perhaps even preventing the need for liver transplant. However, where nontransplant addiction services are called upon to provide post-transplant follow-up to aid in maintaining abstinence, the priorities of the transplant service for their patients (in whom they have invested a great deal in terms of time, effort, money, and organs) may not match those of the addiction service, which will have many more *non*-transplant patients, for whom becoming abstinent in the first place is a more pressing goal.

In addition to the need for programmatic strategies tailored to address the unique needs of ALD/AUD liver transplant candidates, there is additional evidence that the content and theoretical approach to addiction treatment for these individuals may also need to be uniquely tailored to their needs. A main difference may be the motivation for which these liver transplant candidates stop drinking. While it is commonly held in addictions theory that AUD individuals have to have strong and compelling reasons to stop (e.g. "hitting rock bottom") being confronted with a life-threatening illness from which the only possible rescue is a liver transplant and for which sobriety is mandated is a unique "rock bottom" experience. Perhaps these patients stop not through thoughtful intent but by necessity. This is not to say that other "rock bottom" experiences do not force similar abrupt transitions from active drinking to abstinence or that all ALD liver transplant candidates experience this type of transformation.

In addiction theory, the process of changing addictive behaviors has been conceptualized as a series of successive stage phenomena including precontemplation,

contemplation, action, and maintenance. For the ALD patient who becomes abruptly ill, perhaps experiencing a catastrophic life-transforming medical event such as a life-threatening gastrointestinal bleed, the leap from precontemplation (e.g. "don't need to stop drinking") to action ("stopping drinking") could be instantaneous. Whether such a rapid progression through these stages effectively creates the same behavior change that true contemplation and work towards this goal would accomplish is unknown. However, in the field of addiction it has been recognized that patients in the precontemplative phase, even treatment-seeking individuals, differ from those who have achieved the contemplation or action phase by having less guilt or worry over their alcohol use, being less receptive to help, and being less likely to have previously sought help [29]. This profile seems similar to that identified by Weinrieb et al. [25] in their report on ALD liver transplant candidates. They identified that ALD liver transplant candidates who had achieved some abstinence did not perceive a need for addiction treatment and had little motivation for treatment. These individuals were less likely to consider themselves to have an alcohol problem or identify as being "alcoholic," were resistant to treatment, and did not want to take medication for cravings or urges to use alcohol [25].

This is particularly relevant to the question of liver transplant for alcoholic hepatitis, which is currently an absolute contraindication in most units. A recent French study provides evidence to contradict the prevailing view that the early outcomes were poor, both medically and in terms of relapse to alcohol use [30]. However, opening transplantation to candidates who, by definition, are drinking up to presentation, calls into question the need for and validity of the assessments currently undertaken for less acute forms of ALD. This evidence, together with publicity surrounding several cases of young British patients who died from alcoholic hepatitis after being declined transplant, has generated a proposal for a UK pilot project to assess this further, announced in 2014 [31].

Therapies to address these specific nuances in ALD/AUD liver transplant patients may be critical to engage them appropriately in addiction counseling. Accordingly, Weinrieb et al. [25] conducted a randomized controlled study for ALD liver transplant candidates using motivational interviewing techniques to encourage and facilitate engagement in addictions treatment (see Chapter 18

for discussion of the use of motivational interviewing therapies). They found motivational interviewing could overcome the ambivalence towards and improve engagement in addiction counseling, improved recognition of their problem, reduced alcohol use, and prepared individuals for transplantation [25]. However, they also found that the patient's medical illness often interfered with their full participation in all therapy sessions. They suggested the future use of telemedicine to overcome some of these barriers. This could also address logistical issues of transplant candidates living some distance from the transplant program especially if the addiction rehabilitation was not local but was embedded within the transplant program clinic.

Comorbidity is an issue throughout medicine, and no less so in this area. Patients who misuse alcohol are more likely to misuse drugs, and put themselves at risk of hepatitis B and C virus infection via intravenous drug misuse or sexual contact. In addition, rising levels of obesity are leading to dramatic increases in the rates of nonalcoholic fatty liver disease (NAFLD). Some of this comorbidity may be sequential, but transplant units now see increasing numbers of patients who simultaneously have ALD, NAFLD, and hepatitis C cirrhosis. This means that transplant services, and those allied with them, will increasingly be expected to cross specialty borders, and advise patients who have misused alcohol about diet and exercise, even if they are not morbidly obese, or, conversely, to advise overweight patients about alcohol use, even when there is no AUD (Table 24.2).

Conclusions

The first step in moving forward is to acknowledge that, though progress has been made in addressing the consequences of alcohol, preventative measures are lacking. We have focused on the areas of potential clinical interventions in the future to continue building on the extensive knowledge we have of ALD and AUD. On a medical system or payer level, there is the possibility of having nationally set targets or pay-for-performance measures that require questioning about alcohol use and intervention to receive reimbursement, making preventative services billable, and requiring discharge referral appointments to addiction specialists for anyone with an alcohol-related diagnosis code on hospitalization. On an

Table 24.2 Levels of alcohol treatment intervention for patient with comorbid alcohol use disorders (AUD) and liver disease.

Level of intervention	Typical location	Level of disease identification	Intervention	Outcomes
Primary prevention	Outpatient general medical office or primary care	Screening for unhealthy risky alcohol use	Brief behavioral counseling interventions (not intended for those with AUD)	Established efficacy reducing risky or hazardous consumption [3,6]
Secondary prevention	Outpatient specialist office (hepatologist or mental health professional), emergency room, or inpatient medical settings	Alcohol use disorder and/or alcoholic liver disease	Addiction treatment coupled with long-term monitoring (may include monitoring of liver disease and referral to hepatologist)	Unknown, single center studies suggest combined treatment confers benefits
Tertiary prevention	Outpatient or inpatient setting in hepatology or liver transplant unit	End-stage alcoholic liver disease	Addiction treatment, long-term monitoring, liver transplant, addiction treatment embedded within LT care would be optimal	Rate of any alcohol use cumulates with time following LT (~30% at 5 years) but survival is equal to or better than other recurrent diseases. One single center study demonstrated reduced relapse rates with addiction management coupled with LT team care [28]

LT, liver transplantation.

individual level, there are possible interventions at the primary, secondary, and tertiary level. Primary prevention using brief behavioral counseling at the primary care level for those at-risk is the most cost-effective means of preventing at-risk drinking from progressing. There remains a need for increased efficacious and simple screening tools and interventions that can be administered, possibly by ancillary staff at primary care clinics. Additionally, secondary and tertiary prevention interventions will require coordination of care at the gastroenterology or transplant clinic level to ensure increased referral for addiction counseling and evaluation and to ensure medical screening for all patients with AUD. Effective tools to predict, prevent, and monitor recidivism in the setting of transplantation are continuing to be developed. A component of these could be technology-based counseling via telemedicine as well as improved monitoring devices and metabolomics/genomic techniques that could aid in optimizing transplant candidate selection. Beyond direct medical system interventions on a health care system level, potential interventions could include better access to mental health services to prevent people from using alcohol as self-medication and allow access to addiction specialists at an early stage. All of these areas of suggested interventions require further research. This is especially so for the secondary and tertiary interventions where the majority of work is descriptive and single center studies. As no intervention strategies to date have substantially decreased the rates of AUD or related liver disease our field should be compelled to consider and examine this next generation of potential interventions.

References

[1] DiMartini A, Day N, Dew MA, et al. Alcohol consumption patterns and predictors of use following liver transplantation for alcoholic liver disease. *Liver Transpl* 2006; **12**: 813–820.

[2] Beresford TP. Psychiatric assessment of alcoholic candidates for liver transplantation. In: Lucey MR, Merion RM, Beresford TP, eds. *Liver Transplantation and the Alcoholic*

Patient: Medical, Surgical, and Psychosocial Issues. Cambridge University Press, Cambridge, UK; 1994: 29–49.

[3] US Preventive Services Task Force. Screening and behavioral counseling interventions in primary care to reduce alcohol misuse: recommendation statement. *Ann Intern Med* 2004; **140**: 554–556.

[4] Jonas DE, Garbutt JC, Amick HR, et al. Behavioral counseling after screening for alcohol misuse in primary care: a systematic review and meta-analysis for the US Preventive Services Task Force. *Ann Intern Med* 2012; **157**: 645–654.

[5] Department of Health. Healthy Lives, Healthy People. Our strategy for public health in England. UK White paper published by UK Department of Health, Secretary of State for Health Andrew Ashley, November 2010.

[6] Bradley KA, Williams EC, Achtmeyer CE, Volpp B, Collins BJ, Kivlahan DR. Implementation of evidence-based alcohol screening in the Veterans Health Administration. *Am J Manag Care* 2006; **12**(10): 597–606.

[7] Institute of Medicine. *Broadening the Base of Treatment for Alcohol Problems: Report of a Study by a Committee of the Institute of Medicine, Division of Mental Health and Behavioral Medicine.* National Academy Press, Washington, DC; 1990.

[8] Saitz R. Alcohol screening and brief intervention in primary care: absence of evidence for efficacy in people with dependence or very heavy drinking. *Drug Alcohol Rev* 2010; **29**(6): 631–640.

[9] Hasin DS, Stinson FS, Ogburn E, Grant BF. Prevalence, correlates, disability, and comorbidity of DSM-IV alcohol abuse and dependence in the United States: results from the National Epidemiologic Survey on Alcohol and Related Conditions. *Arch Gen Psychiatry* 2007; **64**(7): 830–842.

[10] Blixen CE, Webster NJ, Hund AJ, et al. Communicating about alcohol consumption to nonharmful drinkers with hepatitis c: patient and provider perspectives. *J Gen Intern Med* 2008; **23**(3): 242–247.

[11] Touquet R, Harris D. Alcohol misuse Y91 Coding in ICD-11: rational terminology and logical coding specifically to encourage early identification and advice. *Alcohol Alcohol* 2012; **47**(3): 213–215.

[12] Millett C, Gray J, Saxena S, Netuveli G, Majeed A. Impact of a pay-for-performance incentive on support for smoking cessation and on smoking prevalence among people with diabetes. CMAJ 2007; **176**(12): 1705–1710.

[13] National Institute for Health and Care Excellence. *Alcohol-Use Disorders: Preventing Harmful Drinking.* June 2010 NICE public health guidance 24. Guidance.nice.org.uk/ph24.

[14] Scottish Government. *Changing Scotland's Relationship with Alcohol: A Framework for Action.* 2009.

[15] Scottish Intercollegiate Guidelines Network (SIGN). *Guideline 74: The Management of Harmful Drinking and Alcohol Dependence in Primary Care.* 2003.

[16] NHS Health Scotland. ABI HEAT Standard National Guidance 2013–2014.

[17] Skinner HA. Instruments for assessing alcohol and drug problems. *Bull Soc Psychol Addict Behav* 1984; **3**: 21–33.

[18] Au DH, Kivlahan DR, Bryson CL, Blough D, Bradley KA. Alcohol screening scores and risk of hospitalizations for GI conditions in men. *Alcohol Clin Exp Res* 2007; **31**(3): 443–451.

[19] D'Amico EJ, Paddock SM, Burnam A, Kung FY. Identification of and guidance for problem drinking by general medical providers: results from a national survey. *Med Care* 2005; **43**(3): 229–236.

[20] Saitz R, Freedner N, Palfai TP, Horton NJ, Samet JH. The severity of unhealthy alcohol use in hospitalized medical patients: the spectrum is narrow. *J Gen Intern Med.* 2006; **21**(4): 381–385.

[21] Stoller EP, Hund AJ, Webster NJ, et al. Alcohol consumption within the context of hepatitis C: a quantitative study of non-problematic drinkers. *Alcohol Alcohol* 2006; **41**(5): 546–552.

[22] Blaxter M, Cyster R. Compliance and risk-taking: the case of alcoholic liver disease. *Sociol Health Illness* 1984; **6**(3): 290–310.

[23] Moriarty KJ, Platt H, Crompton S, et al. Collaborative care for alcohol-related liver disease. *Clin Med* 2007; **7**(2): 125–128.

[24] Julapalli VR, Kramer JR, El-Serag HB. Evaluation for liver transplantation: adherence to AASLD referral guidelines in a large Veterans Affairs center. *Liver Transpl* 2005; **11**(11): 1370–1378.

[25] Weinrieb RM, Van Horn DHA, Lynch KG, Lucey MR. A randomized, controlled study of treatment for alcohol dependence in patients awaiting liver transplantation. *Liver Transpl* 2011; **17**(5): 539–547.

[26] Vaillant GE. The natural history of alcoholism and its relationship to liver transplantation. *Liver Transpl Surg* 1997; **3**: 304–310.

[27] Dew MA, DiMartini AF, Steel J, et al. Meta-analysis of risk for relapse to substance use after transplantation of the liver or other solid organs. *Liver Transpl* 2008; **14**(2): 159–172.

[28] Addolorato G, Mirijello A, Leggio L, et al; Gemelli OLT Group. Liver transplantation in alcoholic patients: impact of an alcohol addiction unit within a liver transplant center. *Alcohol Clin Exp Res* 2013; **37**(9): 1601–1608.

[29] Willoughby FW, Edens JF. Construct Validity and predictive utility of the stages of change scale for alcoholics. *J Subst Abuse* 1996; **8**(3): 275–291.

[30] Mathurin P, Moreno C, Samuel D, et al. Early liver transplantation for severe alcoholic hepatitis. *N Eng J Med* 2011; **365**: 1790–1800.

[31] British Liver Trust. NHSBT: transplantation of those with severe alcohol related liver damage. http://www.british livertrust.org.uk/nhsbt-new-pilot-study-transplantation-severe-alcohol-related-liver-damage/ (accessed 13 December 2014).

Index

Note: 'liver disease' in subheadings implies 'alcohol-related liver disease'

Alcohol Abuse and Liver Disease, First Edition. Edited by James Neuberger and Andrea DiMartini.
© 2015 John Wiley & Sons, Ltd. Published 2015 by John Wiley & Sons, Ltd.